Clinical Decision Making
in
Therapeutic Exercise

D0086977

Clinical Decision Making
in
Therapeutic Exercise

Patricia E. Sullivan, PhD, PT
Clinical Consultant Physical Therapy Services
Massachusetts General Hospital
Associate Professor, Physical Therapy Program
Institute of Health Professions
Massachusetts General Hospital
Boston, Massachusetts
Lecturer, Department of Orthopaedic Surgery
Harvard Medical School
Cambridge, Massachusetts

Prudence D. Markos, MS, PT
Senior Physical Therapist, Physical Therapy Services
Assistant Professor, Physical Therapy Program
Institute of Health Professions
Massachusetts General Hospital
Boston, Massachusetts

Photographs by Libba Ingram and Patricia Sullivan

APPLETON & LANGE
Stamford, Connecticut

Notice: The author(s) and the publisher of this volume have taken care that the information and recommendations contained herein are accurate and compatible with the standards generally accepted at the time of publication. Nevertheless, it is difficult to ensure that all the information given is entirely accurate for all circumstances. The publisher disclaims any liability, loss, or damage incurred as a consequence, directly or indirectly, of the use and application of any of the contents of this volume.

Copyright © 1995 by Appleton & Lange
Paramount Publishing Business and Professional Group

All rights reserved. This book, or any parts thereof, may not be used or reproduced in any manner without written permission. For information, address Appleton & Lange, Four Stamford Plaza, PO Box 120041, Stamford, Connecticut 06912-0041.

98 99 / 10 9 8 7 6 5 4

Prentice Hall International (UK) Limited, *London*
Prentice Hall of Australia Pty. Limited, *Sydney*
Prentice Hall Canada, Inc., *Toronto*
Prentice Hall Hispanoamericana, S.A., *Mexico*
Prentice Hall of India Private Limited, *New Delhi*
Prentice Hall of Japan, Inc., *Tokyo*
Simon & Schuster Asia Pte. Ltd., *Singapore*
Editora Prentice Hall do Brasil Ltda., *Rio de Janeiro*
Prentice Hall, *Upper Saddle River, New Jersey*

Library of Congress Cataloging-in-Publication Data
Sullivan, Patricia E., 1946–
    Clinical decision making in therapeutic exercise / Patricia E.
Sullivan, Prudence D. Markos. — 1st ed.
      p.   cm.
    ISBN 0-8385-4045-7
    1. Exercise therapy — Decision making.   I. Markos, Prudence D.,
1940- . II. Title.
    [DNLM: 1. Exercise Therapy. 2. Decision Making.
3. Rehabilitation.   WB 541 S951ca 1994]
    RM725.S837   1994
    615.8'2—dc20
    DNLM/DLC
    for Library of Congress   94-20009
                                      CIP

Acquisitions Editor: Cheryl L. Mehalik
Production Editor: Sondra Greenfield
Designer: Penny Kindzierski

PRINTED IN THE UNITED STATES OF AMERICA

ISBN 0-8385-4045-7
9 780838 540459

The great thing in this world is not
so much where we stand as in what
direction we are moving.

——Oliver Wendell Holmes

To our patients and the professionals dedicated to the
improvement of their care.

Contents

Preface

Therapeutic exercise is the foundation of physical therapy. It continues to be the primary intervention that distinguishes our profession from other health-related fields. The use of exercise as therapy has a long history, from the simple regimens used by construction aides in World War I to the more complex programs of current times. Today the knowledge base and with it the role of the physical therapist continue to expand, as do the expectations for improved quality care. Because of today's health care environment, exercise programs must be cost-effective as well as logical and efficient. Increasingly, patient function is expected to improve within limited time frames. Consequently, the decisions that physical therapists make regarding the type and implementation of therapeutic exercise programs are more crucial than ever.

The purpose of this text is to aid the physical therapist in making the clinical decisions about the choice and progression of exercise procedures. Our first text began this process with the delineation of the components of an exercise procedure: activities, a posture and any movement occurring within that posture; techniques, the type of muscle contraction(s) involved in the movement. This terminology was developed to facilitate identification of similarities among different treatment approaches and promote consistency of thought and logical sequencing of procedures. We are indebted to Mary Alice Minor, who was a major contributor to the formulation of the concepts and terms that are further developed in this text.

In the first section, our procedural terminology is expanded to include parameters of exercise related to muscle *endurance*. Besides focusing on the development of movement control, we have added the dimension of movement *capacity* based on concepts of tissue healing, exercise physiology, and motor learning. We have also proposed empiric principles and rules, which are introduced in beginning chapters and italicized for easy identification. These principles and rules guide the development of the treatment plans in the later sections on patient treatment.

A major addition to this book is a chapter presenting a framework of clinical practice designed to facilitate decisions about the selection of appropriate exercise procedures. This framework consists of both an evaluation and an intervention paradigm and provides the structure for the text. The evaluation model allows identification of deficits in the physical systems and of the interactive effects of multiple internal and external factors on those systems. The intervention model guides the therapist in translating the evaluative findings into movement control and capacity characteristics. Thus it is possible to identify impairments, such as decreased range of motion and limited postural stability, that need to be sequentially addressed in treatment. This process directs the choice of appropriate exercise procedures to rectify individual impairments and achieve functional outcomes. The achievement of function by remedying impairments is the emphasis of the intervention strategies.

Another addition to this text is a chapter on evaluation, which discusses the assessment of various body systems, with a focus on their relationship to therapeutic exercise. The general screening methods discussed in this chapter are applicable to all patients, whereas more specific supplemental information is included in the separate patient treatment sections.

The second section of this book demonstrates use of the framework and the decision-making process through examples of patients with musculoskeletal and neurologic dysfunction. In addition, because of changing demographics, a chapter on exercising the geriatric patient has been included. Advantages and disadvantages of specific treatment procedures are discussed throughout these chapters to further aid the physical therapist in making appropriate selections. Illustrated home exercise programs are located at the end of the clinical chapters. These drawings are distinguished by darkened page edges for easy reader identification.

Other added features include an example of documentation of a patient treatment in various stages and the appropriate overlapping of treatment procedures, which is located in the shoulder chapter; discussions of balance and ankle control, which can be generalized to many patient problems, are included in the geriatric and hemiplegic chapters respectively. A glossary of neurophysiologic, musculoskeletal, and exercise terms used throughout the text is located at the end of the book.

We have chosen to use diagonal movement patterns and techniques described by the originators of the proprioceptive neuromuscular facilitation (PNF) approach because we have found them to be effective with a wide variety of patients. Many of the basic tenets of PNF have been substantiated by studies we and others have conducted, which are referred to in this text. However, emphasis throughout this book is not on the promotion of one particular approach, but rather on the integration of theoretical and empiric knowledge and the choice of correct procedures to rectify impairments and improve function.

It is our hope that academicians, students, and clinicians will all find this book to be of value. We feel we have presented a decision-making strategy by which any problem requiring therapeutic exercise can be approached. Practice with the framework and familiarity with the rules and principles will shape thought processes, minimize trial and error, and foster a logical approach to treatment. There exist many unanswered questions regarding the various components and parameters of therapeutic exercise. These questions can only be answered through continued research and communication between the academic and clinical communities.

Acknowledgments

We thank our families, friends, and colleagues in bringing this process to completion.

For assistance and comments in editing the written and graphic work we thank Nancy DeMuth, Joan Cole, Chris Pickard, Meryl Cohen, Cheryl Maurer, Beth Ratcliff, Emily Smith, and graduate students in the therapeutic exercise and clinical decision-making classes at the Institute of Health Professions at Massachusetts General Hospital. Nancy DeMuth, Bill Markos, Sara Rubin, Elizabeth Ballantine, Viswa Sagar, Jye Wang, Jaime Paz, Elizabeth Falcone, and Lynn Troy were generous with their time in posing for photographs. Kathy Gill-Body, Jim Zachazewski, Rita Popat, Marie Giogetti, and Harriet Wittink provided support in their areas of clinical expertise.

Leslie Portney and Andrew Guccione provided conceptual assistance in the development of the framework and in the integration of clinical decision-making terminology. Joan and Peter Cole helped develop the concept of therapeutic principles as one of the themes of this book.

The photographs were taken, in part, by Libba Ingram. Lannie Therman and Diane Baumrecker assisted with the typing. Graphic illustrations were made by John Deecken.

For time, equipment, and location support we thank Colleen Kigen, Michael Sullivan, and our colleagues in the outpatient unit of the physical therapy department at Massachusetts General Hospital.

We are also grateful to the following specialists for reviewing the manuscript:

Gary Krasilovsky, PhD, PT
Hunter College
New York, New York

Barbara Sanders, PhD, PT, SCS
Southwest Texas State University
San Marcos, Texas

Sharon L. Held, MS, PT
Daemen College
Amherst, New York

Karen Maloney Backstrom, MS, PT
University of Colorado Health Science Center
Denver, Colorado

Tom Schmitz, PhD, PT
Long Island University
Brooklyn, New York

A Framework of Clinical Practice

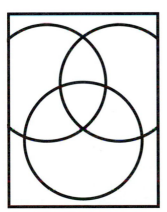

The framework of clinical practice (Fig. 1–1) is a comprehensive practice model that integrates the empirical, scientific, and theoretical foundations of clinical practice with processes of decision making.[1-3] The framework guides patient care decisions by delineating principles that link general clinical models to particular treatment procedures. The evaluation and intervention models within the framework describe the scope of clinical practice and provide a unified perspective from which to test and enhance clinical effectiveness and efficiency.

The framework is based upon four general *principles* (Table 1–1).

1. Functional capability is found in the interaction between environmental demands or restrictions and the individual's abilities.[4] Both the person who enters the therapeutic situation and the environment in which that person functions must be considered during the evaluation and intervention.

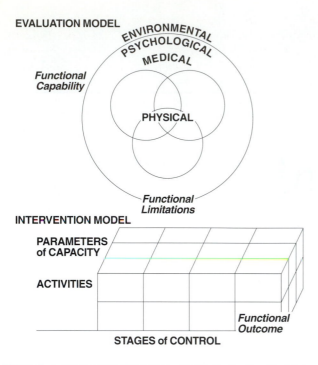

Figure 1–1. Framework of Practice with the Evaluation Model depicting the factors influencing the individual and the Intervention Model depicting characteristics of movement.

2. Functional outcomes can be attained by intervention strategies to: help the individual change if change is possible or appropriate; teach or provide compensatory aids if individual change is not possible or appropriate; and modify the environment to alter the challenge. Intervention develops the individual's abilities most effectively if the environmental constraints are modified to accommodate the patient's resources.
3. Intervention is designed to remedy both the primary and secondary impairments that limit function through a program that enhances movement control and capacity. This program develops the quality and quantity of posture and movement by proceeding through a logical sequence of intervention procedures.
4. Physical therapy includes: the promotion of wellness, the improvement or maintenance of functional abilities, the prevention of limitations, and rehabilitation if impairments are present.[5]

The framework consists of the evaluation model and the intervention model. These models describe the external and internal factors influencing the individual who enters the therapeutic situation. The individual's functional capability is assessed and functional limitations are determined during the evaluation; the functional outcomes are achieved by the intervention

TABLE 1–1. PRINCIPLES OF THE FRAMEWORK OF PRACTICE

Functional Capability =	Environmental Demands + Individual's Abilities
Functional Outcomes achieved by:	Changing the individual Teaching compensatory strategies Modifying the environment
Functional Outcomes an interaction of:	Improved movement control + capacity
Intervention =	Promotion of wellness Improvement or maintenance of function Prevention of limitations Rehabilitation

strategies. The models provide two methods of movement analysis: the evaluation model depicts a systems perspective of assessing movement; the intervention model classifies characteristics of functional movement. These perspectives allow clinically meaningful relationships to be established among functional limitations, impairments, general intervention strategies, specific treatment programs, and outcomes for both the individual patient and groups of patients sharing similar impairments or limitations.

The evaluation model categorizes the relationships among the many factors influencing a person's functional capability including environmental, social, psychological, medical, and physical factors (Fig. 1–2). Although all these factors are important, the primary focus of the physical therapy evaluation is to examine the physical systems that have the greatest impact on physical functioning and upon which physical therapy seems to have the greatest influence. The impairments found to limit function and that are amenable to physical therapy intervention, as well as

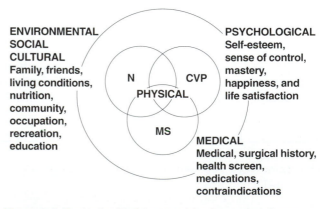

Figure 1–2. Evaluation Model categorizing interaction of many factors that influence physical capability.

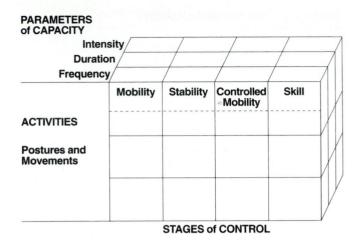

Figure 1–3. Intervention Model classifying characteristics of movement.

those abilities that enhance function, are transposed into treatment goals and functional outcomes incorporated within the intervention model.

The intervention model (Fig. 1–3) classifies the characteristics of functional movement affected by physical therapy. Intervention, as described in this text, achieves functional outcomes by altering the impairments limiting function through incorporation of three intervention strategies: promoting change in the individual, educating and compensating for impaired movement, and modifying the environmental constraints (Table 1–2). As part of the clinical decision-making process the patient's impairments are classified within the intervention model and a treatment plan consisting of a sequence of treatment procedures is developed. Intervention principles guide the application of the model to the particular patient's case by directing the choice and sequence of treatment procedures. The patient's capacity to change, the availability of resources, and the demands and possible modifications of the environment are considered when developing and implementing the intervention strategy.

TABLE 1–2. INTERVENTION STRATEGIES

- Change physical impairments
- Provide compensatory aids
- Modify environmental constraints

EVALUATION MODEL

The evaluation model (Fig. 1–2) is a depiction of the individual. The environmental, social, and cultural factors that describe the external milieu are repre-

sented on the outside of the model. Within the outside circle are factors inherent in the individual including the psychological, medical, and physical factors. The physical systems of most concern to the physical therapist, because of their influence on movement, are delineated in the center of the model. The cardiovascular-pulmonary (CVP), musculoskeletal (MS), and nervous (N) systems are depicted as three interlocking circles. These physical systems have both unique anatomical and common physiological areas. The autonomic nervous system (ANS) encompassing immune functions is shown in the center overlapping portion because of its influence on the other physical systems.

Environmental and Psychological Factors

Relevant environmental social and cultural factors include family, living conditions, nutrition, community, friends, education, occupation, and recreation. Relevant psychological factors include the individual's self esteem, the sense of mastery and control, level of anxiety, and the assessment of happiness and life satisfaction.[6] All these factors influence health in either a positive coping manner or through a negative strain leading to a stress response.

Environmental, social, cultural, and psychological factors have been found to correlate with physical dysfunction, disease, and illness behavior. For example, a happy, supportive partnership, satisfactory employment, a positive outlook, hardy personality, close supportive relatives and friends, as well as caring for others will allow the individual to better cope with adversity, and will result in fewer physical problems.[7-9] However, an accumulation of negative strains as a result of chronic hardship, major life events, and daily occurrences is associated with stress reactions that may manifest psychologically as depression or anxiety and physically as hypertension or low back pain.[10,11] A complex interaction of environmental, psychosocial, cultural, psychological, perceptual, and sensory factors contribute to pain behavior and chronic pain syndromes. Strains, especially when influenced by poverty, race, and gender, may increase vulnerability to disease by altering the ANS and immune system functioning.

A patient's functional status may not improve to the extent expected because of environmental or psychological constraints. These factors are considered throughout the evaluation and course of rehabilitation and may necessitate referrals to other health professionals. Some of these factors cannot be changed, but in some cases additional intervention may modify environmental and psychological strains or provide the patient with more effective coping mechanisms.

Physical environmental strains that are part of the person's occupation or recreation may be the immediate cause of the injury or insult, or may result in repetitive trauma that weakens the tissues. Environmental limitations that restrict the individual's independence may create a negative influence, such as the type of housing and the presence of various architectural barriers in the community.

Physical Systems

The interlocking circles of the evaluation model represent the MS, N, and CVP systems. The anatomical structure of each system is depicted in the unique area. The overlap between the CVP and MS systems denotes the **capacity for movement,** the area between the N and MS systems designates the **control of movement,** and the area between the CVP and N systems indicates **neural perfusion** (Fig. 1–4). Common to all are the physiologic functions of the ANS and the immune system.

A physical therapy evaluation assesses an individual's physical **functional capability** by determining the relative contribution of each of the physical **impairments** to the **functional limitations.** Following this assessment the therapist determines which **functional outcomes** can be achieved by changing the individual's impairments and modifying the environmental constraints. The functions that generally reflect the interaction of the person with the environment are (Table 1–3):

1. Locomotion or ambulation, the ability of the individual to explore and move in the environment including activities necessary for daily living, occupation, and recreation;

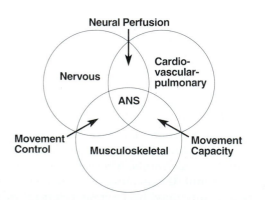

Figure 1–4. Physical Systems of the Evaluation Model depicting the areas most influenced by physical therapy.

TABLE 1–3. FUNCTIONAL CAPABILITY

▶ LOCOMOTION
   Ambulation, Wheelchair, Transfers
   Occupation, Recreation

▶ MANIPULATION
   ADL, IADL, Occupation, Recreation

▶ COMMUNICATION
   Oral motor, Feeding
      Level of Independence, Assistance Required
      Time to Achieve Outcome
      Changes in Person/Modifications in Environment

ADL, activities of daily living; IADL, instruments of activities of daily living.

2. Manipulation of the environment and the performance of activities of daily living (ADL), including the use of the upper body and trunk in occupational and recreational activities; manipulation of instruments or equipment, for example, pushing a vacuum cleaner or the pedals of a car (IADL).
3. Communication, encompassing the motor prerequisites for speech and nonverbal communication as well as other oral motor activities, such as feeding.

The amount of independence possible and the projected time it will take to reach that level is determined, as is the patient's assessment of the reason for the limitations, such as pain on movement, decreased flexibility, diminished strength, poor balance, or poor endurance.

The general factors and specific physical impairments that negatively influence function are examined to determine appropriate interventions. For example, if the patient has poor balance following an ankle fracture, the therapist determines if the associated sensory and motor impairments can be improved, a possibility in most situations. Temporary compensation with an ankle support and cane may be required, however, and grab handles in the bathroom may be necessary. In addition to impairments that limit function, abilities that enhance the person's function also are ascertained, since they may be augmented to improve the outcome.

Evaluation Process

The decision-making process guided by the model includes:

▶ identifying the individual's functional needs and desired outcomes;

▶ gathering of information, including determination of which measures are appropriate, the amount of detail required, and when the information is needed;

▶ assessing the individual's physical impairments and the environmental constraints to determine the contribution of each in limiting functional ability;

▶ examining the limitations and impairments to find a possible source or cause;

▶ determining the appropriateness of physical therapy intervention to enhance functional ability by alteration of the impairments that limit function;

▶ establishing functional outcomes and treatment goals directed toward the patient and the environment;

▶ determining the measures to be used to assess change and the frequency of reassessment;

▶ referring to other practitioners for information or treatment;

▶ documenting and communicating the findings (see Chapter 4).

The gathering of data may include observation of the patient and physical environs, a description of past and current problems and symptoms, and manual or mechanical measurement of movement ability, joint and muscle function, sensation, and cardiovascular and muscle capacity.

A general evaluative strategy begins with an overview of the environmental and psychological factors and the demands of vocational and recreational activities. If the patient is referred by a medical practitioner, the diagnosis that guides the medical intervention is noted. The medical and surgical history are recorded, as well as medications and their effect on physical functioning. This is included within a general health screen.[12]

After this preliminary information is gathered, an in-depth assessment of the physical system(s) is performed. Based on the initial data, the therapist hypothesizes the physical system(s) most involved. Assessment of these areas will probably yield the most pertinent information and link the physical impairments to the functional limitations. To rule out involvement of other systems and reduce the possibility of omitting important data, additional measures to screen the other systems may be performed.[12]

Assessment of the physical systems begins with the ANS. The ANS deserves special consideration during both the evaluation and intervention, for it is affected by environmental and psychological strains and it in turn influences the functioning of the other

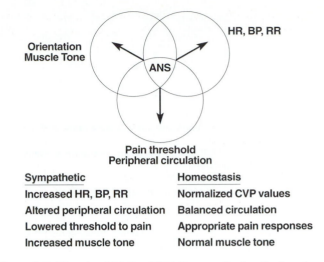

Figure 1–5. Ways in which the ANS influences the functioning of the other systems. BP, blood pressure; HR, heart rate; RR, respiratory rate.

systems (Fig. 1–5). In addition, altered ANS functions may bias the interpretation of the findings from other systems. For example, patients may demonstrate heightened sympathetic function[13] identified by increased heart rate (HR), blood pressure (BP), respiratory rate (RR), altered peripheral circulation, lowered pain threshold, and an increase in pain behavior, muscular tension, muscle tone, and general sensory awareness. The amount of pain reported by a patient may be heightened because of anxiety about beginning physical therapy, and the altered distal and skin temperature may be a physical manifestation of sympathetic activity.

After the assessment of the ANS, the evaluation focuses on the structures of the involved physical system(s) and the functions of the overlapping control and capacity areas (Fig. 1–6). The particular evaluation strategy used with each system varies because each system influences function differently and also responds uniquely to direct and indirect sequelae of injury or disease.[14,15] In addition, the severity, type, and chronicity of dysfunction and the reactivity and healing of the tissue will influence the strategy. Regardless of these differences the evaluation may include measures of range of motion (ROM), the ability to initiate and sustain movement, to maintain and move within and between postures, and to perform functional activities with varying amounts of intensity, duration, and frequency. These assessments measure the capability of the individual and delineate those structures or functions that limit or cause the impairment. Findings are considered in the context of other data and with respect to normal variability, which is influenced by age, sex, and body structure.

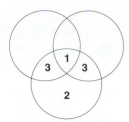

1 = ANS – vital functions and the influence of the ANS on other systems
2 = MUSCULOSKELETAL – the structures of the system directly involved
3 = MOVEMENT CONTROL and MOVEMENT CAPACITY – the systems secondarily or indirectly involved

Figure 1–6. Suggested order of evaluating the systems for a patient with musculoskeletal involvement.

The areas outside the system that is primarily involved may demonstrate secondary or indirect dysfunction that needs to be addressed by preventive and rehabilitative measures. For example, although the nervous system and the control of movement may be directly involved following a cerebral vascular accident (CVA), impairments in the MS system and a reduced capacity for movement equally may limit function.

At the conclusion of the evaluation the therapist determines if physical therapy is appropriate and, if so, the functional outcomes and treatment goals that can be achieved. To make these judgments regarding the impairments that are potentially amenable to change and the functions that can be enhanced, the therapist must know which physical abilities can be improved and what compensatory measures and environmental modifications are possible. Thus, the therapist's interpretation of the evaluation is within the context of the possible interventions and potential responses.

INTERVENTION MODEL

The intervention model (Fig. 1–3) is a three-dimensional matrix that classifies the physical characteristics of functional ability. The classifications encompass the control of and capacity for posture and movement. The model describes a general intervention strategy designed to achieve functional outcomes by sequencing the difficulty of movements. Anatomical and biomechanical principles and theories of motor control, motor learning, and exercise physiology are integral within this strategy and for-

mulate the basis for the principles of physical therapy intervention. The model and principles guide the therapist in designing a specific treatment program to remediate the patient's impairments.

The postures and movements included in treatment are termed activities and are sequenced along the model's vertical axis (see Chapter 2). Movement control, delineated into stages that progress the complexity of motor tasks,[16] constitutes the horizontal axis. Control is enhanced with the use of various techniques (see Chapter 3). The third axis consists of parameters of capacity, which adjust the physiologic, tissue, and learning stress of the movement. By classifying the patient's impairments within the components of the model, the therapist may better be able to analyze the relationship between impairments and function and determine the most appropriate sequence of intervention procedures.

Intervention Process

The intervention process includes these steps:

▶ The physical findings associated with the functional limitation are classified in the intervention model. For example, the patient is functionally limited in walking and with climbing stairs as a result of the impairments of decreased ankle ROM and muscle stability and generalized decreased muscle endurance. These impairments correspond to movement classifications described by the stages of control and parameters of capacity.

▶ Each of the impairments that can be changed are translated into treatment goals. The goals reflect the postures and movements to be achieved and the quality and quantity of that movement. To continue the above example, the goals might include that patient will be able: to achieve full passive ROM, to sustain isometric contractions for 10 seconds, to maintain unilateral weight bearing in standing for 10 seconds, to walk with normal timing and sequencing of movement for one mile, and be able to control stair descent at a normal pace.

▶ The treatment procedures are developed, sequenced, implemented, and progressed to achieve the treatment goals and functional outcomes. The choice of specific activities and techniques depends on the body segment and tissue involved and the general physical capabilities. The movement parameters reflect appropriate physiological and tissue stress and learning requirements. For example, stability control for our patient with ankle dysfunction is first developed in postures that limit the amount of weight-bearing stress. If stability can be maintained in low-level postures without pain or swelling, the activity is advanced by increasing the amount of weight bearing. More difficult techniques are added to each of these postures. If the patient has difficulty learning the movement, the frequency of the task may be altered, and verbal or visual inputs may be varied.

▶ The home program, teaching compensatory strategies, modifying the environment, and providing education, in this example, regarding safe ambulation are ongoing throughout the rehabilitation program.

▶ The objective and subjective changes in the specific impairments and functional abilities are continually noted so that appropriate modifications to the general strategy and specific procedures can be made.

▶ The impairments that cannot be changed by physical therapy are determined and appropriate referrals made.

Components of the Model

Activities: Postures and Movements

The sequence of postures and movements to be included in treatment is determined by relating anatomical, biomechanical, neurophysiological, and physiological principles to the patient's impairments and abilities. These principles relate to the size of the base of support, the height of the center of mass, the range of movement emphasized, and the effect of various resistive forces. The relevance of these factors will vary according to the patient's dysfunction, body proportion, and desired functional outcome.

Stages of Control

The stages of control[16] provide a schema for analyzing the quality of normal and abnormal movement and sequencing intervention strategies (Fig. 1–7). The stages are a descriptive classification of motor abilities, beginning with simple tasks and progressing to the timing and sequencing of movement required for the functional outcomes of locomotion, manipulation, and communication. Included in each category are: the motor abilities, and tissue and movement characteristics described by that stage; the criteria for measuring the patient's response; and the therapeutic techniques, including exercise, mobilization, physical modalities, and sensory or thermal inputs, appropriate to enhance

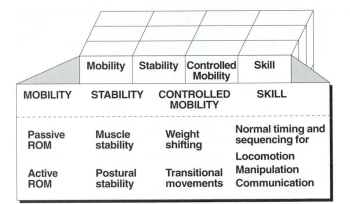

Figure 1–7. The Intervention Model highlighting the Stages of Movement Control.

those abilities. The stages are: **mobility,** which encompasses passive ROM and the initiation of active movement; muscle and postural **stability; controlled mobility,** encompassing movement within and between postures; and **skill,** including the timing and sequencing of movement required for functional activities.

Parameters of Capacity

The third axis of the model, the parameters of movement capacity, describes the frequency, duration, intensity and, if appropriate, the speed of the movement. These parameters that describe the quantity of movement are varied according to: the physiological stress that is appropriate for the patient; the healing and tissue reactivity that occurs in the process of recovering from an insult or injury; the schedule and amount of reinforcement, feedback, and other sensory input needed to learn; and the acuity or chronicity of the impairment (Fig. 1–8). For example, patients experiencing involvement of the CVP system may require that the treatment parameters be adjusted pri-

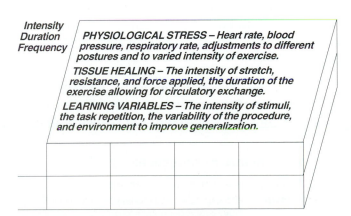

Figure 1–8. Parameters of Movement Capacity and the considerations for patients with involvement of different systems.

marily according to the physiological stress clinically measured by the heart rate, blood pressure, and respiratory rate responses and reports of fatigue.[17]

With patients recovering from an insult or injury, the parameters are modified according to principles of tissue healing[14] and the patient's report of pain. During early phases of healing, tissues mainly tolerate low-intensity levels of passive or active procedures; in addition, the integrity of the local circulation may limit duration and frequency. As healing occurs, increasing the intensity of the resistance and the frequency and duration of the muscle contraction will modify the challenge of the total procedure.

If a patient has difficulty with learning motor tasks, the parameters may be altered according to principles of learning; for example, the frequency and duration of the task can reflect mass or distributed practice schedules, and varying the intensity will affect the internal and external feedback or reinforcement. Initially the intensity of additional input may be increased to enhance learning of the task and then be progressively decreased to encourage internalization of the response.[18]

Strength or muscle force is not designated in one particular category of the model but rather is functionally defined within each of the control and capacity classifications. Strength, from this perspective, encompasses the motoric ability to maintain, move within and assume various postures, and perform limb movements with the intensity, duration, and frequency needed for function.

Intervention Strategies Directed Toward the Patient

Treatment procedures combine the three components of intervention: **activities;** postures and movements; **techniques** to achieve the stages of movement control, and **parameters** of movement capacity. Each procedure is designed to achieve specific treatment goals prerequisite to the functional outcome (Table 1–4).

Treatment always begins with procedures the patient can perform and progresses in difficulty toward the functional outcome. The challenge of each

TABLE 1–4. TREATMENT PROCEDURES

A–ACTIVITY:	the posture and movement
T–TECHNIQUE:	the exercises and modalities to achieve the stages of movement control
P–PARAMETERS:	the variations in movement capacity to influence physiological stress and learning

procedure may be altered by changing any component of the procedure. For example, the **activity** can be made more difficult by advancing from supine, to sitting, to standing—a progression down the vertical axis. Within each activity the stage of control can be advanced by changing **techniques,** for example by progressing from mobility techniques to those that enhance stability. This progression is depicted by horizontally moving across the model. Within each procedure the **parameters** of frequency, duration, and intensity can be adjusted. The progression and regression of difficulty can be modulated according to the patient's responses in keeping with the general intervention strategy and the particular treatment plan. The patient's responses to the specific procedures and to the plan in general are compared with the expectation so that treatment can be appropriately modified to achieve the stated goals, or the goals or outcomes adjusted.

Most procedures can employ various types of equipment and be modified for a home or group program. To enhance patient education and to ensure incorporation of motor skills into daily life, the setting, type of feedback, and reinforcement need to vary. As improvements occur, external stimuli are removed to increase the patient's automatic movement and internal motivation.

Intervention Strategies Directed Toward the Environment

Specific evaluative and intervention strategies vary according to the goals, the setting, the type of patient, the experience of the therapist, and whether the emphasis of intervention is directed toward the individual or toward modifying environmental conditions. The availability and cost of diagnostic and intervention options and the amount of information available also are variables needing consideration.

The environmental constraints on activities of daily living and on vocational and recreational activities can be analyzed according to the same parameters used to analyze the individual's physical ability. Task analysis includes: the postures incorporated, the type of movement control required, and the repetition, speed, and intensity requirements. These findings direct interventions. For example, altering the height of a step, cabinet, or toilet seat changes ROM (mobility) requisites; modifying the support and the shock absorption of a chair, car seat, or surface will alter alignment and tissue stress during maintenance of a posture (stability). The therapist evaluates both the environmental constraints and individual impairments that contribute to the functional limitation and directs intervention toward changes of either or both so that the functional outcome can be achieved most efficiently and effectively.[19]

Some impairments and limitations can be anticipated, such as decreased walking speed and reduced flexibility in the elderly,[20] the decreased movement capacity experienced in sedentary individuals, or the indirect deficits following most insults to the physical systems. In many cases, preventive measures may be the most effective and efficient means of maintaining or enhancing the attributes of movement required for function.

In many occupational, recreational, and community situations, modifying the environment may be the primary method of intervention and may be the main consideration when numerous persons share common impairments or functional limitations. For example, many elderly people have difficulty crossing intersections in the allotted time because of reduced walking speed; those with other ambulatory deficits have difficulty with stairs or curbs. The status of many of these individuals cannot be changed; therefore, modification of the environment by reducing architectural and community barriers may be the most effective strategy to achieve the functional outcome. Modifying the environment is also important for those experiencing occupational and recreational strains and injuries. Alteration of the work station, education in proper movement technique, varying the playing field, or even changing rules, such as eliminating some gymnastic maneuvers, may result in a widespread reduction of physical impairments. Therapist's efforts can be combined with the efforts of professional and community groups such as the organizations representing athletes or the elderly to encourage these changes.

DECISION-MAKING CONSIDERATIONS

Consistent with the modified Nagi definitions,[4,21] the framework guides the therapist in categorizing functional limitations and classifying physical impairments. This structure facilitates the association between these levels of deficit, the proposed intervention strategy, and the anticipated functional outcomes. To complete the circle, the functional outcomes achieved by the intervention should match the therapist's determination of the individual's functional capability.

To effectively evaluate the patient's potential for change, a knowledge of the possible interventions is required and, conversely, implementing the intervention is based on an understanding of the interaction

of the physical systems. Progressing from the evaluation to the intervention is termed *forward reasoning*, whereas determining the intervention and the evaluation strategy based on the anticipated functional outcome is *backward reasoning*. Combining these processes improves the effectiveness of decision making.[22]

The sequence of the evaluation strategy follows an adapted breadth and depth perspective. The breadth of factors that can influence physical functioning are screened with an in-depth assessment made of the involved physical system(s). Measured are the movement control and capacity characteristics, the categories of the intervention model that can be altered by physical therapy. These considerations encourage the efficient assessment of all probable causes of the limitations, rather than inefficiently assessing all possible causes, and as well ease the transformation between the evaluative findings and the intervention procedures.

The evaluation should yield physical findings that can be clustered into logical classifications or physical diagnoses. Findings that are not expected, or do not cluster, must be considered carefully, for they can reflect problems beyond the scope of physical therapy, requiring referral. The tendency to close the assessment too soon once an impairment has been found and to overlook relevant data is also avoided.[23] Once one abnormal finding is obtained, a definitive conclusion should not be made without exploring other tissues or functions that may contribute to that impairment. In addition, other characteristics of movement that are indicative of other impairments may be found. Although one impairment may account for the facts, this does not mean that it is the only impairment, nor does it mean that it is the finding most related to the functional limitation.[24] For example, one impairment common in patients with low back pain is limited range during active movements. Many tissues at different segments may limit range, and these all need to be assessed before a conclusion is made about the tissue limitation. In addition, before range is increased, its relation to other findings and to function needs to be determined.

The general models link the patient's impairments to the intervention strategy and particular procedures to the functional outcomes, thus allowing the therapist to better analyze the decision process and determine the most effective and efficient intervention. However, the framework cannot describe, explain, or predict all the particular characteristics of a patient, especially in each environmental context.[24] This discrepancy between the general, theoretical model and the specific, clinical application requires a thoughtful and skilled application by the clinician.

▶ **SUMMARY**

The framework of clinical practice integrates scientific and empirical theories into a unified, clinically applicable construct. The framework consists of models that describe clinical practice and depict the primary areas of physical therapy expertise. The evaluation model, built on a systems approach, depicts the many factors influencing physical capability, emphasizing the physical systems upon which our practice seems to have the most effect. The treatment planning process continues as the patient's impairments and functional limitations are classified within the intervention model. This model describes the characteristics of functional movement. From these classifications, general intervention strategies and particular procedures of treatment are developed. Principles that guide the clinical application of the models are integrated with decision-making strategies.

The categories of the physical systems and classifications of the movement parameters help develop the relationships among functional limitations, physical impairments, treatment interventions, and functional outcomes. The models of the framework establish a context within which to set and solve both common and unique clinical problems and relate clinical rules and principles to the process and outcomes of intervention.

▶ **REVIEW QUESTIONS**

1. What are the three categories of function that reflect the patient's ability to interact in the environment?

2. What are the levels of factors that need to be assessed when determining the patient's functional limitations? Describe a situation that highlights the interactive effects.

3. What is the influence of the ANS on the other physical systems? How might the ANS be affected by the other factors inherent in the evaluation model?

4. What are the three general intervention strategies? Give an example of how each may be implemented to achieve the functional outcome.

5. You are working with an elderly patient with a Colles' fracture. What are some of the secondary or indirect problems that you would anticipate? What preventive measures may be implemented in addition to the treatment procedures directed at the primary impairments?

REFERENCES

1. Watts NT. Clinical decision analysis. *Phys Ther.* 1989; 69:569–576.

2. Schon D. *The Reflective Practitioner: How Professionals Think in Action.* New York, NY: Basic Books Inc; 1983.

3. Schwartz S, Griffin T. *Medical Thinking: The Psychology of Medical Judgment and Decision Making.* Philadelphia, Pa: Springer-Verlag; 1986.

4. Guccione AA. Physical therapy diagnosis and the relationship between impairments and function. *Phys Ther.* 1991;71:499–509.

5. Philosophical statement on physical therapy (HOD 06-83-03-05). In: *Applicable House of Delegates Policies.* Alexandria, Va: American Physical Therapy Association; 1989:26.

6. Levine S, Croog SH. What constitutes quality of life? A conceptualization of the dimensions of life quality in healthy populations and patients with cardiovascular disease. In: Wengen NK, Mattson ME, Furberg CD, eds. *Assessment of Quality of Life in Clinical Trials of Cardiovascular Therapies.* New York, NY: Le Jacq Publishing Co; 1984:46–66.

7. Thoits PA. Dimensions of life events that influence psychological distress: an evaluation and synthesis of the literature on psychosocial stress. In: Kaplan HB (ed). *Psychosocial Stress: Trends in Theory and Research.* New York, NY: Academic Press Inc; 1983.

8. Trumbull R, Appley MH. A conceptual model for the examination of stress dynamics. In: Appley MH, Trumbull R. *Dynamics of Stress.* New York, NY: Plenum Press; 1986.

9. Kobasa S. The Hardy Personality: Toward a Social Psychology of Stress and Health.

10. McClelland DC, Floor E, Davidson RJ, et al. Stressed power motivation, sympathetic activation, immune function and illness. *J Hum Stress.* 1980;6:11–19.

11. Biering-Sorenson F. Physical measurements as risk indicators of low back trouble over a one-year period. *Spine.* 1984;9:106–119.

12. Boisonault WG: Examination in Physical Therapy Practice: Screening for Medical Disease. New York, NY: Churchill Livingstone; 1991.

13. Hoskins TM, Troy L, Dossa A. Effect of slow stroking on the autonomic nervous system. Unpublished research conducted at the New England Medical Center, 1984.

14. Harris BA, Dyrek DA. A model of orthopedic dysfunction for clinical decision making in physical therapy practice. *Phys Ther.* 1989;69:548–553.

15. Shenkman M, Butler RB. A model for multisystem evaluation, interpretation, and treatment of individuals with neurologic dysfunction. *Phys Ther.* 1989;69:538–547.

16. Stockmeyer SA. An interpretation of the approach of rood to the treatment of neuromuscular dysfunction. *Am J Phys Med.* 1967;46:900–956.

17. Cohen M, Hoskins TM. *Cardiopulmonary Symptoms in Physical Therapy Practice.* New York, Churchill Livingstone; 1988.

18. Winstein CJ. Motor learning considerations in stroke rehabilitation. In: Duncan PW, Badke MB, eds. *Stroke Rehabilitation—The Recovery of Motor Control.* Chicago, Ill: Year Book Medical Publishers Inc; 1987.

19. Bryan JM, Geroy GD, Isermagen SJ. Nonclinical competencies for physical therapist consulting with business and industry. *J Orthop Sports Phys Ther.* 1993;18:673–681.

20. Himann JE, Cunningham DA, Rechnitzer PA, et al. Age-related changes in speed of walking. *Med Sci Sports Exerc.* 1988;161–166.

21. Nagi S. Disability concepts revisited: implications for prevention. In: Pope A, Tarlov A, eds. *Disability in America: Toward a National Agenda for Prevention.* Washington, DC: National Academy Press; 1991.

22. Kleinmutz B. The processing of clinical information by man and machine. In: Kleinmutz B, eds. *Formal Representation of Human Judgment.* New York, NY: John Wiley & Sons Inc; 1968.

23. Voytovich AE, Rippey RM, Suffredini A. Premature conclusions in diagnostic reasoning. *J Med Ed.* 1985; 60:302–307.

24. Gorovitz S, MacIntyre A. Toward a theory of medical fallibility. *J Med Philos.* 1976;1:51–71.

Activities: Postures and Movement Patterns

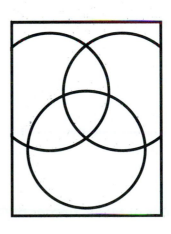

The postures and movements incorporated into treatment are termed *activities* and are sequenced on the vertical axis of the intervention model (Fig. 2–1). As part of the clinical decision-making process the therapist determines which postures and movements should be included in the treatment program to achieve the treatment goals and functional outcomes and when to progress the difficulty. To make these decisions, biomechanical, neurophysiological, and physiological principles are considered in conjunction with the patient's physical needs and abilities (the reader is referred to the bibliography in the appendix for additional pertinent readings). These principles are described in the first section of this chapter. In the second section the particular postures and movements are analyzed according to the influence of these principles. The clinical advantages and disadvantages of each activity related to common patient uses are delineated in this section.

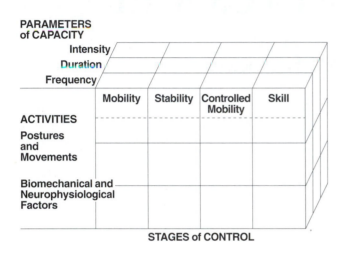

Figure 2–1. Intervention Model.

BIOMECHANICAL EFFECTS ON POSTURE

Base of Support

The base of support (BoS) refers to the amount of the body in contact with the supporting surface and the size of the area within the base. For example, sitting with upper extremity support has a larger base than sitting unsupported, and standing with the feet apart has a larger base than standing with the feet in tandem. A large BoS reduces the difficulty of maintaining the posture. *The progression is usually from a large BoS to one that is smaller.*

Center of Mass, Center of Gravity

When analyzing postures, the term *center of gravity* (CoG) is used to refer to the center of the mass that is raised from the BoS.[1,2] For example, when the center of mass (CoM) or CoG is on or near the supporting surface, less muscular control is required to support the body or segment than when the CoM is raised from the BoS. For example, the CoM is closer to the BoS in the supine posture than in sitting and even fur-

ther away in standing, making supine and sitting more stable and less difficult postures for the patient to maintain. *The progression is from a low CoG to one that is higher.*

Number of Joints or Segments Involved

The number of joints involved refers to the number of segments participating in the activity. An activity can involve the total body, such as walking, or can be isolated to a specific area, such as the lower lumbar spine. In weight-bearing postures, joint involvement usually refers to the weight-bearing segments; for example, prone on elbows does not require participation of the forearm and hand or of the lower body, as compared to quadruped. The placement of the therapist's manual contacts or addition of other external forces also will influence the number of segments involved. For example, contacts placed on the scapula and pelvis in sidelying will promote involvement of the entire trunk, whereas contacts positioned on the lumbar spine and pelvis will result in more isolated activity of the lower trunk. *If segments other than the involved segment are included in the activity, the amount of motor unit activation in the involved area may increase.*[3] This increased activation is a result of overflow from stronger parts. In developing procedures to promote muscle strengthening, overflow is desirable. For example, to increase activation of weak lower-trunk extensors, stronger upper-trunk segments can be incorporated into the activity, thus increasing the number of segments involved and increasing overflow to the involved area.[4] In contrast, *isolating the activity to one area will reduce total muscular activation by limiting overflow.*

When a new movement is learned, many of the segments not directly involved in the movement may be rigidly stabilized to reduce the amount of control required at those joints. This allows the focus of learning to be on the specific task and on those segments that require precise, dexterous control. When that specific portion of the total task is learned, attention then may be focused on improving control of the entire body so that the total task can be performed more efficiently. In his analysis of movement, Bernstein discussed controlling the many degrees of freedom that occur during functional tasks.[5] According to Bernstein, a functional task is a composite of each joint's movement, which can vary between two and six motions, with ongoing readjustment to control the force and timing of each prime mover and synergist. In addition to each of these internal variables, adjustment must be made to the changing external stimuli. From this perspective, the number of segments dynamically involved while a movement is learned begins with those directly participating in the task while the other segments are statically stabilized and progresses to the involvement of the entire body, with dynamic stabilization providing greater adaptability but requiring more control.

Weight Bearing On or Through a Joint

Weight bearing on or through a joint refers to how body weight or external forces are transmitted; body weight can be transmitted **through** a joint, causing approximation of joint surfaces, or weight can be borne **on** a particular joint, with the segment in contact with the supporting surface. *Weight bearing on a joint requires sufficient range of motion of that joint to assume the particular posture.* For example, in prone on elbows, weight bearing occurs on the elbow. Sufficient range of elbow flexion must be present to allow for assumption of this posture. *Weight bearing through a joint requires stability of the joint to maintain the posture.* In quadruped, weight bearing occurs

through the elbow. The stability, enhanced by approximation forces, can be provided by joint alignment, or ligamentous, fascial, capsular, muscular, or external supports such as an orthotic device or air splint. If in quadruped the elbow is hyperextended, the congruity of joint structures and noncontractile tissue may provide the stability; however, if the elbow is maintained in a straight but not hyperextended position, muscular stability maintains the elbow position. *Stability provided by dynamic muscle forces reduces strain and protects joint structures.*[6] Stability, although predominantly dependent on the extensor musculature, requires coordinated contraction of all muscles around the joint.

Extremity Movements

Trunk Combinations

The extremity movements can be differentiated into trunk, bilateral, and unilateral combinations.[7] In trunk patterns the limbs are in contact with each other, closing the kinematic loop. In the upper extremities the contact can be at the elbows,[8] the forearm,[7] or at the hands[9] (Fig. 2–2). In the lower extremities the contact comes from the limbs touching each other. *The primary focus of the trunk combinations is on trunk and proximal limb segments.*

Bilateral Combinations

In the bilateral combinations the two limbs are separated, but both are involved in the activity. The limbs

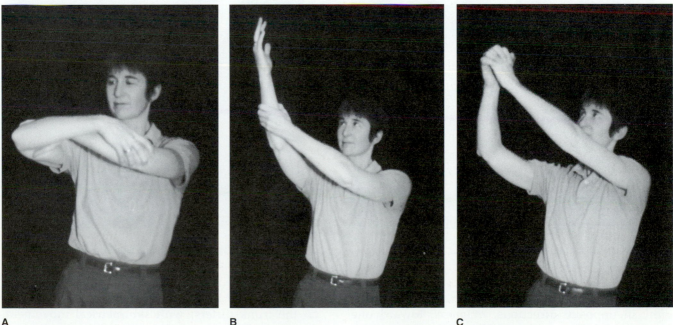

A   B   C

Figure 2–2. Upper-extremity trunk pattern: **(A)** with contact at the elbows; **(B)** contact at the forearm; **(C)** contact at the hands.

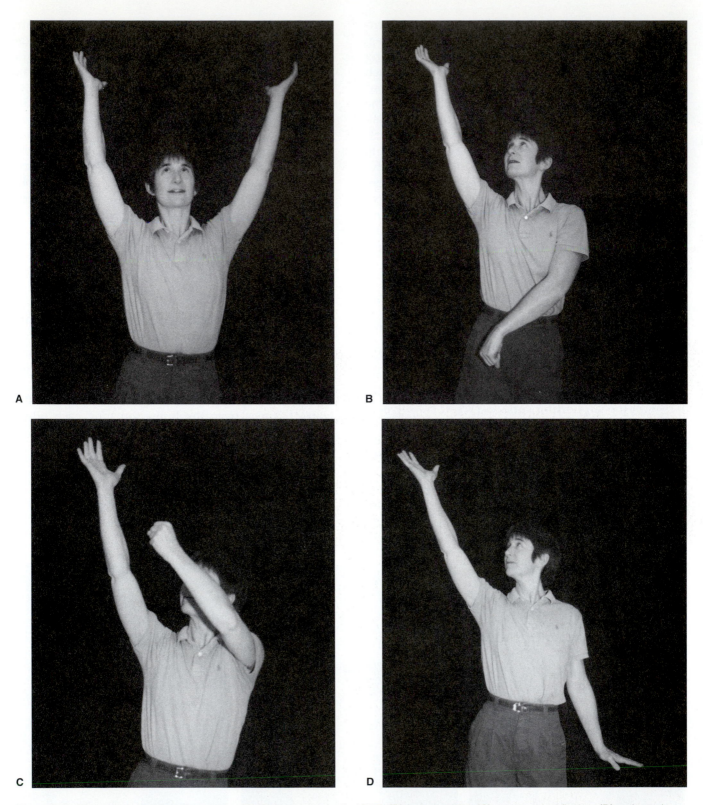

Figure 2–3. Bilateral upper-extremity patterns: **(A)** bilateral symmetrical D2F; **(B)** reciprocal D2; **(C)** asymmetrical flexion; **(D)** reciprocal asymmetrical or cross diagonal.

may be moved in the same direction, termed *symmetrical;* in opposite directions, *reciprocal;* toward one side of the body, *asymmetrical;* or, toward opposite sides of the body, *cross diagonal* or *reciprocal asymmetrical* (Fig. 2–3).[7] With each limb movement the effect on the trunk differs: with symmetrical movements the trunk flexes or extends, with reciprocal movement the trunk rotates, with asymmetrical movement the trunk combines flexion or extension with rotation and lateral bending, and with cross diagonals the opposite limb movements produce a stabilizing force in the trunk. *The focus of the bilateral patterns is usually on the proximal limb segments.*[10] Some upper extremity swimming strokes can be likened to the bilateral combinations. For example, the breaststroke and butterfly are symmetrical movements, the freestyle and backstroke are reciprocal movements, and the sidestroke is a cross diagonal motion.

Unilateral Patterns

During unilateral patterns a single limb moves independently. *With unilateral combinations any joint within the limb can be emphasized, allowing for a variety and specificity of movement.*

Primitive Patterns

The lower extremities can be moved or be positioned in primitive, mass, or advanced combinations. Primitive movements are stereotyped actions similar to those movements that may dominate movement in patients with an abnormal central nervous system (CNS). In the lower extremity the primitive flexion movement, analogous to the flexor synergy, combines hip, knee, and ankle flexion, with hip abduction, external rotation, and foot inversion. The extension pattern combines hip and knee extension and ankle plantarflexion with hip adduction, internal rotation, and foot inversion.[8] Because of their stereotyped nature and minimal functional carryover, *the primitive patterns are avoided if mass or advanced combinations are possible.*

Mass Patterns

Mass patterns combine hip, knee, and ankle flexion or extension (Fig. 2–4).[11] In contrast to the primitive movements, however, the rotation and abduction–adduction components can vary, depending on the desired motion or muscle activation. Mass patterns can be performed as non-weight–bearing open-

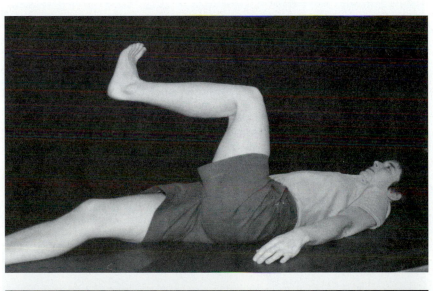

A

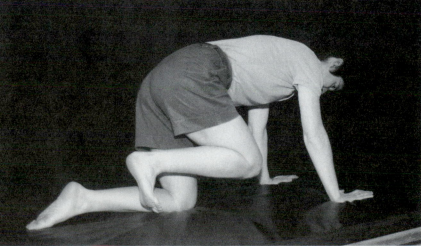

B

Figure 2–4. Mass patterns in the lower extremity: **(A)** mass flexion in supine; **(B)** mass flexion in quadruped.

chain movements, for example, mass flexion–extension in supine or sidelying. Mass patterns also occur in weight-bearing, closed-chain postures, such as the mass lower extremity flexion that occurs when positioned in quadruped. *Mass patterns are chosen when the goals of treatment are to increase joint range of motion (ROM), to initiate movement, to strengthen a muscle or movement pattern, or to enhance overflow from stronger to weaker muscles.* For example, if a patient has isolated weakness of the anterior tibial muscle, a mass flexion movement may enhance overflow from the hip and knee flexors to the ankle dorsiflexor muscle.[12]

Advanced Patterns

Advanced movements combine hip extension, knee flexion, and plantar flexion, or hip flexion, knee extension, and dorsiflexion[11] (Fig. 2–5). During these movements the two joint muscles are simultaneously shortening at both joints, a difficult task as neither end of the muscle is stabilized and active insufficiency may occur. On the other side of the limb, the two joint antagonist muscles are lengthening over both joints and may limit the total excursion of motion through passive insufficiency.[13] Advanced combinations, which can be performed as open- or closed-chain movements, are incorporated into postures, such as bridging and kneeling, and in many functional tasks, such as ambulation. *Advanced movements are chosen to promote the proper timing and sequencing of motor activity and the control of specific segments after strength and general control have been gained with mass patterns.* Advanced combinations are used to further integrate abnormal synergistic movement once the patient can perform mass patterns. Continuing with the previous example of a patient experiencing difficulty with dorsiflexion, the movement progresses from mass flexion to an advanced combination of hip flexion, knee extension, and ankle

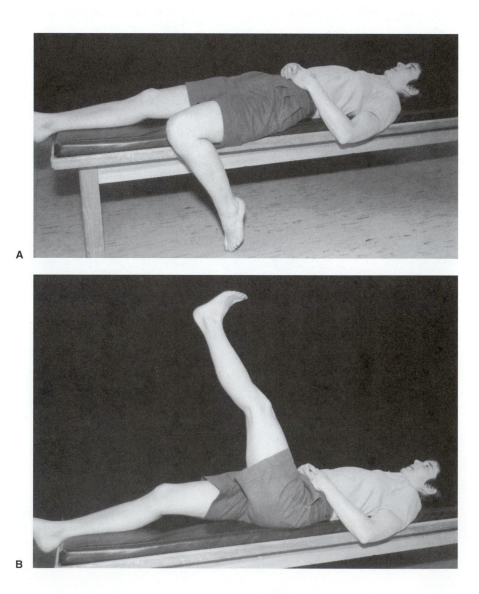

Figure 2–5. Advanced patterns in the lower extremity: **(A)** hip extension, knee flexion, plantar flexion; **(B)** hip flexion, knee extension, dorsiflexion.

dorsiflexion. These movements can be performed in supine or sitting and also are incorporated into modified plantigrade.

Diagonal and Anatomical Patterns

Combinations of movement can be performed in diagonal patterns, which incorporate three planes of motion,[7] as well as in individual anatomical planes. Diagonal patterns combine two or three muscle actions and may be more effective and efficient in enhancing functional range and movement than straight plane motions (see Glossary). In addition, rotational movements, which are inherent in all diagonal patterns, are essential to all levels of movement control, especially skilled upper extremity movement. Diagonal patterns have three degrees of freedom at the proximal joints[1] and combine various distal movements that may require greater control but at the same time allow for the most diversity and freedom of movement. *By choosing the appropriate movement patterns and performing them in different combinations and in different postures, the complex movements needed for functional activities can be achieved.*

FACTORS INFLUENCING THE POSTURE AND MOVEMENT _____

Reflexes and reactions are automatic responses to particular stimuli. Mediated at various neuronal centers within the CNS, their influence may dominate motor behavior during development and be evident later in life, depending on many factors including the normalcy of the CNS.[14-16] Some reflexes adversely affect functional movement, whereas others seem to support function. Although reflexes have been categorized in different ways, this text classifies them according to the response produced: a phasic or tonic reflex, a righting reaction, or a postural control or balance response.

The effects of reflexes and reactions should be considered when one is choosing an activity or progressing the difficulty of the program. For patients with neurological involvement, abnormal reflex dominance may interfere with normal movement; for those with either neurological or musculoskeletal deficits, improving righting reactions or postural control responses may enhance function.[17]

Phasic Reflexes

Phasic reflexes are stereotyped responses to exteroceptive or proprioceptive stimuli. The receptors are located primarily in the hand or foot but also within the limb. The dominance of many of these reflexes, common during the first year of development, gradu-

ally diminishes, but vestiges of these responses can emerge under stressful conditions throughout the life-span. The response is a phasic or movement response, usually within a limb or between two upper or two lower extremities.

Phasic reflexes include the extensor thrust, flexor withdrawal, or grasp reflex and may be stimulated when the foot or hand is lightly touched or in contact with the supporting surface, as occurs in bridging, quadruped, or standing. The phasic response may hinder a sustained holding response and interfere with the development of stability in weight-bearing postures.[18,19] *Activities that facilitate abnormal phasic reflex responses are avoided when the goal of the procedure is to initiate or facilitate voluntary control and stability in a posture.* If the patient cannot initiate voluntary movement, the use of phasic reflexes to produce a response may be necessary.

The stretch reflex, even though categorized as a phasic response, can be elicited throughout life and is part of the regulatory system for normal motor behavior, including postural control.[20,21] The receptor for the stretch reflex is the Ia ending of the muscle spindle. The stretch reflex may be diminished or exaggerated and is a common measure of the status of the CNS and the integrity of the neural supply to the muscle. *The stretch reflex can be used to facilitate movement when the patient has difficulty initiating movement or to reinforce weak movements.*

Tonic Reflexes

The tonic reflex is a sustained posturing in response to the position of the head or neck.[14] The receptors for tonic reflexes are located in the labyrinths and the upper cervical spine. The response encompasses more of the total body than the within- or between-limb response of the phasic reflexes. The tonic reflexes are named according to the receptor location: the tonic **labyrinthine** reflex or tonic **neck** reflex and the type of limb response, **symmetrical** or **asymmetrical.** In supine, the symmetrical tonic labyrinthine reflex (STLR) increases extensor tone, and in prone extensor tone is reduced. In sidelying, the asymmetrical labyrinthine reflex (ATLR) increases flexion of the uppermost limbs and extension of the limbs in contact with the supporting surface. Neck flexion or extension stimulates the symmetrical tonic neck reflex (STNR): the upper extremities perform flexion or extension motions in combination with neck flexion or extension respectively, while the lower extremities perform movement in the opposite direction. Neck and trunk rotation have an asymmetrical influence on the limbs: the response to neck rotation (ATNR) is extension of the upper extremity toward which the head rotates, chin side, and flexion of the upper extremity on the skull side.

As with phasic reflexes, the tonic reflexes may be dominant during development and demonstrated as extremity movements in response to changes in the head or body position.[14] A child with an intact CNS should be able to overcome the response, indicating that the reflex is not obligatory.[16] These reflexes are normally integrated within the first year of life. Subsequently the response may be seen as a change in muscle tone or variations within normal strength. Where pathology exists the tonic reflexes, like the phasic reflexes, may exert either a dominant or obligatory influence on behavior. *Postures are chosen to reduce, avoid, or eliminate those responses that interfere with voluntary movement. Whenever possible, postures or movements are incorporated into the treatment plan to enhance reflex integration.* For example, if the patient has a dominant STLR, the sidelying posture may be chosen to promote muscular control of the abdominals and back extensors before moving toward supine or prone, which are postures where the reflex influence may be greater.

Righting Reactions

Righting reactions are automatic responses of the head, neck, and trunk to maintain alignment within the body and orient the body to the environment.[14] Righting reactions, which normally persist throughout life, contribute to function by enhancing the ability to maintain a posture and to move within and between postures. The stimuli emanate from visual and labyrinthine receptors, and from proprioceptors in the neck and trunk. The **optical, labyrinthine,** and **body-on-head** righting reactions align the head, neck, and trunk to the horizontal and vertical in the flexion, extension, and lateral directions. For example, if the body tilts backward in sitting, the righting reactions promote head, neck, and trunk flexion to maintain the eyes horizontal, the head vertical, and the lower body in relation to the superior segments. If the body tilts to one side, the head rights or laterally flexes away from the tilting motion, and the trunk curves with the head motion. The **neck** and **body-on-body** righting reactions result in orientation within the transverse plane with log and segmental rolling respectively. When the neck turns, the entire body follows, neck righting; when either the upper or lower body rotates, the rest of the body follows, body-on-body righting.

Both the tonic and righting reactions are stimulated by head and neck movements but result in totally different responses. Righting reactions facilitate body movement in the direction opposite the sustained response of the tonic reflexes. For example, the tonic response to the prone position is flexion of the head and limbs, but the righting reaction in prone enhances head, neck, and body extension; the tonic response to neck rotation is retraction at the scapula on the skull side, while the righting response facilitates trunk rotation in the same direction as the neck rotation. Analysis of motor behavior during development and of patients with neurological deficit has not clearly delineated the relationship between the maturity of the CNS, the area of lesion, and other central facilitory and inhibitory influences. Thus conditions that result in a predominance of tonic reflexes or righting reactions cannot accurately be predicted. Empirically, righting responses provide more support to functional activities such as rolling than do phasic or tonic reflexes, although the dominance of righting responses also can be detrimental.[22] For example, patients with leg length differences may demonstrate spinal curvatures because the eyes and head will right to the upright position. Cervical asymmetries and temporomandibular joint dysfunction may be related to the predominance of righting reactions.

Righting reactions contribute to the control of functional movements such as rolling, the assumption of various postures, postural alignment, and orientation in upright positions.

Postural Control

Postural control is a complex interrelationship among sensory inputs and motor responses needed to maintain and move within and between postures.[23,24] Postural control, also termed *balance* and *equilibrium reactions,* has been analyzed from many perspectives: a biomechanical analysis may describe the position of the center of pressure within the BoS,[25] whereas a neurophysiological analysis may emphasize visual, labyrinthine, proprioceptive, and tactile inputs and muscular responses under various conditions.[26] Cardiovascular–pulmonary support for the assumption and maintenance of various postures measured by heart rate and blood pressure is a physiological perspective.[27]

The extent of a person's functional independence depends on the ability to maintain, assume, and move within and between postures. During functional activities, postural control is challenged as an individual sways in standing, walks, or lifts a limb, as in reaching for a doorknob, or while dressing. During these self-directed, frequently performed activities the change in the CoG is anticipated and an automatic stabilizing muscular contraction precedes the functional movement.[23,27] The initial postural activity occurs automatically with little or no peripheral modulation. In other situations posture may be disturbed externally or the situation may not be correctly anticipated, as occurs, for example, during walking on uneven surfaces or lifting an object of unanticipated weight. Under these conditions the person must respond to the unexpected feedback[28] in time to maintain or adjust the posture.

The initial postural response that occurs to maintain and move the body within the position commonly occurs in the segment in contact with the surface; for example, in standing, normal sway occurs primarily at the ankle, termed an **ankle strategy**.[29] However, if sensory input, ROM, or strength in the ankle is deficient, the response may be observed in superior segments, such as the knee, hip, trunk, or upper extremities.[30] When the response occurs in segments away from the BoS, closer to the CoG, a greater magnitude of response results. For example, someone with poor ankle control may respond with exaggerated hip or trunk movements as they balance in standing.[31] Because the hip movement is larger, the potential to fall may be greater. Another strategy includes extremity movements that occur to counter the direction of the displacement and move the CoM within the BoS. The extremities also can change position on the support surface, to extend or enlarge the BoS,[32] termed **protective extension**. For example, if the person sways backward in standing, a sequence of strategies may include ankle dorsiflexion, quadriceps contraction, then hip flexion, then upper extremity flexion, all in an attempt to maintain the CoG within the BoS. If these strategies are unsuccessful, one limb moves posteriorly to extend the BoS under the new position of the CoM.

Many factors can influence the speed and accuracy of the postural response, including: receptor threshold, the speed of transmission from the receptor to central mechanisms, the central interpretation of the situation, the centrally controlled feed-forward mechanism, the activation of an adequate motor response, and the appropriate execution of that response. If problems exist at any of these levels, the patient may not adequately maintain the posture and may fall. For example, a patient with an anterior cruciate ligament sprain may experience knee buckling while walking at night on uneven ground. This may be due to diminished visual input and delayed feedback from peripheral receptors in the muscle and joint, as well as a slowed and weak quadriceps response. Proprioceptive feedback from the muscle spindle normally combines with the input from joint receptors to provide continuous information regarding position and movement.[33,34] In weight-bearing postures, this input helps to maintain the posture. Thus, if the feedback from the spindle or joint to higher centers is diminished, postural control will be compromised. Another common example is that of a patient with a chronic sprained ankle, who has decreased feedback from the ankle coupled with weakness, particularly of the everters.[35,36] Postural problems will be accentuated if the patient is older, diabetic, has poor vision, vestibular disturbances, or has neurological involvement, with less acute position sense, delayed nerve conduction velocity, stiffness in the involved tissues, and weaker muscle responses. Persons with diminished peripheral input may have to increase reliance on vision or vestibular input. However, when vision also is impaired, as when walking in the dark, the risk for falls may increase.[37] In new or unusual situations, feedback from the periphery may be needed to augment the feedforward automatic responses.[38,39]

Treatment may be directed at enhancing the effectiveness of the involved system, compensating with an intact system if change will be delayed or not possible, and modifying environmental conditions. In a therapeutic or research environment the following can be altered to modify the challenge to postural control (Table 2–1):

▶ The size of the base can be altered. For example, in standing, difficulty can progress from bilateral to unilateral weight bearing or to forefoot or hind foot support.[40] The base can be enlarged by using the parallel bars or narrowed by standing on a balance beam or in tandem[38] (Fig. 2–6).

TABLE 2–1. POSTURAL CONTROL VARIABLES

Surface	Displacement	Awareness	Type	Stimuli	Condition	Strategy
Wide	Self	Anticipated	Static	Visual	Congruent	Ankle
Narrow	External	Unanticipated	Dynamic	Vestibular	Diminished	Hip
Stable				Proprioceptor	Conflicting	Trunk
Mobile				Tactile		Extremity
						Protective extension

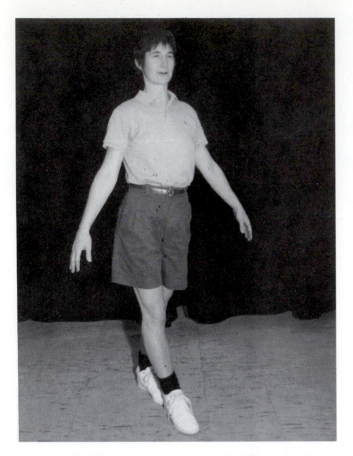

Figure 2–6. Altering the base of support to challenge postural control; standing in tandem.

conditions, for example, when lifting an object that is heavier than anticipated.

▶ The magnitude, velocity, direction, and placement of the disturbing force can be altered. A small, slow force will result in a different disturbance of the CoM from that produced by a fast, large input. If the force is applied near the BoS, the lever arm is of a different length compared to that when the force is applied near the CoG. The direction of the force will vary the compensatory responses that occur as the CoM is adjusted to stay within the BoS. For example, when a force is posterior, the response is anterior; when the force is diagonal, the response is also angular.[39]

▶ In common clinical situations visual, proprioceptive, and tactile inputs can be manipulated.[41] If the eyes are closed, visual input is eliminated, leaving the vestibular, proprioceptive, and tactile receptors to detect any disturbances. The visual condition can be altered by moving part of the visual environment or by changing the common vertical and horizontal alignments to a diagonal orientation. The tactile and proprio-

▶ The stability of the support surface can be progressed from a static or stable surface to a mobile base, such as a balance or wobble board or a trampoline. Maintaining the CoM on a stable BoS is usually less difficult than controlling the CoM on a movable base (Fig. 2–7).

▶ The CoM can be self-displaced or externally disturbed.[28,31,39] Self-displacement usually is less difficult for the patient to control and may be more functionally relevant than external displacement. For example, self-displacement occurs if the patient reaches for an object while sitting or standing; external displacement occurs if the therapist or other external force disturbs the CoM or the BoS (Fig. 2–8).

▶ The disturbance can be anticipated or unanticipated.[26,28] Anticipated input results in feedforward preemptive motor responses, unlike unanticipated disturbances, where the person has to respond to the feedback of postural disturbance. In anticipated conditions, the movement of the CoM within the BoS is less. Self-disturbance is primarily anticipated except when the expected conditions are not the actual

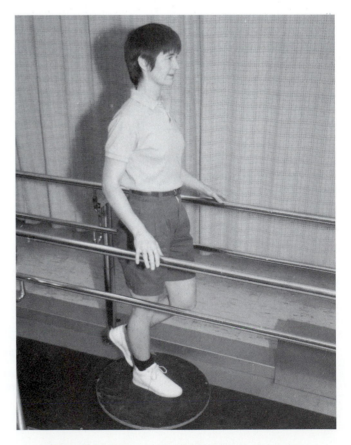

Figure 2–7. Standing unilaterally on a balance board.

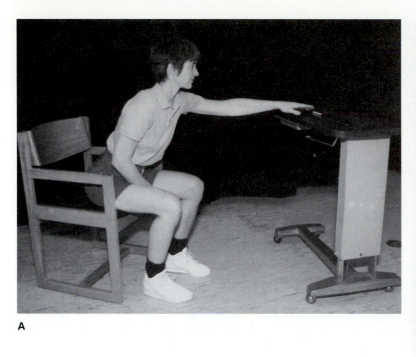

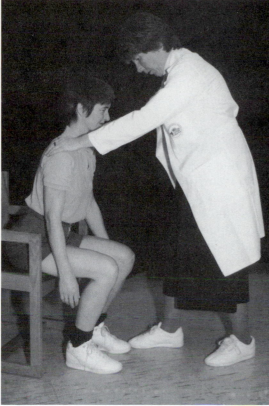

Figure 2–8. Self- and external displacement: **(A)** sitting and reaching for an object; **(B)** therapist challenging postural control.

ceptive input can be varied by standing on soft foam.[5]

▶ These sensory inputs can be congruent, diminished, or conflicting.[26] Under most normal environmental conditions input is congruent, meaning that the sensory inputs from the different receptors are anticipated within the CNS and "describe" an environmentally logical event. In some situations, however, the inputs are diminished or conflict, as for example, when part of the environment moves unexpectedly, or when proprioceptive changes occur in isolation. This occurs in standing on a balance board when the ankles dorsiflex but the body position remains upright. An imbalance in input from matched receptors may occur with unilateral vestibular dysfunction, a cerebral vascular accident (CVA), or with abnormal position sense, as commonly occurs with lower-extremity musculoskeletal involvement.

Postures that have a low CoG and a wide BoS minimize the need for postural control and are utilized when the goals of treatment are increasing mobility and ROM, improving the initiation of movement, and strengthening. These stable postures allow the patient to focus atten-

tion on these treatment goals. Performance of functional activities in progressively less stable postures requires increasing control over postural responses.

Resistance

Resistance is an internal or external force that alters the difficulty of moving. Internal resistive forces include tissue stiffness, tightness, and reflexive influences; external forces may be provided manually, mechanically, and by the gravitational resistance of body weight. Resistance alters the weight of the segment and thereby increases the difficulty of movement; however, it also provides an external stretch to muscles that increases feedback from muscle and joint receptors and enhances the response.[20,21]

Resistance may effect alpha–gamma coactivation, central–peripheral motor coordination, the actin-myosin bonding of muscle fibers, and the circulatory bed of the muscle. Resistance has an interactive effect on the three physical systems and on movement control and capacity. Therefore with the application of resistance many goals can be accomplished including improvement of: initiation of movement, muscle and postural stability, the timing, sequencing and recruitment of responses, motor learning, total body and specific muscle endurance, and muscle strength and hypertrophy.[42,43] The patient's ability to move against various types and amounts of resistance needs to be considered when choosing activities. *The amount of resistance provided will vary depending on treatment goals but should always allow for a smooth, controlled contraction of movement and must always be within the physiologic capability of the patient.*

Types of Resistance

Manual resistance applied by the therapist can be more finely graded than any other means of resistance. Transitions between resistance and assistance can be made depending on the patient's abilities and needs. Refinement and control of resistance are especially important when the manual muscle test (MMT) grade is less than 4/5.[44] To apply resistance in a skilled manner the therapist must have a sense of the desired goal and be able to respond according to the patient's efforts.[7] The therapist's manual skill is challenged when resisting a very weak muscle; the resistance must be adequate to provide appropriate muscle facilitation and feedback, but not so intense that the response is inhibited. Manual resistance can be used to indicate the direction of movement, termed *tracking resistance.* The contact is placed in the direction of the intended movement to provide a tactile guide. In contrast, manual resistance has limited value when the goals are increased general body endurance and improved strength and hypertrophy with muscles above 4/5. In such cases mechanical resistance may be more appropriate.

Mechanical resistance provided by equipment such as free weights,[45] elastic bands, pulleys,[7] and isokinetic devices[46] can be particularly effective in reaching the goals of increasing muscular endurance, improving general aerobic capacity, and improving strength or anaerobic ability in muscles with grades of 4/5 to 5/5. The visual feedback provided by some devices can be useful to improve patient motivation and the objective data comparing certain measures of strength can be useful. However, as discussed, resistive equipment is limited in its ability to provide the fine gradations of resistance needed for patients with very weak musculature or when isolated portions of muscles are the focus of treatment. Patients with imbalances of strength often will perform the movement with the strongest muscles, especially after a few repetitions when the weaker muscles fatigue. Mechanical resistance must be used carefully with some patients with neurological involvement who exhibit poor muscle control or with those patients with pain or a fragile skeletal system.

Reflexive influences will provide resistance to any activity if they dominate motor behavior.[16] Their influence may be greatest in patients with neurological deficits or with decreased ability to voluntarily activate muscles. For example, trunk flexion is resisted by the STLR when rolling from supine toward prone, necessitating that the movement be initiated in sidelying or semisupine in some patients. In contrast, the effect may be minimal in those with an intact CNS and normal muscle strength.

Gravitational or body resistance can be altered by changing vertical–horizontal alignment and the length of the lever arm. Gravitational resistance is maximized when the segment is extended and horizontal. For example, active trunk extension is maximally resisted in prone; angling the upper trunk on a wedge reduces resistance.

With all forms of resistance the amount of muscle force required to match or overcome the external force is dependent on the **length of the lever arm,** which includes both the length of the segment and the point of application of the resistive force.[13] A short lever arm keeps the CoM, or the resistive force, closer to the joint's center of rotation and reduces the muscle action needed to counter the force. *To reduce the amount of effort required, activities are chosen in which the length of the lever arm is short. As control or strength improves, the difficulty of the activity can be increased by lengthening the lever arm.* This can be accomplished by extending the elbow or knee or by positioning the resistive force farther from the center of rotation.

Movement can be passive, active assisted, active, or resisted. During passive movement the segment is externally moved with instructions to relax. To stay below the threshold of muscle excitation, movement must be either slow and rhythmical, or fast and unexpected. Rarely, however, is the movement actually passive, or without contractile activity. Normally innervated muscle will automatically assist with the movement, termed a *shortening response.*[47] This normal response is incorporated into some techniques designed to initiate movement (see Chapter 3, Techniques-rhythmic initiation). The terms *active assisted, active,* and *resisted* refer to the relationship between external resistive forces and the weight of the segment. With active assisted movement, the applied force reduces the weight of the segment; with active movement, no additional external force is provided; and with resistive movement, external manual or mechanical forces are added to the weight of the segment.

Appropriate grading of resistance is a major factor in determining a muscle's response. In general, if too little resistance is provided, the limb may move too quickly for appropriate alpha–gamma coactivation and actin–myosin bonding,[48] resulting in improper feedback and an ineffective response. However, the application of excessive resistance, particularly to weakened postural muscles, may tend to increase inhibitory influences and may produce insufficient actin–myosin bonding. In addition, excessive resistance may result in muscle microtearing, especially during eccentric contractions, when muscle force generated can be greater than that occurring during isometric or concentric contractions.[49] *The amount of patient effort resulting from the activity chosen and the amount of resistance applied should be consistent with the therapeutic goals.* For example, a patient with neurological dysfunction may demonstrate an increase in unwanted tonal patterns or nonfunctional synergistic movements if resistance is increased or if too difficult a posture is attempted; patients with cardiovascular–pulmonary involvement may demonstrate an increase in physiological stress, including increases in heart rate and blood pressure; for those with musculoskeletal involvement, excessive resistance may be inconsistent with the goal of tissue healing.

To increase strength and to maximize facilitatory influences of a muscle graded less than 3/5, postures should be chosen in which (1) gravity and reflexes provide assistance so that manual resistance can be applied, or (2) gravity is eliminated or resists the movement, and manual assistance is provided. If the muscle grade is 3/5, gravity-assisted and manually resisted activities may be indicated so that repetitive exercise can be per-

formed. When the muscle grade is 3+/5 or greater, gravity plus manual or mechanical forces are appropriate. For example, if the hip abductors are less than 3/5, manual resistance may be provided in supine. A progression would be gravitational resistance in sidelying, or manual or elastic resistance in bridging.

Both the direction of resistance and the angle at which it is applied will influence the response. The use of pulleys best illustrates this principle. Changing the patient's position relative to the pulley will allow resistance to be applied in a diagonal direction (Fig. 2–9A and B). Maximum resistance occurs when applied at a 90° angle to the limb (Fig. 2–9C). When the angle is more acute, compression is combined with resistance (Fig. 2–9D) and when more obtuse, traction occurs.[13]

Overflow

Overflow can be defined as the spread of facilitation as increased effort alters the excitatory threshold level at the anterior horn cell (AHC)[50]. Under normal conditions overflow usually occurs into those mus-

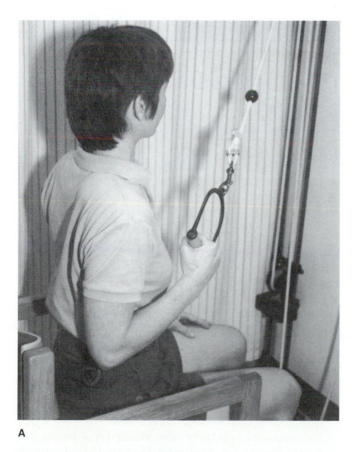

A

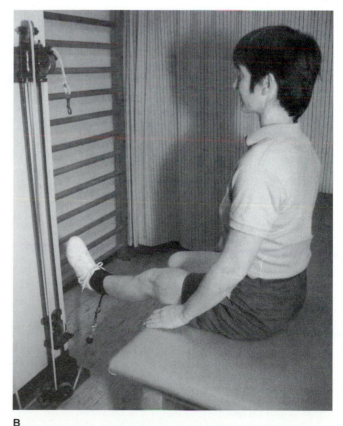

B

Figure 2–9. Direction of resistance and angle of maximum resistance: **(A)** diagonal resistance to shoulder extension and abduction; **(B)** diagonal resistance to knee extension. (Continued)

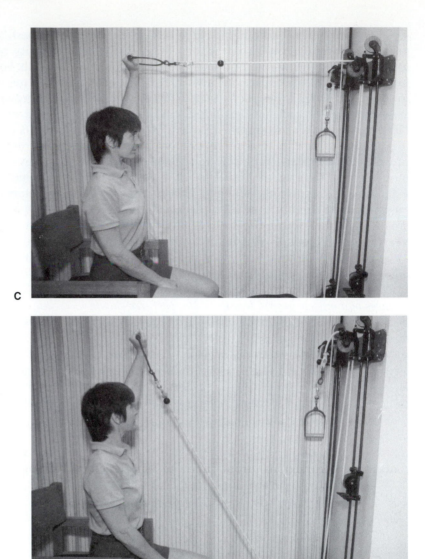

Figure 2–9 (Continued). (C) maximum resistance at 90° of shoulder flexion; **(D)** shoulder compression at approximately 180°.

cles that act in a biomechanically stabilizing manner[3] or that synergistically support the prime mover. Persons with an intact CNS can volitionally inhibit or modify the pattern of overflow, also termed an **associated movement**. When many segments are included in the activity, such as with trunk and bilateral combinations, overflow is increased.[4] The increased peripheral feedback that occurs when more than the involved segment participates in the activity may enhance the ability to respond and to learn the motor task. Overflow also occurs when the intensity of an action is great. *Overflow from stronger segments may enhance the motor unit activation of the involved or weaker segment and promote strengthening of the involved area.*[51,52]

In contrast, specific control is best obtained with low-intensity activation of the specific segment.[21] This can be achieved with less resistance to particular segments performing unilateral patterns. *Overflow is*

avoided when the goals are to reduce excessive muscular activity and to promote specific control. Overflow is used cautiously when patients are experiencing pain with muscle activation.

Persons with abnormal inhibitory control may not be able to modify or inhibit the spread of excitation, and the overflow may be consistently directed to a particular muscle group or pattern of motion. This stereotyped response is termed an **associated reaction**.[9] *When an associated reaction occurs, the therapist needs to determine the cause of the stress that produced the reaction. If the response interferes with the therapeutic goals, some aspect of the procedure may need to be altered to reduce the level of stress.*

Associated reactions may occur for a variety of reasons, including: excessive stimulation of visual, auditory, exteroceptive, or proprioceptive receptors, attempts to maintain a difficult posture or cope with excessive resistance, increased velocity of movement, or movement that occurs through too wide a range. Any or all of these factors can produce overstimulation and abnormal responses in a system that cannot easily integrate stimuli.

Range of Initiation, Range of Emphasis

The range in which movement is initiated and the range that is emphasized during treatment differ according to whether one-joint, postural extensor muscles or two-joint flexor muscles are emphasized. The facilitatory and inhibitory neurophysiological influences affect the optimal range of activation for these muscles differently. Furthermore, functional tasks are performed by extensors and flexors in different ranges.

Extensor, Postural Muscles. For both neurophysiological and functional reasons, postures and movement patterns that allow the extensors to be activated in the shortened range, where they provide postural support, are employed. To promote extensor muscle control, a sequence may consist of isometric contractions in or near the shortened range, eccentric contractions from shortened to mid ranges, then concentric contractions from mid to shortened ranges. Concentric contractions into the shortened range may be difficult as a result of decreased alpha–gamma coactivation as the tension on the muscle spindle decreases. Clinically this may be observed as an active lag.

Clinical observations suggest that weak postural muscles appear to become weaker or inhibited when they are maintained and resisted in the lengthened range. Inhibitory influences have been shown to have a greater effect on tonic versus phasic muscle groups.[53] To counteract these inhibitory influences and increase facilitation, *the muscle spindle stretch sensitivity in postural muscles needs to be enhanced in shortened ranges with isometric contractions* (see Chapter 3, Stability).

When extensor muscles are weak, postures and movement patterns that emphasize the shortened range are chosen. Once the muscle can sustain an isometric contraction in shortened ranges, treatment is progressed by increasing the length of the muscle from the shortened to the mid and then to the lengthened range in conjunction with manual, mechanical, or gravitational resistance. For example, quadriceps activity is first isometrically promoted in shortened ranges in non-weight bearing with a progression to supported standing before bridging, quadruped, or kneeling are introduced. These postures increase the amount of weight bearing and stretch on the quadriceps.

Flexor Muscles. Unlike the extensors, flexor or phasic muscle groups appear less affected by peripheral inhibitory influences even in lengthened ranges. In addition to the neurophysiological influences, the physiology of the two-joint flexor muscles favors contractions in lengthened ranges. Multijoint muscles have a longer excursion and become actively insufficient in the shortened range, reducing actin–myosin bonding. Functionally, flexors act primarily in the lengthened to mid ranges; thus, treatment for flexors can begin with and emphasize the lengthened, then mid, then the shortened range.[13] For example, the hamstrings are functionally most important in lengthened to mid ranges as they provide posterior support and flex the knee. *When flexor muscles are weak, postures and movement patterns that emphasize lengthened to mid ranges are chosen.*

Both flexors and extensors can be facilitated by a quick stretch in the lengthened range. In addition to Ia facilitation, the external stretch elongates the passive elements in the muscle. Because the slack in the noncontractile tissues has been absorbed by the stretch, the effectiveness of the initial contractile force in moving the segment is enhanced.[49] However, quick stretch to an extensor in the lengthened range must be immediately followed by resisted movement into the shortened range to optimize strength in the range in which the muscle commonly functions. In contrast, repeated quick stretch in the lengthened range is incorporated into techniques to facilitate flexors (See Chapter 3, Repeated Contractions).

Approximation and Traction Forces

Approximation, or **compression,** into or through a joint stimulates the joint receptors and may facilitate extensor muscles and stability around the joint.[54] Approximation occurs with weight bearing through the joint, also termed *closed-chain activities,* or can be manually or mechanically applied. For example, in prone on elbows, weight bearing occurs through the shoulders and scapula; in modified plantigrade, both the upper and lower extremity joints are approximated. Additional weight-bearing force can be applied manually or with equipment such as weighted belts to increase the activation of muscular stability forces (Fig. 2–10). *Approximation is included when the goal of the procedure is to increase extensor activation and postural stability control.*

Traction, or distraction, separates the joint surfaces. Traction is most commonly applied manually, although it can be applied by various types of equipment (Fig. 2–11). Traction is incorporated if increasing ROM around the joint is desired.

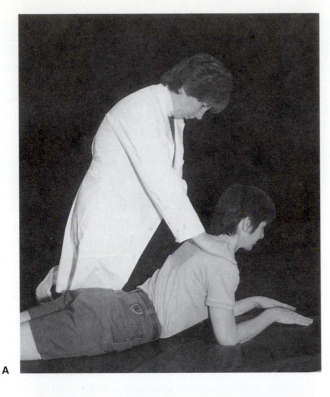

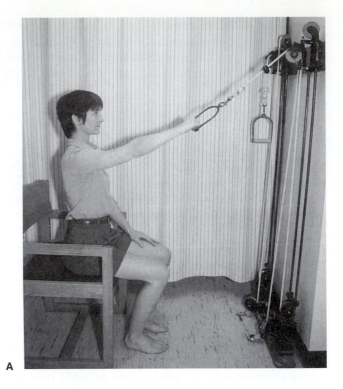

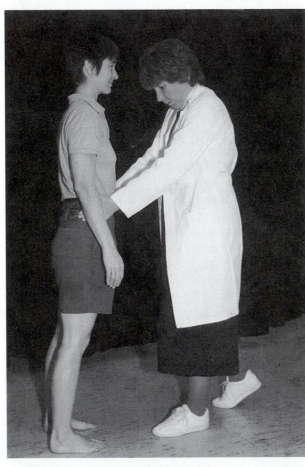

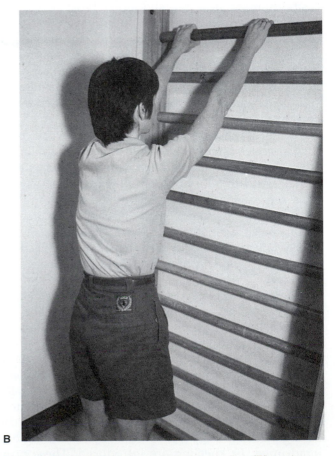

Figure 2–10. (A) Approximation applied at the shoulders in prone on elbows; **(B)** standing with approximation.

Figure 2–11. (A) Traction force applied by a pulley; **(B)** traction with stall bars.

Cutaneous and Pressure Input

The placement of manual contacts and various types of cutaneous and proprioceptive stimuli can alter muscle responses. Prolonged pressure on long tendons, such as the quadriceps, biceps, hamstrings, or finger flexors, seems to inhibit responses.[19] The pressure can be applied by the weight-bearing surface, for example, weight bearing on the quadriceps tendon in quadruped, on the triceps tendon in prone on elbows, or with manual pressure directly applied, such as on the biceps tendon.

The placement of manual contacts is critical to facilitate the desired response. Contacts are placed in the direction toward which the segment is to move. For example, if shoulder flexion is desired, the contact should be such that the limb tracks into that direction (Fig. 2–12).

In summary, the relationships between muscle type, strength, the factors of resistance, stretch, and postural control are important clinical factors to be considered when choosing postures and movements. Many questions regarding these parameters still exist and warrant continued investigation.

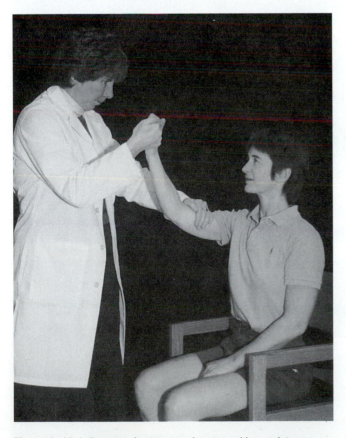

Figure 2–12. Influence of cutaneous input: tracking resistance on the flexor surface of the limb.

POSTURES AND MOVEMENT PATTERNS

The biomechanical and neurophysiological factors and principles discussed above are the basis for determining treatment postures and movement patterns. In the following discussion common clinical applications and the advantages and disadvantages of each posture are delineated. Certain factors have a greater influence on particular patient groups than others. For example, patients with nervous system involvement may be affected more by reflexive influences than those with primarily musculoskeletal impairments. These factors are addressed further in the chapters guiding patient care. The order of presentation of the activities does not indicate an order of importance or a hierarchical interpretation of the material.

Supine Progression: Supine, Sidelying, Rolling

Common Factors

The BoS is large, the CoG, is low making the postures inherently stable. Weight bearing occurs on but not through the trunk segments. The placement of resistive forces, including the positioning of manual contacts, will determine the length of the lever arm. Depending on the goals to be achieved, the focus of the procedures can be on the trunk or extremities.

Phasic reflexes are not facilitated unless the hands or feet are stimulated or are contacting the surface. In supine, the STLR increases extensor tone of the trunk and limbs. Righting reactions, if dominant, may result in neck, trunk, and limb flexion, termed withdrawal or supine flexion.[19] If the neck rotates, the ATNR influence may increase extensor tone in the chin arm and flexor tone in the skull arm. In contrast, head and neck rotation in supine or sidelying may stimulate the neck righting reaction of log or total trunk rolling. In sidelying, the uppermost limbs may exhibit decreased extensor tone, and the limbs in contact with the surface an increase in extensor tone, which is most commonly attributed to the ATLR. Also noted in supine and sidelying is the body-on-body righting reaction of trunk segmental rotation, which contributes to the rolling activity. The body-on-body response is evident when the upper body or lower body is rotated and the other body segments follow with a rolling motion. If the patient can overcome the tendency to always roll when the head or trunk segment is rotated and if trunk counterrotation can be performed, the body-on-body reaction is considered integrated.

Supine

The trunk and extremity extensor muscles are in shortened ranges whereas the flexor musculature is lengthened. Most of the trunk, bilateral, and unilateral upper- and lower-extremity movement combinations can be performed in any direction. For example, to increase range and control of trunk extension and rotation, a sequence of combinations might be upper trunk extension to the right, a bilateral symmetrical or reciprocal, and a unilateral diagonal 2 (D2) pattern (Fig. 2–13). This sequence would be useful for many elderly patients and those with parkinsonism. For patients with weakness in the gluteus medius, a sequence might be lower trunk extension toward the involved side, bilateral symmetrical diagonal 1 extension (D1E) and unilateral D1E (Fig. 2–14). Elongation of tight back extensors or of the quadratus lumborum can occur when the lower trunk flexion pattern is maintained in the shortened range. Unilateral lower extremity mass patterns can be used to initiate muscle activation and to improve strength. The advanced lower extremity combination of hip extension with knee flexion must be performed with the leg off the

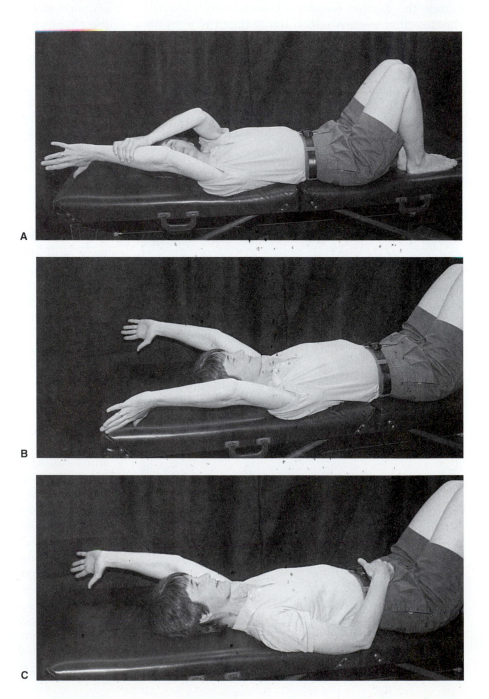

Figure 2–13. Sequence of upper-extremity combinations: **(A)** upper-trunk extension to the right; **(B)** BS D2 flexion; **(C)** unilateral D2 flexion.

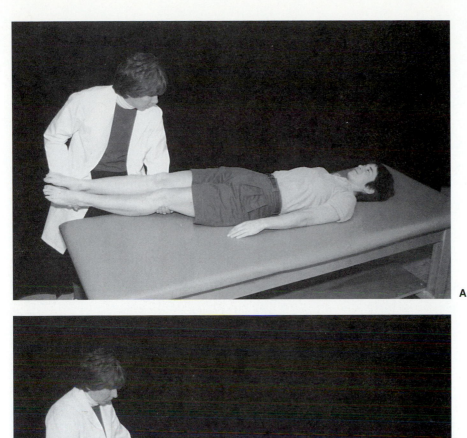

A

Figure 2–14. Sequence of lower-extremity movements to strengthen the gluteus medius: **(A)** lower-trunk extension toward the involved right side; **(B)** bilateral D1E, LE; **(C)** unilateral D1E, LE.

B

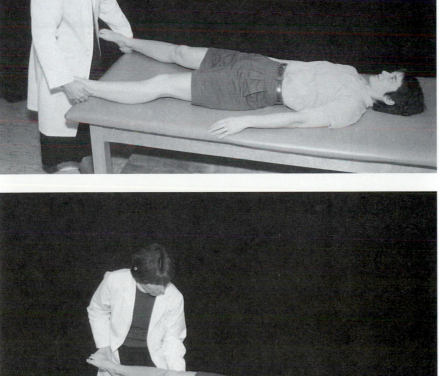

C

Figure 2–15. Advanced lower extremity movement in supine.

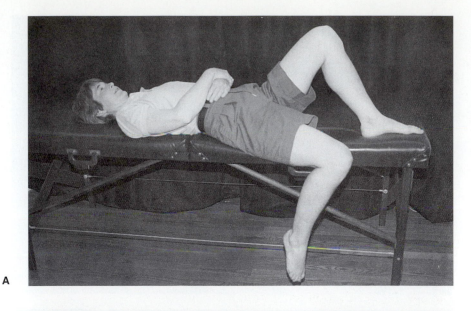

A

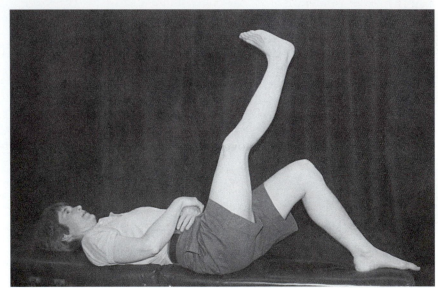

B

supporting surface to allow full movement (Fig. 2–15).

Gravity and the tonic reflexes resist flexion of the head, trunk, and the limbs to 90°; extensor movements are assisted. Because the BoS is large and stable and the CoG is low, no postural balance responses are needed to maintain the posture.

Advantages. The large BoS and low CoM make supine a stable posture. Supine is a good position in

which to achieve the treatment goals of increased relaxation, increased ROM, and the initiation of active movement, all encompassed within the mobility stage of control. The reflexive and gravitational influences are beneficial when improving strength of weak extensors in the trunk and proximal limbs. Initial holding of the postural extensors may be achieved in the shortened range by positioning the patient supine with a pillow or bolster under the knees. A "quad and glut set" may be performed in

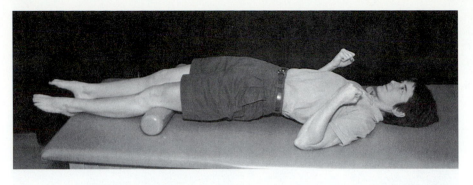

Figure 2–16. Quadriceps and gluteal sets combined with upper-body extension.

conjunction with contraction of the lower and upper trunk extensors (Fig. 2–16).

Disadvantages. Flexion and rotation are resisted by both reflexive influences and gravity, making these movements difficult for patients dominated by tonic reflexes or those with strength below 3/5. Movement into the range of hip and shoulder hyperextension is limited by the supporting surface, a concern with patients who are supine for prolonged periods (see Chapter 8). Because the scapula is contacting the supporting surface and is not easily accessible, it may not move with the glenohumeral joint during ROM exercises, resulting in abnormal movement or impinge-

ment. Supine may be difficult for some patients with cardiovascular–pulmonary (CVP) dysfunction, requiring elevation of the top of the bed.

Sidelying

The size of the BoS can vary depending on the placement of the extremities. If the uppermost limbs are flexed and in contact with the surface, the BoS is increased; if these limbs are extended the BoS is smaller (Fig. 2–17). In contrast to supine, sidelying has a smaller BoS and higher CoG. Unilateral control of the uppermost proximal limbs can be performed with gravity resisting abduction, assisting with adduction, and eliminated during flexion and extension move-

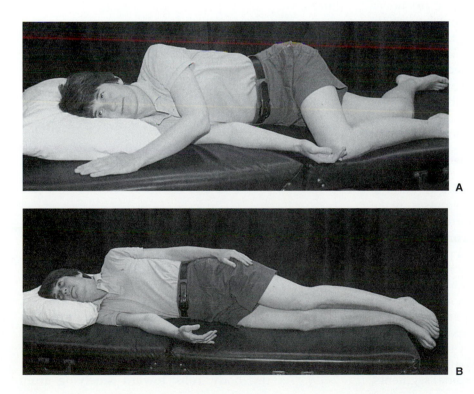

A

B

Figure 2–17. Limbs positioned to alter the base of support.

Figure 2–18. Sidelying, lower-trunk flexion combined with lower-extremity flexion.

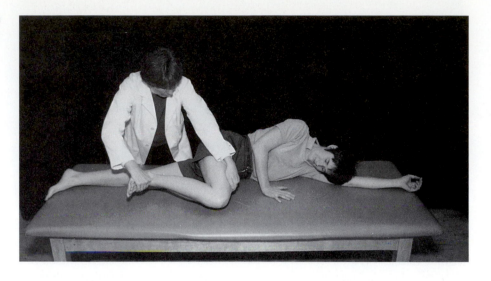

ments (Fig. 2–18). Within the trunk, total body control or control of specific spinal segments may be the focus. When the trunk and hip are positioned in extension and the scapula adducted, control of these muscles can be promoted in shortened ranges; antagonistic flexor muscles can be initiated and emphasized from lengthened ranges assisted by the ATLR influence. Segmental lumbar motions and pelvic tilt can be combined with mass lower-extremity (LE) flexion and extension motions (Fig. 2–18). A sequence of trunk movements incorporated into treatment might be: upper or lower body motions to initiate muscle contractions, isometrics to promote stability, log rolling for controlled movement, segmental rotation to strengthen trunk muscles and to promote body-on-body reactions, and trunk counterrotation to improve the control needed for ambulation. This series of movements may be useful in promoting trunk control with many patients, including those with hemiplegia, parkinsonism or spinal dysfunction.

Advantages. The BoS is large, the CoG low, and the requirement of minimal postural responses make sidelying, like supine, a useful posture to increase ROM, to initiate movement, and to promote stability and rotational control in the trunk and proximal segments of the uppermost limbs. Sensory awareness may be increased in the lowermost limbs by weight bearing and body contact on the supporting surface, a consideration with hemiplegic patients. When rolling is initiated in sidelying, as compared to beginning in supine or prone, the effects of tone, reflexes, and gravity may be diminished. For patients who require mobility or stability of specific spinal segments,

such as those with back dysfunction, manual contacts can be placed to enhance the control at specific levels. In contrast, if a patient has poor trunk stability resulting from weakness or decreased motor control, the therapist's contacts may be positioned on the scapula and pelvis to enhance activity of the entire trunk before attempting a specific focus. Trunk rotation is easily promoted with log rolling, segmental motion, or counterrotation. Flexion, extension, and sidebending of particular levels and of the entire trunk can be emphasized.

Disadvantages. In sidelying, the primary emphasis is on the uppermost limbs and segments. The weight bearing on the lowermost shoulder or hip may cause pain in some patients. Trunk and bilateral extremity combinations are not performed in sidelying because of the restrictions of the supporting surface. Circulatory perfusion and aeration of one lung may be diminished in sidelying and must be taken into account with patients who have CVP involvement.[55]

Rolling

Rolling is the transitional activity between supine and sidelying.

Trunk, bilateral, and unilateral upper-extremity movement combinations and unilateral lower-extremity patterns can augment the trunk movement. With the upper-trunk combinations the limbs can make contact at the elbows, forearms, or hands;[7–9] varying the point of contact will change the number of joints involved and the length of the lever arm (Fig. 2–19). As the body rolls toward sidelying from

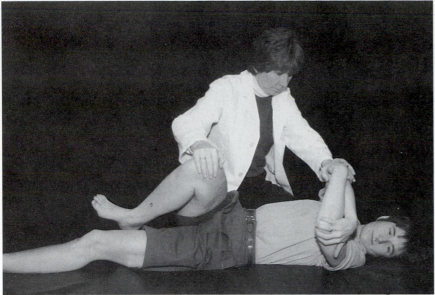

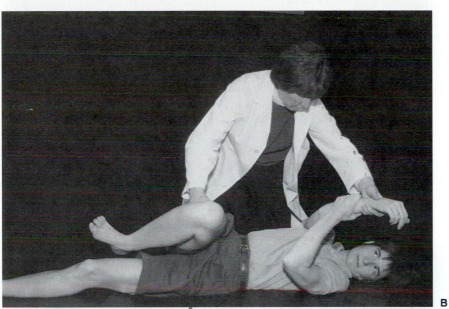

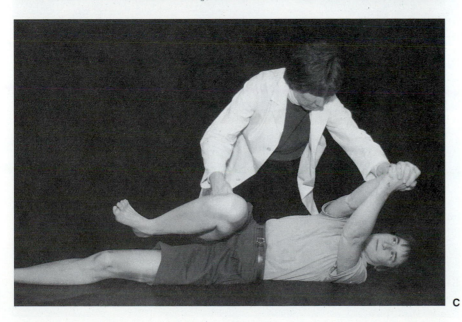

Figure 2–19. Rolling with various upper limb combinations: **(A)** contacting at the elbows; **(B)** contacting at the forearms; **(C)** contacting at the hands.

Figure 2–20. Rolling with the limbs flexing and adducting.

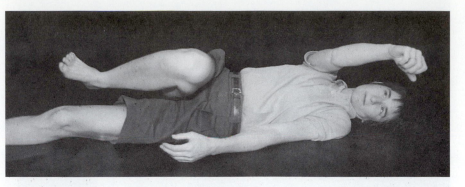

supine, the ipsilateral limbs flex and adduct across the midline (Fig. 2–20). If the patient has one-sided weakness, the involved limb may be assisted by the uninvolved side. For example, when rolling toward the right, the head and trunk flex with rotation to the right, the left upper and lower extremities flex and adduct to or across the midline. The left lower extremity can push off with extension and abduction prior to the flexion–adduction motion.

Because the BoS is large and the CoG low, minimal postural control responses are needed; however, the body reacts to the self-imposed change of the CoM within the BoS.

The initial flexion motion from supine is resisted by gravity and the STLR; adduction of the ipsilateral limbs is resisted by the ATNR. In addition, the ATNR may interfere with rolling by increasing the extensor tone in the limb toward which the patient is moving.[16] The limb may act as an immobile strut, reduc-

ing the person's ability to roll toward that side. To reduce gravitational and reflexive resistance, rolling may be initiated from a semisupine position with the body supported by pillows and one lower extremity crossed over the other (Fig. 2–21).

Rolling movements provide an initial way of coordinating extremity with trunk motions in a posture with a large BoS and low CoG. For example, a college-age pitcher is receiving therapy following a right Bankhart shoulder repair. To enhance the contribution of his trunk to the pitching motion, upper-trunk flexion and rotation to the left is combined with diagonal 2 extension (D2E) of the right upper extremity (UE) (Fig. 2–22). Maximizing the trunk contribution to the throwing motion is important to enhance the force of the throw and to minimize stress on the shoulder complex. Rolling provides a means of integrating these motions while learning to use them in standing.

Figure 2–21. Initiation of rolling from semisupine.

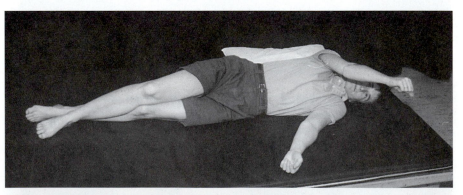

Figure 2–22. Rolling with an upper extremity D2E movement.

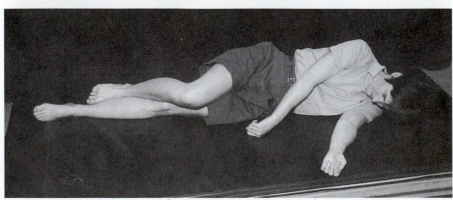

Advantages. Rolling is a functional activity important for bed mobility, pressure relief, and assumption of sitting; for some patients it is a prerequisite for dressing (see Chapter 8). The large BoS, low CoG, and the involvement of varying segments make rolling a useful activity to balance tone and initiate trunk and proximal movement. Rolling in both directions is desirable to promote a normal variety of movement.

Disadvantages. Patients with dominant tonic reflexes will have difficulty initiating flexion while in the supine position and may attempt to compensate with abnormal reflex-dominated movements. Rolling onto an involved side may increase pain, particularly in the shoulder.

Prone Progression: Pivot Prone, Prone on Elbows, Prone on Hands, Quadruped

Common Factors

In these prone positions the STLR reduces extensor tone, resulting in increased flexion of the trunk and proximal limbs. Gravity and the STLR resist extension of the head, trunk, and limbs. The hand contact with the surface may stimulate the grasp reflex. If the patient is dominated by tonic reflexes, head extension may stimulate the STNR, enhancing the symmetrical upper-extremity extension position. Rotation of the head will tend to flex the skull elbow, and flexion of the head will tend to flex both elbows. The optical, labyrinthine, and body-on-head righting reactions increase the tendency toward trunk extension.

The progression within these prone postures is toward decreasing the size of the BoS, raising the height of the CoG, and increasing the number of joints involved in supporting the body weight.

Pivot Prone

The size of the BoS will vary with the number of segments raised from the surface. The head, neck, upper- and lower-trunk, and hip extensor musculature are performing isometric contractions in the shortened range against gravity.[19] Varying the length of the lever arm, for example, flexing or extending the elbow, changes the CoM of the limb. The arms can be unilaterally or bilaterally extended by the side or flexed overhead. The elbow variation, coupled with a change in position of the shoulder joint, alters the challenge to the upper-body extensors. When the shoulders extend and scapulae adduct, the middle trapezius, rhomboids and posterior deltoid are active; when the shoulders flex and the scapulae upwardly rotate, the lower trapezius and middle deltoid are more active[56] (Fig. 2–23). In the lower extremities, the gluteus maximus and medius extend and abduct the hip, reducing any abnormal tendency of hip extension with adduction. The extremity combinations can be varied to alter the difficulty of the activity and to achieve specific therapeutic goals. For example, if all the limbs are maintained in bilateral symmetrical patterns, symmetrical activation of the trunk extensor musculature, including the deep extensor muscles, occurs. Raising the limbs in a contralateral pattern, for example the left upper extrem-

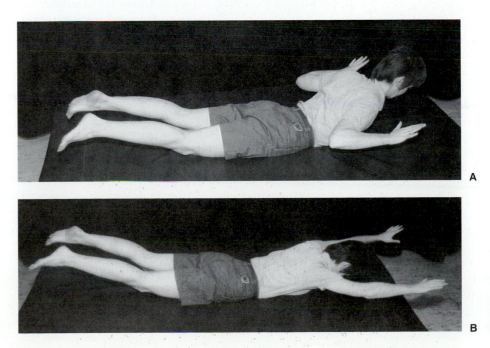

A

B

Figure 2–23. Pivot prone with different symmetrical patterns: **(A)** shoulders extended; **(B)** shoulders flexed.

Figure 2–24. Pivot prone with contralateral limb combination.

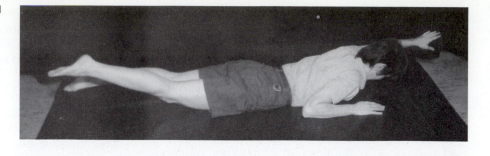

ity with the right lower extremity, produces an asymmetrical activation of the upper- and lower-trunk musculature (Fig. 2–24). This pattern of muscular activation, which crosses the thoracolumbar junction, stabilizes the trunk against the rotating forces of the limb weight. No weight occurs through the joints, although compression in the posterior lumbar spine may occur with the extensor muscle activity (see Chapter 7).

Phasic reflexes are not stimulated, provided that the palm of the hand and sole of the foot are not contacting the surface. The ability to extend in prone indicates integration of the STLR and the STNR and sufficient range and strength to move into the extended position. Vestibular input may be enhanced if the body is tilted slightly downward. Increased vestibular stimulation facilitates postural extensors when the body is linearly accelerated, for example, in a hammock or with a child supported in the therapist's arms.[57] Postural responses may be evident if the supporting surface is tilted or unstable, such as occurs when extending over a ball. The resistance of gravity can be altered by angling the trunk using a prone board, wedge, or a ball.[16]

Advantages. The sustained contractions of the head, neck, trunk, and proximal limb extensors are performed against body-weight resistance promoting both muscle stability and endurance. Stability control in the postural extensors is enhanced by the increase in muscle spindle stretch sensitivity, which occurs as the contraction is maintained for about 10 seconds.[9] Muscle stability is a prerequisite to postural stability, which occurs when weight-bearing positions are maintained. Endurance is improved as the person contracts against the resistance of gravity with the same intensity but for longer durations. The intensity, of approximately 40% of a maximum contraction, is within the aerobic boundary.[42,48] This contraction should be maintained for a prolonged duration, for example, from 20 seconds to 1 minute, although the duration will vary among individuals. The type I, slow-twitch, oxidative fibers needed to improve stability and endurance are activated by this low-intensity, long-duration contraction. To better ensure aerobic activity, the person should breathe with normal depth and speed of respirations. The duration of the exercise can be measured by the number of breaths: for example, maintaining the contraction for 3 breaths and progressing up to 10 breaths, which is approximately 30 seconds.

For some patients with low-back dysfunction and radiating pain to the lower extremity, lying prone on a firm surface may reduce symptoms.

Disadvantages. The inability to move into pivot prone may indicate decreased range, dominance of the tonic reflexes, ineffectual righting reactions, or weakness of the extensor muscles, below 3/5. For those with hip flexor tightness or ROM limitations in the lumbar spine or anterior body, a pillow under the chest and abdomen will allow the patient to maintain prone more comfortably. If the resistance from the tonic reflexes and gravity is too difficult to overcome, positions such as sidelying, semisitting or supported prone can be substituted. To reduce the resistance of limb weight, upper and lower body extension can be performed in supine before progressing to prone.

For patients with compromised cardiopulmonary status, the position may be difficult or contraindicated. The weight bearing on the chest wall can decrease the excursion of the rib cage. Patients with weakness of the respiratory muscles, including patients with spinal cord injury (SCI), may find prone too difficult in the early stages of the rehabilitation process.

The compression that occurs in the posterior vertebral joints may be uncomfortable or contraindicated for some with low-back pain; for others, the active muscular contraction may be consistent with the goal of increasing range into lumbar extension.

Prone on Elbows

The CoM of the head and upper trunk are raised slightly off the supporting surface while the lower body remains in contact. The upper extremities are held in a bilateral symmetrical position with the scapulae in mid range between protraction and re-

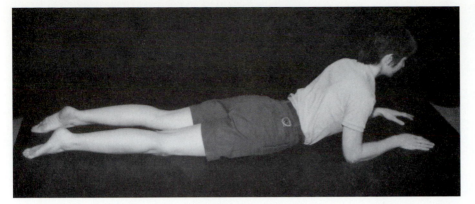

Figure 2–25. Prone on elbows.

traction, the shoulders flexed to 30 to 45°, and the elbows flexed to 90° (Fig. 2–25). Weight is borne on the elbow, which must have sufficient range to assume the posture. Because no weight occurs **through** the elbow joint, stability is not required. Weight bearing occurs through the scapulothoracic and shoulder joints, requiring stability at these joints. When unilateral arm movements are performed, increased weight bearing on and through the supporting limb occurs.

The neck extensors are positioned in mid range, rather than the shortened range that occurs in pivot prone.[19] This slight stretch facilitates contraction of the short and long neck extensors and flexors. The position of the upper arm will influence the amount of activity in the shoulder musculature: if the elbows are positioned directly under the shoulders, the position is mechanically stable and little shoulder activity is needed; resistance applied anteriorly, posteriorly, or laterally will require increased proximal muscle activation to maintain the posture. Weight shifting anteriorly and posteriorly promotes symmetrical shoulder flexion and extension; lateral weight shifting promotes asymmetrical scapular and shoulder abduction and adduction.

If the hand contacts the supporting surface, the grasp reflex may be stimulated. Head extension may increase extension in the upper extremities, especially at the elbows via the STNR. Rotation of the head can result in an ATNR response, which is extension of the chin arm and flexion or a collapse of the skull arm (Fig. 2–26).[14] This response may, however,

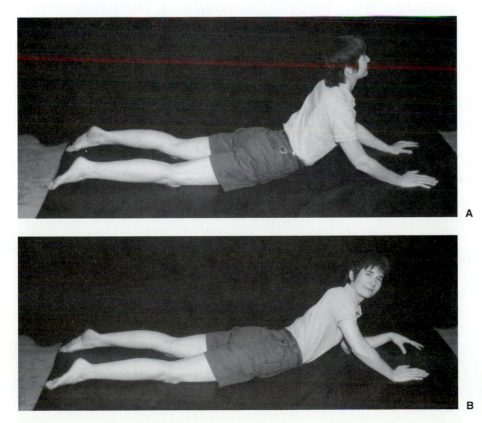

A

B

Figure 2–26. The influence of the tonic neck reflexes in prone on elbows: **(A)** STNR; **(B)** ATNR.

Figure 2–27. Unilateral weight bearing in prone on elbows.

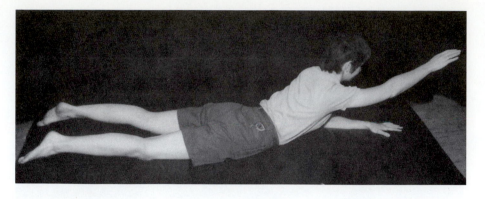

be dampened by the weight bearing through the proximal upper extremities. The amphibian reflex, which can facilitate lower extremity flexion if no other response is possible, is stimulated by rotating one side of the pelvis backward, resulting in flexion of the ipsilateral lower extremity. The optical, labyrinthine, and body-on-head righting reactions help maintain the head and body position.[58] However, if dominant, the response may increase upper-body and shoulder extension. Postural responses help maintain the position and control movement of the CoM during weight shifting. If one upper extremity is lifted from the supporting surface to reach for an object or in preparation for crawling, the CoM shifts toward the supporting BoS, increasing the activation of supporting musculature (Fig. 2–27). As the raised limb moves, the supporting segments need to respond in a dynamic stabilizing manner to counter the changing CoM. This proximal dynamic stability can be further challenged and enhanced by isometric resistance provided to the supporting limb and by resistance to the moving limb.

Gravity and tone resist head, neck, and trunk extension, most movements of the shoulder, and movement of the hip into extension and the knee into flexion. The serratus anterior contracts with the trapezius and rhomboids to maintain mid range of the scapulothoracic joint. Because the elbows are flexed, the length of the upper extremity lever arm is short in comparison to other weight-bearing postures, such as quadruped. A wedge or other support under the upper chest can further reduce the body weight resistance imposed on the upper extremities.

Advantages. The large BoS and low CoM reduce the need for postural control responses, making prone on elbows useful for patients with diminished ability to control more biomechanically challenging postures. The short lever arm in the upper extremity and the decreased need for elbow stability allows treatment to be focused on the proximal scapula and shoulder

(see Chapter 8). Unlike pivot prone, the range of lumbar spine extension can be passively maintained, which may be beneficial when the goal is to increase range into lumbar extension (see Chapter 7). Knee flexion can be promoted either passively or actively with the thigh well supported. However, active range may be limited by insufficiency of the hamstrings and passive range limited by insufficiency of the two joint quadriceps (see Chapter 6). With the knee extended, ankle dorsiflexion lengthens the gastrocnemius over the knee and ankle.

Disadvantages. As with the pivot prone posture, weight bearing occurs on the abdomen, resisting chest wall expansion and increasing the difficulty of breathing. This may make prone on elbows contraindicated for patients with CVP involvement and for some elderly patients.

Extension in the lumbar spine and hip may be difficult if the trunk or hip flexors are tight, although the effect of this tightness can be reduced by a pillow placed under the abdomen (Fig. 2–28). Patients with low back involvement may experience either a decrease or increase in pain, depending on the etiology of their condition, and may require modifications in the posture (see Chapter 7).

Patients with neuromuscular dysfunction may demonstrate an increase in abnormal tone in the shoulder internal rotators, elbow flexors, and wrist and fingers flexors, an indication that the posture may be too difficult. If this abnormal posturing interferes with the patient's functional or therapeutic use of the posture, an alternative position should be chosen, such as modified sitting (Fig. 2–29).

Because the upper extremity is flexed both at the shoulder and elbow, the triceps is maintained in a lengthened position. This stretch, coupled with the weight-bearing pressure on the triceps tendon, tends to increase inhibitory influences, making prone on elbows contraindicated if the treatment goals include increasing triceps control. To reduce the tendency to-

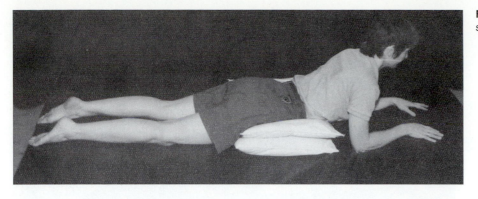

Figure 2–28. Prone on elbows with pillow support.

ward hip and knee extension with adduction, a pillow can be placed between the thighs and under the lower legs.

Prone on Hands

The upper body CoM is raised from the BoS. Weight is borne through the elbow in addition to the proxi-

mal joints, and on the wrist. The upper extremities remain in a symmetrical pattern with a long lever arm.

More body weight resistance occurs through the upper extremities than in any of the previous postures. The head, neck, and thoracic and lumbar spine are extended, the shoulders are flexed to about 60°, and the triceps are holding in the shortened ranges at

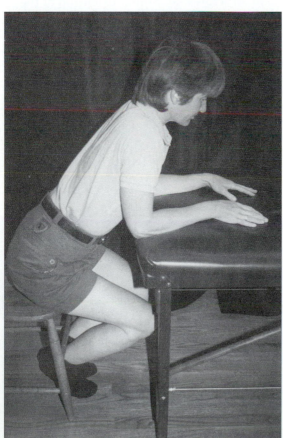

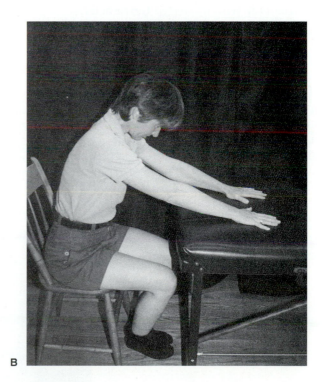

Figure 2–29. Modified sitting for upper limb control.

Figure 2–30. Prone on hands.

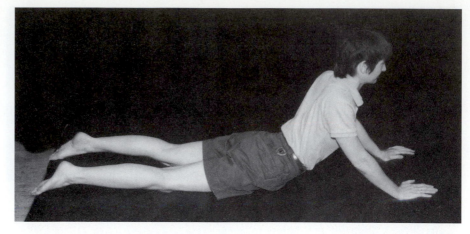

the elbow. The hips and the lower extremity joints are extended (Fig. 2–30).

Because the CoM is raised higher off the BoS in comparison to prone on elbows, some postural control in the upper body and limbs is required.

Advantages. The elbow is held in an extended position, which may be appropriate for patients with hyperactivity of the biceps or weakness of the triceps. Pressure on the finger flexor tendons increases inhibitory influences to these muscles and is indicated for patients with increased flexor activity.

The fully extended position of the lumbar spine may increase mobility for some patients with lumbar spine dysfunction (see Chapter 7).[59]

Disadvantages. The extended head and symmetrical pattern of the upper extremities may reinforce a dominant STNR, especially in children. As with the previous prone postures, the extension of the lumbar spine and hips may be painful for some patients. Children are usually more flexible than adults and can maintain this posture more easily.

Quadruped

Quadruped has a smaller BoS, a higher CoM and more joints are involved with increased weight bearing as compared to prone on elbows or on hands (Fig. 2–31). Upper extremity weight bearing occurs through the elbow and on the wrist and hand. The elbow must be stabilized to support the body weight. If the elbow is hyperextended and the shoulder externally rotated, the congruence of the bony structures provides passive stability. Contraction of the triceps and biceps provides stability to reduce stress on the joint structures. ROM into extension at the wrist and hand must be complete to bear weight on the wrist. In the lower extremity, weight bearing occurs through the hip and on the knee. Pressure on the patellar tendon can increase inhibition to the quadriceps and weight bearing on the knee can be painful for some patients.

Rocking can be performed in flexion and extension or in diagonal directions, promoting dynamic trunk control and straight plane or diagonal limb movements. Unilateral diagonal upper extremity patterns enhance trunk movements of flexion or exten-

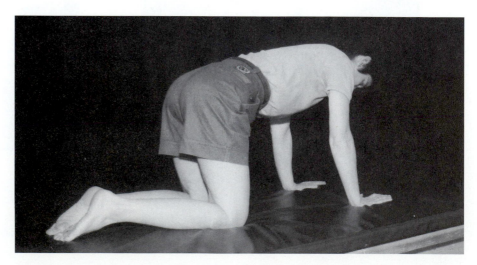

Figure 2–31. Quadruped.

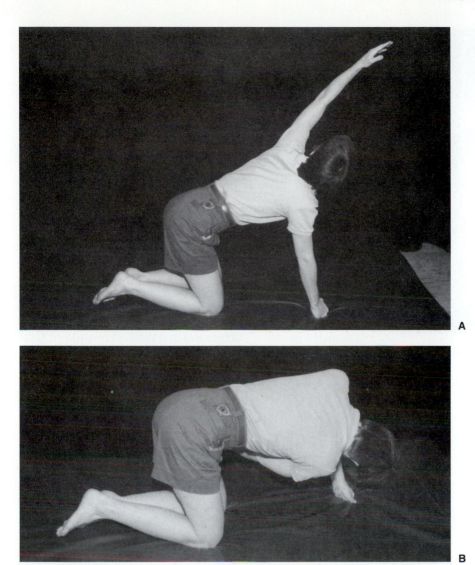

A

B

Figure 2–32. Quadruped with unilateral upper-extremity movements to enhance trunk movements: **(A)** D2F for upper trunk extension with rotation; **(B)** D2E for upper trunk flexion with rotation.

sion combined with rotation and lateral sidebending (Fig. 2–32). Lifting one limb or contralateral limbs decreases the BoS and increases the challenge to pos-

tural responses (Fig. 2–33). The limbs that remain in contact with the supporting surface provide the dynamic stability needed to adjust the CoM within the

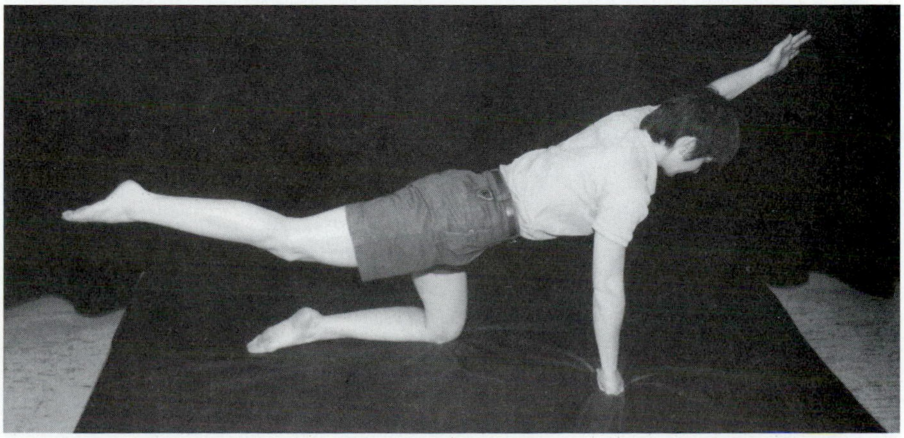

Figure 2–33. Quadruped contralateral limb lifts.

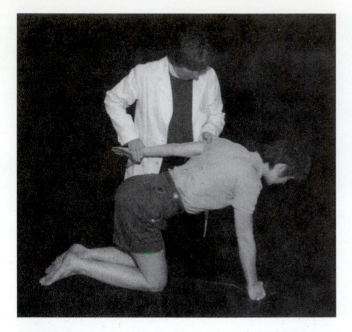

Figure 2–34. Quadruped manual resistance to upper extremity D1E.

BoS. This control is further challenged when the non-supporting limbs actively move, are resisted, or if the body weight shifts (Fig. 2–34). Postural control also can be challenged by placing the person on a movable surface such as a balance board or a pliable surface such as foam. With the eyes closed, visual input is eliminated and more reliance put on the labyrinthine, proprioceptive, and tactile inputs.

The weight of the trunk tends to extend the spine. This force is countered by abdominal contraction, with the back extensors providing additional stability. Controlled movements into trunk flexion, sidebending, or rotation can occur as a total body motion or can be promoted at specific spinal segments, depending on the combinations performed. A ball placed under the abdomen can support some of the body weight and also provide dynamic support as the limbs are raised.

The lower extremities are in mass flexion and can move from the surface toward mass extension or flexion (Fig. 2–35). A mass flexion pattern is assisted from the lengthened range by both tonal influences and gravity. To activate the flexors manual or mechanical resistance can be provided. Extension movements into the shortened range are resisted by gravity and

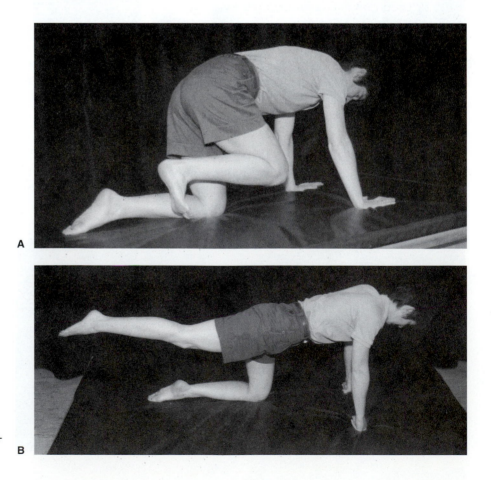

Figure 2–35. Quadruped lower-extremity movements: **(A)** mass flexion; **(B)** mass extension.

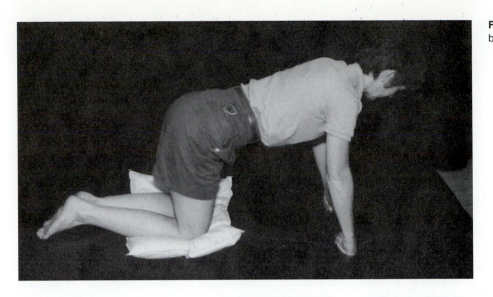

Figure 2–36. Quadruped altering weight-bearing forces.

tone with mechanical resistance or assistance added depending on the patient's ability. When the hip is in the shortened range of extension, the flexors are lengthened. If the hip flexors are tight, this position may increase lumbar extension if the abdominals cannot dynamically stabilize the trunk. An eccentric contraction of the hip extensors will lower the limb from the shortened range. D1E in the lower extremity promotes a normal synergistic action of the gluteus medius and maximus, a muscle combination required for the stance phase of gait.[60]

Advantages. In quadruped, the upper extremity is weight bearing with the shoulder at about 90° of flexion. This 90° usually is emphasized toward the latter phase of rehabilitation in patients with shoulder pain (see Chapter 5). Less compression occurs through the spine than in sitting and standing,[61] and the trunk can easily be maintained in a neutral position, which can be of benefit for patients with low back pain. Postural stability and dynamic control of the trunk can be promoted as well as controlled movement of particular spinal segments in all directions (see Chapter 7). Because of the assistance provided by tonal influences and gravity, weak hip flexors can be easily facilitated. Therefore, for those with increased extensor tone in the trunk and lower extremities, quadruped may be an appropriate posture in which to promote a balance of muscular activity.

Disadvantages. The range and the amount of weight bearing in the upper extremity, and the pressure on the knee may make quadruped too difficult for some patients to assume or maintain. The hand may be moved to the edge of the supporting surface or the posture can be modified by weight bearing on a fist.

Such wrist modifications decrease the range of wrist extension but increase the amount of muscular stability required. The supporting surface can be cushioned with towels or pillows, which may disperse pressure and change range at a painful wrist or knee (Fig. 2–36).

The mass flexion in the lower extremity may be in conflict with the goals of promoting advanced combinations in patients with neurological involvement.

Lower Trunk Sequence: Hooklying, Bridging, Kneeling, Half-Kneeling

These activities are included in the intervention program when the treatment goals include improved lower trunk and lower extremity control. An indirect effect is improved upper trunk stabilization, which occurs to counter the movement of the lower body.

In all of these activities, movement of the lower trunk can be performed in all three planes and in combined diagonal movements; flexion and extension occurs with a flattening and arching of the back or a posterior and anterior pelvic tilt; rotation is accomplished by rolling the pelvis from one side to the other; lateral flexion is performed by alternate hip hiking. The position of the pelvis and lower trunk requires sufficient tissue flexibility to assume the posture and a balance of muscular control to maintain and then move within the posture. Muscular control is provided by an interaction of the intrinsic rotatores and multifidi coupled with the erector spinae and oblique lower abdominals.

Hooklying and **bridging** have a large BoS and low CoM. The foot contact with the supporting surface may stimulate the extensor thrust or the flexor

Figure 2–37. Hooklying: altering sensory input.

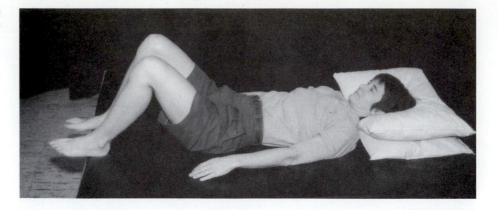

withdrawal reflex. The supine position increases extensor tone through the STLR. The increased extensor tone that occurs from both reflexes can make hip and knee flexion difficult to maintain. To reduce reflexive input, the forefoot contact can be altered by shifting weight onto the heel, and the head can be flexed with pillows; to decrease the knee extensor response, knee flexion can be increased (Fig. 2–37). The length of the lever arm in the lower extremity varies, depending on the position of the limbs and the placement of the therapist's contacts at the pelvis, knees, or ankles. If the limbs are positioned in more extension or if the therapist's contacts are placed more distally, the activation of the hip and knee musculature is increased. Hip flexor activity tends to extend the lower trunk and pull it into lordosis, which is counteracted by increased abdominal contraction (Fig. 2–38). When the lower extremities are held together, the activity of a weaker limb may be enhanced by the body-on-body contact and the tactile input. When the limbs are sep-

arated, tactile support is diminished and, although the BoS is widened, the challenge to lower trunk and hip control is increased.

Because the head is supported, vestibular input is not challenged. Therefore, these postures are appropriate when enhancing proprioceptive feedback in patients with vestibular dysfunction.

Hooklying

The lower extremities are in mass flexion, with the hips and knees usually flexed to approximately 60°, although the angle can be altered. The CoM of the lower extremity is partially raised off the BoS. Positioning the hips and knees in varying amounts of flexion alters the range in which control of these joints can be promoted. The abdominals, hip flexors, adductors, and hamstrings maintain the lower extremity position against gravitational and reflexive resistance.

Lower trunk rotation occurs when the knees

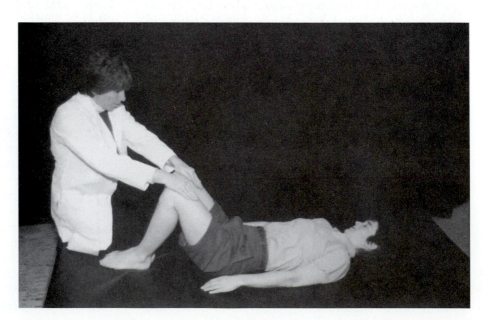

Figure 2–38. Hooklying: resistance to hip flexor and abdominal contractions.

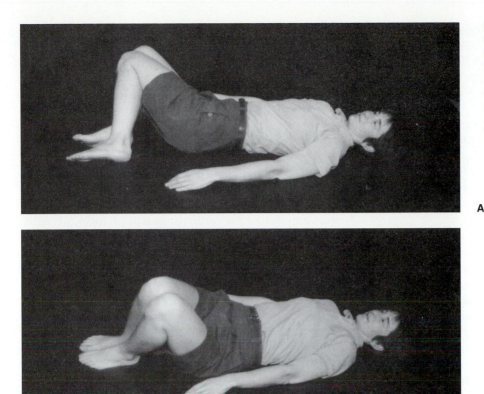

A

Figure 2–39. Hooklying: muscle activity in various portions of the range: **(A)** abdominal and hip flexors concentrically contract to midline; **(B)** abdominals and hip flexors eccentrically contract from mid to lengthened range; **(C)** abdominals and flexors manually resisted to mid range; **(D)** back and hip extensors manually resisted into the shortened range.

B

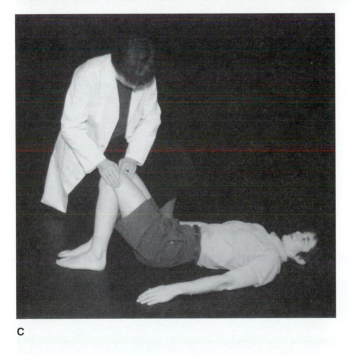

C

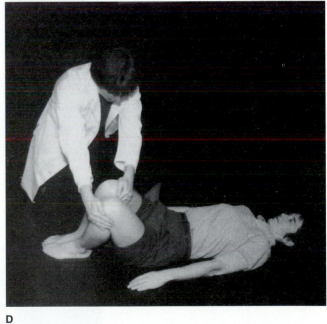

D

move from side to side. As the trunk moves from the lengthened range toward the mid position the abdominals, flexors, and abductors of the leading hip and adductors of the following hip concentrically contract. If these muscles are weaker than 3/5 grade, assistance must be provided. As the extremities lower from midline to the opposite side, the abdominals and hip flexors and adductors of the leading limb and abductors of the following limb eccentrically contract. If external resistance is provided, the muscle activity when coming to midline remains the same; however, when moving away from the midline, the extensors of the lower trunk and hips, with the abductors of the lead limb and adductors of the following limb, concentrically contract into their shortened ranges[62] (Fig. 2–39). Manual resistance promotes a reversal of antagonists; mechanical resistance, such as pulley or elastic bands, promote concentric–eccentric contractions. If the lower trunk and hip extensor response is strong enough to raise the hips from the supporting surface when resistance is applied, a progression to bridging is indicated.

During lower trunk rotation, unwanted upper body rotation may occur if a dominant body-on-body righting reaction or decreased ROM in the trunk are present. Input from the lower body proprioceptors stimulate the postural responses that help maintain the lower extremity position.

Advantages. The large BoS and low CoG support the treatment goals of increasing ROM, initiating movement, improving lower body stability, and promoting controlled movement in a posture with minimal weight bearing. In comparison to the promotion of lower trunk control in sidelying, more segments are involved, the length of the lever arm is increased, and the effect of gravity is varied. These factors make lower-trunk rotation (LTR) a logical progression from sidelying in a treatment sequence. Rotation of the lower trunk is needed during ambulation and commonly needs to be promoted in patients with parkinsonism or those with musculoskeletal tightness.

As the limbs rotate, a slow, maintained stretch can be applied to antagonistic quadratus lumborum and lateral trunk flexors. This stretch may reduce excessive muscular activity found in some patients with low back dysfunction or hemiplegia. The lower body is not weight bearing, which is particularly important when compression in the disc or facet increases pain[61] (see Chapter 7). The amount of abdominal activity may be increased by altering placement of manual contacts from the knees to the ankles and by moving the feet further from the buttocks.

In hooklying, the contraction of the pubococcygeal muscles can be enhanced with overflow from contraction of the hip adductors and abdominals.[63]

Increased awareness of and control over the pelvic floor muscles may be indicated postpartum and for patients experiencing incontinence.

Activating and controlling quadriceps and hamstring activity as the knee nears full extension is included in the treatment plan for many patients with neuromuscular or musculoskeletal dysfunction. Promoting muscular stability in more extended ranges in hooklying may precede promotion of postural stability in closed-chain positions that involve more weight bearing through the knee. In addition to its promotion of muscular control, this position allows performance of osteokinematic range and arthrokinematic glides of the knee (see Chapter 6).

Disadvantages. Maintaining the lower extremity position may be too difficult for some patients because the foot contact with the surface may stimulate an extensor thrust, or less commonly, a flexor withdrawal. Strength of approximately 2+/5 of the abdominals and hip and knee flexors and hip adductors is needed to maintain this posture. The horizontal position of the upper body may be contraindicated for some patients with CVP dysfunction.

Bridging

The bridging posture has a smaller BoS and a higher CoM than hooklying. The base can be widened by separating the feet, or narrowed by lifting one limb. More segments are involved than in hooklying: the lower trunk, hips, and knees serve a supportive weight-bearing function. The bridging position is correctly performed when the hips are at 0° of extension with the lumbar spine in a neutral position (Fig. 2–40). The hip is extended and the knee flexed, an advanced combination.[7] When the BoS is further narrowed by weight bearing on one limb, the challenge to stabilize with the lower trunk and supporting limb

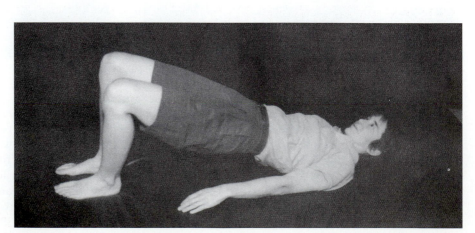

Figure 2–40. Bridging: hips at 0° extension with spine in a neutral curve.

increases. Trunk and hip control can be promoted in all three planes and in diagonal directions. When the knees are flexed to 90°, the hamstrings are in a position of active insufficiency; hip extension, therefore, is maintained primarily by the gluteus maximus.[64]

Because the body does not need to orient to the environment, righting reactions are minimized. Postural responses, primarily from proprioceptive stimuli, will maintain the lower body CoG within the BoS. The challenge can be increased by weight bearing on one extremity or a ball.

Gravity resists as the lower trunk and hip extensors hold in their shortened ranges. When the feet move more distally, the length of the lever arm and the range of knee extension is increased, resulting in progressively increased hamstring activity as ranges closer to knee extension are achieved.[65] The lever arm also lengthens when resistive forces are applied at the pelvis, knees, or ankles. Quadriceps as well as hamstring activity is dependent on the knee range. When the knees are flexed to 90°, the lengthened quadriceps demonstrate minimal activity. When the knees are more extended, the quadriceps activity increases.

Advantages. Bridging is a useful posture to promote the static and dynamic control in the lower trunk and hip needed during standing and for gait. The alignment of the lower trunk and hips segments is similar to upright postures, and many components of gait can be promoted, including pelvic forward progression, pelvic rotation, and hip extension combined with knee flexion with the ankle in dorsiflexion or plantar flexion. These components and the combination of hip extension with lateral stabilization can be practiced without the resistance of the upper body weight and the balance control required while standing. For patients with abnormal synergistic movements, the advanced lower extremity combination promotes hamstring activity and counteracts the excessive quadriceps contraction.

The hamstring activation, which increases as the knee extends, is important for patients with stability impairments of the posterior knee, including those with anterior cruciate ligament (ACL) dysfunction, posterior capsule laxity, and hamstring weakness. The lower body challenge can be increased various ways: bilateral to unilateral support, walking in place, and use of different surfaces, including foam, a balance board, or a ball (Fig. 2–41).

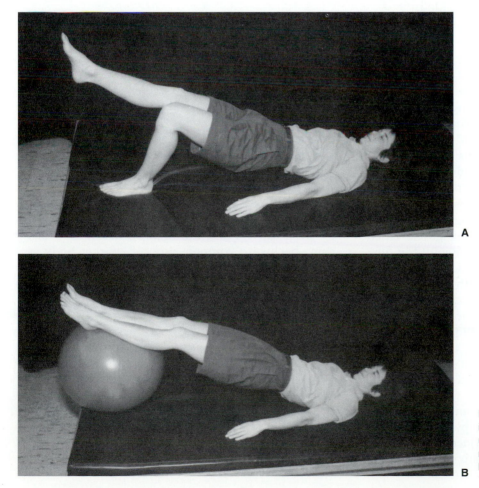

Figure 2–41. Bridging: limbs positioned to increase proximal dynamic stability: **(A)** unilateral weight bearing with the knee in more extension; **(B)** weight bearing on a ball.

For patients with decreased position sense, static and dynamic activity in bridging can be used to stimulate the proprioceptive and tactile receptors. This peripheral input from the lower body is also important for patients experiencing sensory conflict among visual, vestibular, and proprioceptive inputs.

Disadvantages. The supine position and the isometric contraction needed to maintain bridging may be difficult or contraindicated for some patients with CVP involvement. Patients with neurological involvement may be unable to overcome the phasic and tonic reflex influence to assume or maintain the posture. Head position may be altered, however, and weight can be borne on the heel rather than on the entire foot to discourage abnormal extension. If these modifications do not reduce the challenge, other postures, such as sidelying and hooklying, may be more beneficial in promoting a balance of tone and reducing reflex dominance. If the lower trunk and hip extensor muscles are weaker than 3/5, bridging may be too difficult; less demanding activities such as lower trunk rotation or lower trunk extension in the gravity assisted posture of supine may be indicated. Bridging performed with excessive extension of the hips or low back can result in discomfort in the lumbar spine or sacroiliac (SI) joint and should be avoided.

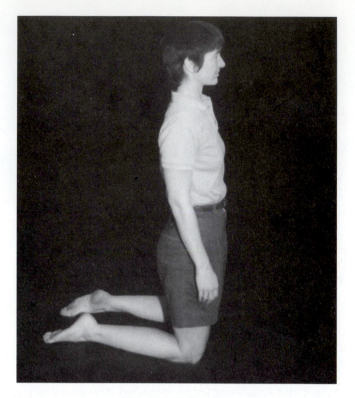

Figure 2–42. Kneeling.

Kneeling and Half-Kneeling

Kneeling and half-kneeling are upright postures in which the knees are flexed and weight bearing occurs through the hip and lower trunk and on the patellar tendon and proximal tibia. The prolonged stretch and maintained pressure on the quadriceps tendon will tend to increase inhibitory influences. In comparison to bridging, kneeling postures have a smaller BoS, a higher CoM, and more joints are involved. The hip(s) is(are) extended and the knees flexed, an advanced combination. The lower extremity position results in the one-joint hip extensors contracting in their shortened ranges, with the two-joint hamstrings shortened at both the hip and knee; both the one-joint hip flexors and the quadriceps are lengthened.

Because the body is aligned with the CoM over the BoS, minimal gravitational forces challenge maintenance of the posture; however, movement of the trunk or limbs from the neutral position is resisted by gravity. In addition, the CoM is high, involving many segments. The movement of therapist's contacts from the pelvis to the shoulders or head will alter the length of the lever arm.

The non-weight–bearing foot can be positioned off the edge of the mat if ROM into plantar flexion is limited or painful. The plantar surface of the foot is not contacting the surface minimizing phasic re-

flexes. The tonic reflex influences are not stimulated, provided the head remains upright. If the head rotates, flexes, or extends this reflex influence may become evident. The optical and vestibular righting reactions will help maintain the upright position. Postural responses help control the CoG within the BoS. As upper trunk movements are performed, dynamic stability in the trunk is promoted.

In kneeling, the BoS is under and posterior (Fig. 2–42). Because of the lack of support anteriorly, any forward movement of the CoM must be counteracted by the posterior trunk and hip musculature or by some backward compensation of another body segment. If neither occurs, the CoM will move anteriorly beyond the BoS and the patient must respond with protective extension or fall.

In half-kneeling, the BoS is angled between the anteriorly flexed limb and the posterior supporting limb (Fig. 2–43). The anterior limb is flexed at the hip, knee, and ankle, and there is no compression on the patellar tendon. Although the one-joint quadriceps of the forward limb are stretched, they are not inhibited by pressure on the tendon, making this limb position relatively easy to maintain. Thus, half-kneeling with the involved limb placed anteriorly can be performed before the kneeling position is introduced. The resis-

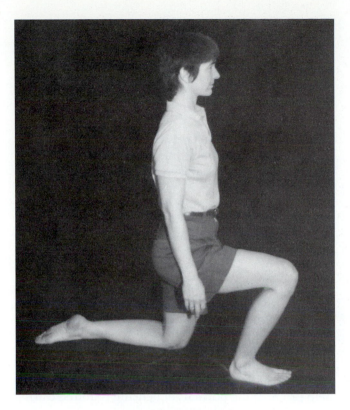

Figure 2–43. Half-kneeling.

tance, however, to the posterior limb is increased by the additional amount of body weight, compared to that which occurs in kneeling, thereby increasing the challenge to the supporting musculature. For these reasons, half-kneeling with the involved limb posterior may follow kneeling in a treatment progression.

Advantages. Kneeling and half-kneeling are transitional activities in the assumption of standing from supine and are therefore functionally useful. For patients with increased quadriceps tone, the inhibitory influences of pressure on the tendon and the maintained stretch, in combination with body weight resistance, are appropriate. When the sole of the foot is not in contact with the supporting surface, hyperactive plantar flexors are not stimulated. Weight shifting in all directions can be performed through increasing ranges. From kneeling or half-kneeling, heel sitting can be assumed by flexing at the hips to lower the CoM within the BoS, or the hips can remain extended while the knees flex, which moves the CoM posteriorly (Fig. 2–44). Both movements are controlled by an eccentric contraction of the quadriceps. The hip extended movement, however, is more difficult because the lever arm is longer and the rectus femoris is lengthened over both joints. Therefore it is included only toward the end of rehabilitation when patients can return to vigorous activity.

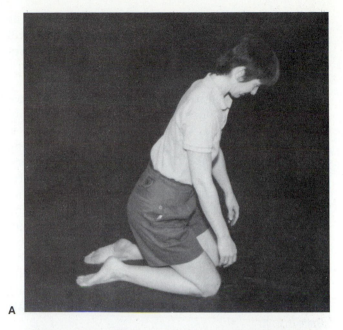

A

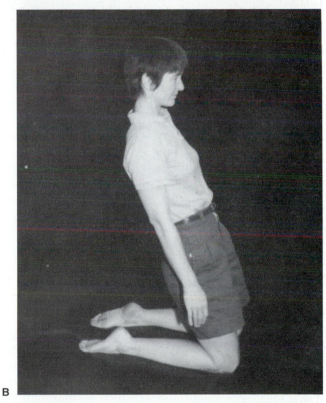

B

Figure 2–44. Two methods of moving from kneeling to heel sitting: **(A)** flexion of hip, with CoM near the center of the BoS; **(B)** hip extended with CoM moved posteriorly.

In kneeling, postural alignment is controlled by the trunk, hip, and knee. For some patients, lower body and hip control can be promoted without weight bearing through the ankle.

In half-kneeling, with the involved leg anterior,

movement of the tibia on the talus can be increased as the patient's weight shifts forward. Eccentric control of the quadriceps and soleus are simultaneously promoted.

Disadvantages. Because the BoS is under or posterior to the CoG in kneeling, the position is very unstable anteriorly; in half-kneeling the position is unstable in the diagonal opposite to the supporting limbs. For patients with tightness of the hip flexors, weakness of the hip extensors, or poor balance responses, these positions are difficult to maintain. They should not be emphasized with patients having quadriceps strength below 4/5, to avoid the inhibitory influences, although they may be incorporated at a later stage to challenge quadriceps control. These positions may be painful for those with degenerative joint disease in the knee or following surgery. Weight bearing on a pillow may alleviate discomfort.

For the hip extensors to react to an anteriorly directed postural disturbance, they first must be able to hold a contraction in the shortened range. If the muscle spindles of the hip extensors are not sensitive to stretch they cannot respond to postural challenges and the patient may fall forward. Tightness in the hip flexors may increase the tendency of the trunk to flex forward, moving the CoM anterior to the BoS. To counter this tendency, the person may flex the hips to change alignment and lower the CoM. When moving from kneeling to heel sitting, if the hips remain extended, the increased passive and active tension may excessively strain or cause microtears in the rectus femoris. Cautious use of this method of lowering is advised.

Upright Progression: Sitting, Modified Plantigrade, and Standing

The functional outcomes of manipulation of the environment, activities of daily living (ADL), and ambulation can be achieved in the sitting and standing postures. To reach these outcomes the patient must have sufficient range and stability to maintain the posture adequately and to control changes in the CoM as weight is shifted during walking and during movement of the limbs to perform tasks.

Contact of the hands or feet with the surface may stimulate grasp, withdrawal, or thrust reflexes. The upright posture minimizes the influence of tonic reflexes. Righting and postural responses provide the automatic control to maintain and move within the posture.

Sitting

The size of the BoS will vary, depending on whether the patient is sitting on a mat or in a chair, and whether and to what extent the upper and lower extremities are providing support. Postural alignment will depend on flexibility and stability in the hips, trunk, and head and neck. For example, if the posterior hip structures are stiff, full hip flexion may be limited. This forces the pelvis into a posterior tilt with flexion in the lumbar spine and a compensatory thoracic kyphosis.

Trunk, bilateral and unilateral extremity combinations can be performed in sitting (Fig. 2–45). In contrast to these combinations performed in supine, the resistance of gravity is altered. In the lower extremity, knee and ankle movements can be emphasized with the hip maintained in flexion (Fig. 2–46). During knee extension, the rectus is shortening at both joints, the hamstrings are lengthening, and maximal gravitational resistance to the quadriceps occurs with the knee fully extended. Advanced combinations of knee extension with ankle dorsiflexion and the reversal movements of knee flexion with plantar flexion can help promote the normal sequencing required during postural responses in standing.

Resistance to improve endurance or strength in the limbs or trunk can easily be provided manually, by pulleys or free weights, or by other mechanical devices.

Advantages. Sitting is an activity that is easily assumed by most patients and is incorporated into many daily activities. Supported sitting in a chair can be incorporated into treatment before the patient is able to maintain the posture independently. Movement of the head and neck can be promoted with gravity assisting flexion. The patient can be supported in a forward-leaning position on the side of a plinth to allow relaxation and palpation of the head and neck muscles and other structures.

Proper sitting posture is a common goal with patients having musculoskeletal or neurological involvement. Trunk extensors and abdominals can be strengthened by direct application of manual resistance or strengthened indirectly by resistance to limb movement. Trunk movements in all directions and in combined diagonal movements are easily performed. The proximal component of the upper limb movements can be observed, palpated, and controlled. In contrast to supine, the scapula is not confined by the surface, eliminating this restriction to full movement of the limb. Bilateral and unilateral movements can be performed as well as upper trunk patterns. For example, to promote upper trunk extension, trunk ex-

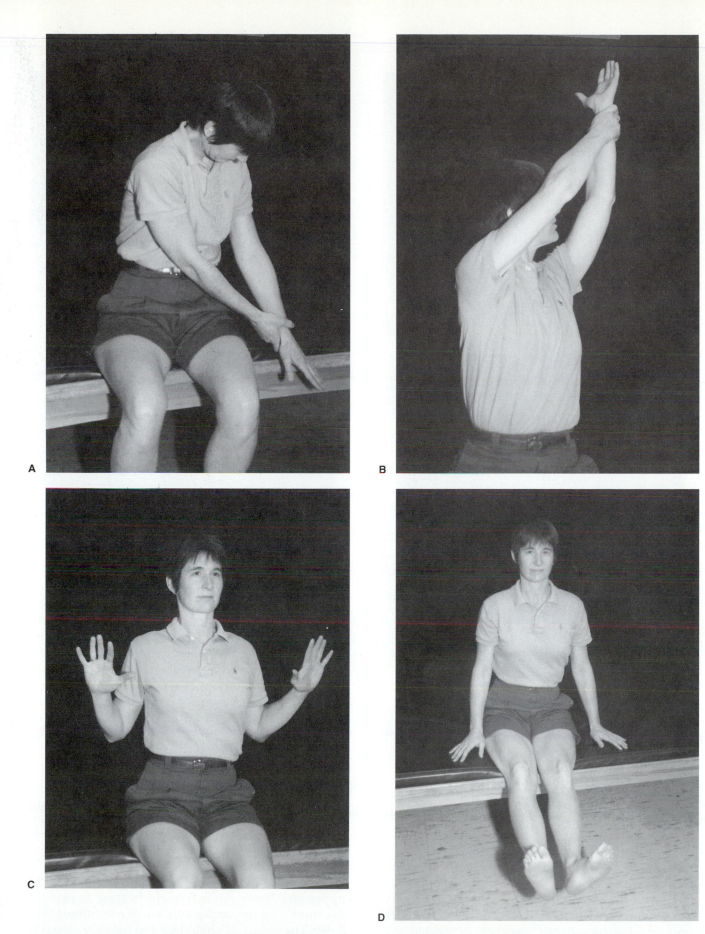

Figure 2–45. Sitting with upper extremity movements: **(A)** upper trunk flexion with rotation combined with shoulder extension; **(B)** upper trunk extension with rotation combined with shoulder flexion; **(C)** bilateral symmetrical withdrawal; **(D)** sitting with lower extremity movements.

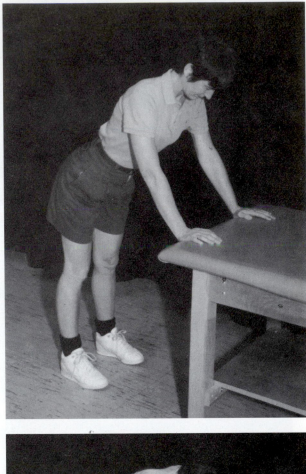

A

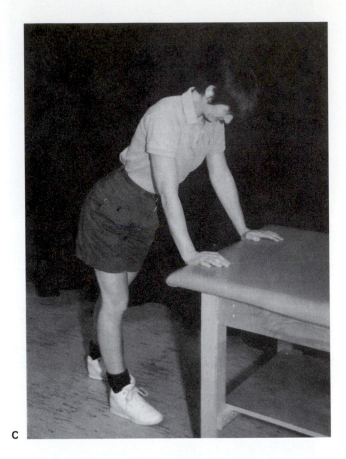

C

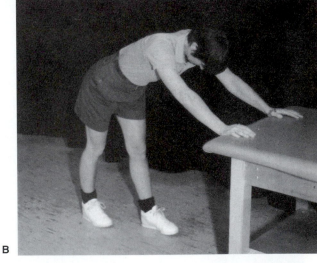

B

Figure 2–46. Modified plantigrade with varied limb position: **(A)** feet symmetrical; **(B)** weight shifting to increase range into shoulder flexion; **(C)** feet in stride.

tensor patterns or bilateral flexor patterns of the arms can be performed.

Knee extension is resisted by gravity in the most shortened range where the rectus is actively insufficient and the hamstrings passively elongated over both joints.

Disadvantages. Weight bearing occurs through the spinal segments which may be painful for some patients with low back dysfunction. Limitation of movement into hip flexion and stiffness in the lumbar region may make assuming correct postural alignment difficult. Decreased postural stability in the trunk musculature reduces the ability to maintain the posture and may result in complaints of fatigue and increase stress on the joint structures. Prolonged sitting can result in adaptive shortening in hip flexors and hamstrings. Abnormal visual, vestibular, or proprioceptive input may decrease the patient's ability to maintain a midline posture. Gravity maximally resists shoulder flexion at 90° which is also the range that maximally challenges rotator cuff control.

Modified Plantigrade

Upper limb, lower body, and trunk control can be promoted in modified plantigrade. It is a transitional posture in the assumption of standing from supine, prone, and sitting and can be incorporated into any of the progressions.

The CoG is high and the BoS is provided by the upper and lower limbs. Weight bearing is through the trunk and the upper and lower extremities (Fig. 2–46). The proximal shoulders and hips are flexed to about 45°; the angle will vary with the distance the feet are positioned from the table (Fig. 2–46B). Weight is borne through the extended elbow and knee joints and on the extended wrist and fingers. The number of joints involved increases when weight is borne through the ankle by rising on the ball of the foot or when weight bearing occurs through the wrist or fingers. The lower extremities can be positioned symmetrically or in stride, which alters the weight bearing through the limbs during rocking movements (Fig. 2–46C).

The scapula and shoulder musculature are contracting in mid range; the extensors of the intermediate joints, the quadriceps and triceps, are in shortened ranges. The lower extremity is in an advanced combination of hip and ankle flexion with knee extension. If the trunk flexes forward, the two joint hamstrings move toward a position of maximum stretch.

Weight bearing on the sole of the foot and the palm of the hand may facilitate the grasp reflexes and the lower extremity extensor thrust. In this relatively upright posture the tonic reflexes are minimally facilitated. Righting reactions will help to maintain the head upright. Postural control is needed to maintain and move within the posture, and many segments can respond to postural challenges.

The abdominals and trunk extensors support the slightly inclined position of the trunk against the resistance of gravity and the limbs support the body weight.

Advantages. Modified plantigrade is a useful position for many patients because postural stability and dynamic control can be promoted in the trunk and all four extremities. Patients with shoulder dysfunction of musculoskeletal or neurological origin can increase static and dynamic weight bearing through the scapula and shoulder and enhance rotator cuff activity.

At the elbow and knee, isometric control can be followed by eccentric and concentric movements through increments of range. Improving muscular control while weight bearing with the knee in or near extension may enhance the patient's awareness of limb position during gait. ROM of the ankle and eccentric plantar flexor control needed during the stance phase of gait can be promoted during weight-shifting activities and as the patient raises and lowers body weight by shifting onto the ball of the foot. Care must be taken during all of these activities that the patient avoids knee hyperextension. Dorsiflexion and plantar flexion and later inversion–eversion control can be enhanced following ankle sprain, tibial fracture, or CVA and can benefit patients with poor postural control.

Weight bearing through the wrist will promote isometric control of the wrist extensors and flexors, a goal with hemiplegic patients or those with lateral epicondylitis or healed wrist fracture. Weight bearing more distally on the fingers facilitates contraction in the intrinsic muscles, appropriate for those with ulnar nerve involvement. The upper extremity weight bearing is important to appropriately stress the bones of those with osteoporosis, a condition common in an older population.

The trunk is supported in a mid position between horizontal and vertical. Patients with back dysfunction may be able to stabilize the trunk in modified plantigrade with less difficulty as compared to other postures. Limb movements can be performed in unilateral or contralateral combinations (Fig. 2–47). It is a posture easily incorporated into a home program. For some, particularly the elderly, postural stability can be challenged.

Disadvantages. The distal segments are in contact with the supporting surface, which may increase an abnormal reflex response. If the patient cannot stabilize the intermediate joint, for example, the elbow, an alternative posture such as weight bearing on elbows can be used. (see Chapter 8). If the patient has poor proprioception and poor control of the quadriceps and hamstrings, hyperextension of the knee can occur in an attempt to stabilize. This abnormal positioning increases the stress on the ligaments and joint capsule.

Standing

The CoG is high and the BoS small. All the joints of the trunk and lower extremities are weight bearing; postural stability is provided via the postural extensors holding in their shortened ranges.

Weight bearing on the sole of the foot may stimulate the positive support reflex or a crossed extension response. Righting reactions will help maintain the head and trunk alignment. Postural control responses will keep the body erect as it normally sways, weight shifts, or responds to internal or external disturbances. The postural responses can be focused at any of the segments. For example, during anterior–posterior sway, the plantar flexors and knee flexors, and the dorsiflexors and knee extensors, respectively, respond to maintain the CoM within the BoS. These muscle patterns are advanced combinations and are the most common strategy for balance maintenance.[66] However, if the more distal proprioceptive receptors do not transmit the sensory changes or if the distal muscles do not respond, balance responses may occur at more proximal segments such as the hip, trunk, or upper extremities. The challenge of maintaining and weight shifting in standing can be increased by narrowing the base, standing on a balance board, soft or

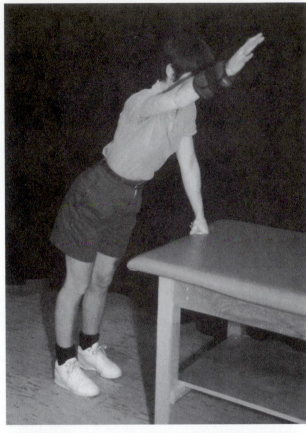

A

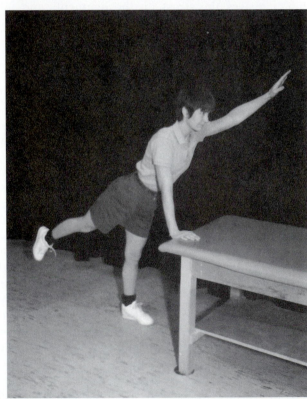

B

Figure 2–47. Modified plantigrade with decreased BoS: **(A)** one upper extremity resisted by a cuff weight; **(B)** contralateral limbs lifted.

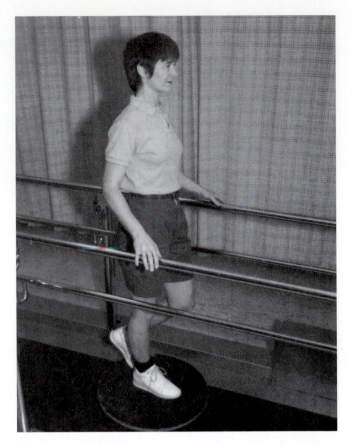

Figure 2–48. Standing: unilateral weight bearing on a balance board.

uneven surfaces, or on a mini trampoline (Fig. 2–48).

All extremity movements from the neutral position are resisted by gravity. Active upper trunk movements are controlled by eccentric contractions.

Advantages. Standing is a functional activity required for many ADL, occupational tasks, and ambulation. The patient's ability to control these tasks in standing can serve as an evaluative measure to guide treatment procedures.

Disadvantage. The high CoG and small BoS make standing a difficult posture for some patients to maintain.

▶ **SUMMARY**

Activities refer to the posture or position of the patient and the movements performed within that posture. Many factors can affect the difficulty of an activity and the patient's performance. An understanding of these factors and how they can be manipulated will aid the therapist in choosing the most appropriate sequence of activities to accomplish the treatment goals and functional outcomes.

▶ *REVIEW QUESTIONS*

1. How can biomechanical factors be altered to increase the difficulty of an activity?

2. How are extremity movements sequenced in increasing order of difficulty?

3. Rolling from supine to prone is a treatment goal for one of your patients. Which reflexes may hinder the patient's abilities; which reactions would facilitate the movement? What muscles will perform the primary trunk motion; what is the influence of gravity on this movement? If the patient has difficulty rolling, what modifications can be made to reduce the influence of these factors?

4. What are the postural control variables that need to be considered during the assessment of the following activities: (1) sitting and reaching for shoes, and (2) standing and walking on uneven surfaces.

5. a. What are the various ways that resistance can be applied? Under what conditions would each type of resistance be appropriate?

   b. Your patient has difficulty lifting his arm in sitting. What are all of the resistive factors that could be making this movement difficult? What can you do to reduce the difficulty?

6. Compare bridging to kneeling and quadruped to modified plantigrade by discussing all the factors that can influence the choice of these activities.

7. You are working with a patient who has a very weak gluteus medius. What range should be emphasized during initial treatment sessions? What sequence of extremity movements and postures would be appropriate? What are the factors that could inhibit the performance of this muscle?

REFERENCES

1. Brunnstrom S, Clinical Kinesiology, 3rd ed. Philadelphia, PA: FA Davis; 1972.

2. Norkin CC, Levangie PK. Joint Structure and Function: A Comprehensive Analysis, 2nd ed. Philadelphia, PA: FA Davis Co; 1992.

3. Portney LG, Sullivan PE. EMG Analysis of Ipsilateral and Contralateral Shoulder and Elbow Muscles During the Performance of PNF Patterns. Presented at the Annual Conference of Behavioral Kinesiology. Boston, Mass; 1980.

4. Michaels, JA. Exercise Overflow: An EMG Investigation of a Clinical Procedure for Indirectly Eliciting Contractions of the Gluteus Maximus and Vastus Medialis. Boston, Mass: Sargent College of Allied Health Professions, Boston University; 1978. Thesis.

5. Toller B, Fitch HL, Turvey MT. The Bernstein perspective: the problems of degrees of freedom and context-conditioned variability. In: Kelso JAS, ed. *Human Motor Behavior*. Hillsdale, Ind: Lawrence Erlbaum Associates; 1982.

6. Murray MP, Peterson RM. Weight Distribution and Weight Shifting Activity During Normal Standing Posture. *Phys Ther*. 1973; 53:741–748.

7. Knott M, Voss DE. Proprioceptive Neuromuscular Facilitation, 2nd ed. New York: Harper & Row Pub Inc; 1968.

8. Brunnstrom S. Movement Therapy in Hemiplegia. New York, Harper & Row Pub Inc; 1970.

9. Bobath B. Adult Hemiplegia: Evaluation and Treatment, 3rd ed. London, England: Butterworth & Heinemann; 1990.

10. Francis NJ. EMG Activity of Shoulder Muscles During Upper Extremity Unilateral and Bilateral PNF Patterns. Boston, Mass: Sargent College of Allied Health Professions, Boston University; 1980. Thesis.

11. Voss DE. Proprioceptive Neuromuscular Facilitation. *AMJ Phys Med*. 1967;46:838-898.

12. Partridge MJ. Electromyographic Demonstration of Facilitation. *Phys Ther Rev*. 1954;34:227–233.

13. Soderberg GL. Kinesiology: Application to Pathological Motion. Baltimore: Williams and Wilkins; 1986.

14. McGraw MB. The Neuromuscular Maturation of the Human Infant. New York, NY: Hafner; 1962.

15. Fiorentino MR. Reflex Testing Methods for Evaluating CNS Development. Springfield, Ill: Charles C Thomas; 1973.

16. Bobath B. Abnormal Postural Reflex Activity Caused by Brain Lesions. London, England: Heinemann Medical Books LTD; 1965.

17. Connolly B, Montgomery P. *Therapeutic Exercises in Developmental Disabilities*. Chattanooga, Tenn: Chattanooga Corp; 1987.

18. Twitchel TE. Normal Motor Development. *J Am Phys Therap A*. 1965;45:419–423.

19. Stockmeyer SA. An Interpretation of the Approach of Rood to the Treatment of Neuromuscular Dysfunction. *Am J Phys Med*. 1967;46:900–956.

20. Gordon J, Ghez C. Muscle Receptors and Spinal Reflexes: The Stretch Reflex. In Kandel ER, Schwartz JA, Jessell TM, eds. *Principles of Neural Science,* 3rd ed. Norwalk, CT: Appleton & Lange; 1991.

21. Brooks VB. Spinal Segmental Control: The Neural Basis of Motor Control. New York: Oxford Univ Press; 1986.

22. Bobath B, Bobath K. Motor Development in the Different Kinds of Cerebral Palsy. London: William Heinemann; 1975.

23. Bouisset S, Zattara M. A Sequence of Postural Movements Precedes Voluntary Movement. *Neurosci Lett*. 1981; 22:263–270.

24. Nashner LM. Adapting Reflexes Controlling the Human Posture. *Exp Brain Res*. 1976;26:59–72.

25. Horak FB. Clinical Measurement of Postural Control in Adults. *Phys Ther*. 1987;67:1881–1885.

26. Woolacot MA, Shumway-Cook A, Nashner LM. Aging and Posture Control: Changes in Sensory Organization and Muscular Coordination. *Int J Aging Hum Dev.* 1986; 23:97–114.

27. Poliner ZR, Dehmer GJ, Lewis SE, et al. Left Ventricular Performance in Normal Subjects: A Comparison of the Response to Exercise in the Upright and Supine Position. 1980;62:528.

28. Dietz V, Quintern J, Berger W, et al. Cerebral Potentials and Leg Muscle EMG Responses Associated with Stance Perturbation. *Exp Brain Res.* 57:348–354.

29. Forssberg H, Nashner LM. Ontogenetic Development of Postural Control in Man: Adaptation to Altered Supported Visual Conditions During Stance. *J Neuro Sci.* 1982;5:545–552.

30. Horak FB, Esselman P, Anderson ME, et al. The effects of movement velocity, mass displaced and task uncertainty on associated postural adjustments made by normal and hemiplegic individuals. *J Neurol Neurosurg Psychiatry.* 1984;47:1020–1028.

31. Nashner LM, McCollum A. The Organization of Human Postural Movements: A Formal Basis and Experimental Synthesis. *Brain Behav Evol.* 1985;8:135–172.

32. Chandler JM, Duncan PW, Studenski SA. Comparison of Postural Responses in Young Adults, Healthy Elderly and Fallers Using Postural Stress Test. *Phys Ther.* 1990;70:410–415.

33. Johansson H, Sjolander P, Sojka P. A sensory role for the cruciate ligaments. *Clin Orthop.* 1990;288:161–178.

34. Cordo PJ. Kinesthetic Control of a Multijoint Movement Sequence. *J Neurophysiol.* 1990;63:161–172.

35. Garn S, Newton R. Kinesthetic Awareness in Subjects with Multiple Ankle Sprains. *Phys Ther.* 1988;11: 1667–1671.

36. Gross MT. Effects of Recurrent Lateral Ankle Sprains on Active and Passive Judgments of Joint Position. *Phys Ther.* 1987;67:1505–1509.

37. Blake AJ, Morgan K, Bendall MJ, et al. Falls by Elderly People at Home: Prevalence and Associated Factors. *Age Aging.* 1988;17:365–372.

38. Pedotti A, Crenna P, Deat A, et al. Postural Synergies in Axial Movements: Short and Long Term Adaptation. *Exp Brain Res.* 1989;74:3–10.

39. Keshner EA. Controlling Stability of a Complex Movement System. *Phys Ther.* 1990;70:844–854.

40. Frank JS, Earl M. Coordination of Posture and Movement. *Phys Ther.* 1990;70:855–863.

41. Shumway-Cook A, Horak F. Assessing the Influences of Sensory Interaction on Balance. *Phys Ther.* 1986; 66:1548–1550.

42. Astrand PO, Rodahl K. Neuromuscular Function: Textbook of Work Physiology. New York: McGraw Hill; 1986.

43. Astrand PO, Rodahl K. Physical Training: Textbook of Work Physiology. New York: McGraw Hill; 1986.

44. Kendall FP, McCreary EK. Muscles: Testing & Function, 4th ed. Baltimore, MD: Williams & Wilkins; 1993.

45. DeLorme T, Watkins A. Techniques of Progressive Resistance Exercise. New York: Appleton-Century; 1951.

46. Hislop H, Perrini JJ. The isokinetic concept of exercise. *Phys Ther.* 1967;47:114.

47. Sarhmann SA, Norton BJ, Bomze HA, et al. Influence on the site of the lesion and muscle length on spasticity in man. *Phys Ther.* 1974;54:1290–1297.

48. Astrand PO, Rodahl K. The Muscle and Its Contraction: Textbook of Work Physiology. New York: McGraw Hill; 1986.

49. Komi PV. Neuromuscular performance: factors influencing force and speed production. *Scand J Sports Sci.* 1979;1:2–15.

50. Sherrington C. The Integrative Action of the Nervous System. New Haven: Yale University Press; 1961.

51. Kabat H. Studies on Neuromuscular Dysfunction. In Payton O, Hirt S, Newton RA, eds. Neurophysiologic Approaches to Therapeutic Exercise: An Anthology. Philadelphia, PA: FA Davis; 1977.

52. Hellebrandt FA. Application of the Overload Principle to Muscle Training in Man. *Am J Phys Med.* 1958; 37:278–283.

53. Crutchfield CA, Barnes MR. The Neurophysiological Basis of Patient Treatment, 2nd ed. Atlanta, GA: Stokesville Publishing; 1975.

54. Johansson H, Sjolander P, Sojka P. A Sensory Role for the Cruciate Ligaments. *Clin Orthop.* 1990;228:161–178.

55. Cohen M, Hoskins TM. *Cardiopulmonary Symptoms in Physical Therapy Practice.* New York, NY: Churchill Livingstone; 1988.

56. Kendall FP, McCreary EK, Provance PG. Muscles: Testing and Function, 4th ed. Baltimore, MD: Williams & Wilkins; 1993.

57. Ayres JA. Integration of Information. In Henderson A, ed. *The Development of Sensory Integration Theory and Practice.* Dubuque, IA: Kendall Hunt; 1974.

58. Barns MR, Crutchfield CA, Heriza CB, et al. *Reflex and Vestibular Aspects of Motor Control.* Atlanta, Ga: Stokesville Publishing Co; 1990.

59. McKenzie RA. The Lumbar Spine: Mechanical Diagnosis and Therapy. Waikonae, New Zealand: Spinal Publications; 1981.

60. Perry J. Basic Functions: Gait Analysis Normal and Pathological Function. Thorofare, NJ: Slack, Inc; 1992.

61. Nachemson A. Lumbar Interdiscal Pressure. *Acta Orthop Scand.* 1960 Suppl 43:1.

62. Konecky CM. EMG Study of Abdominals and Back Extensors During Lower Trunk Rotation. Boston, Mass: Sargent College of Allied Health Professions, Boston University; 1980. Thesis.

63. Herman H. *EMG and Torque Analysis of the Pubococcygeal Muscle.* Boston, Mass: Sargent College of Allied Health Professions, Boston University; 1982. Thesis.

64. Langham T. EMG Analysis of Hip Muscles During Bridging When Techniques Are Applied. Boston, Mass: Sargent College of Allied Health Professions, Boston University; 1981. Thesis.

65. Troy L. EMG Study of Quadriceps and Hamstrings During Bridging. Boston, Mass: Sargent College of Allied Health Professions, Boston University; 1981. Thesis.

66. Nashner LM. Sensory, neuromuscular, and biomedical contributions to human balance. In: Balance: Proceedings of the APTA Forum, Nashville, Tenn, Duncan PW, ed. June 1989; Alexandria, VA.

CHAPTER 3

Techniques to Achieve the Stages of Movement Control

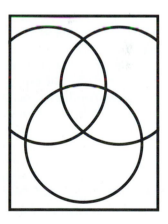

Techniques are an integral part of every procedure and are applied to promote the stages of control (Fig. 3–1). Certain active exercise techniques incorporate the use of isometric and isotonic muscle contractions, while other techniques promote passive tissue stretch. Many adjunctive techniques, such as ultrasound or electrical stimulation, can be used to prepare tissues for function; others, such as icing, may be used after exercise to decrease tissue reactivity. Few techniques are ever used in isolation. Passive and adjunctive techniques are used in combination with those that produce active movement to promote muscle control, strengthening, endurance, and achievement of functional outcomes. Because

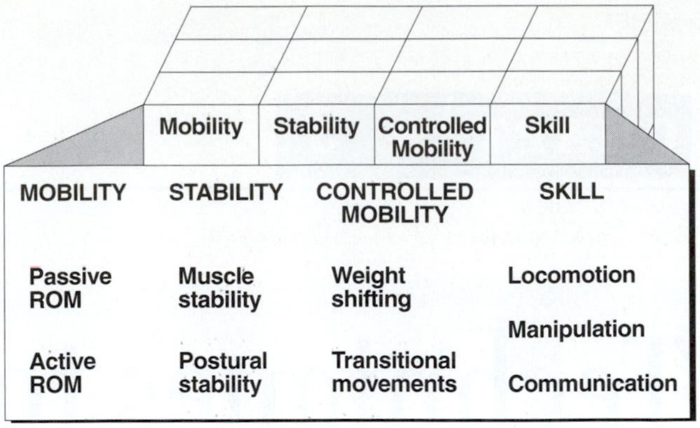

Figure 3–1. Intervention model emphasizing stages of control.

MOBILITY	STABILITY	CONTROLLED MOBILITY	SKILL
Passive ROM	Muscle stability	Weight shifting	Locomotion
			Manipulation
Active ROM	Postural stability	Transitional movements	Communication

this is a text on therapeutic exercise, this chapter will focus on the description and discussion of active exercise techniques and only briefly address other measures that can be applied concomitantly to help achieve a particular stage of control.

The greatest number and variety of techniques are used to achieve the mobility stage of control. The need for using passive and adjunctive techniques in treatment should gradually be decreased as higher levels of control are promoted. Thus the treatment program for an individual working on dynamic stability and skill should emphasize active exercise techniques to increase timing, strength, and endurance and minimize those passive and adjunctive measures that may have been beneficial at earlier stages of treatment.

Many of the active exercise techniques discussed in this section were originally described by Knott and Voss.[1] The purpose of this chapter is not only to instruct the reader on the application of these techniques but, more importantly, to help the reader choose the most appropriate techniques to attain the different stages of control. Although some of these techniques can achieve more than one stage of control, the in-depth description will be included under the particular stage for which it is most commonly used or appears to be most effective clinically.

This chapter also presents some of the underlying mechanisms that may be responsible for the efficacy of the techniques. Most neurophysiological research has been conducted on isolated motor units of animals or humans under controlled conditions. Extrapolation of these findings to function is extremely difficult. Both facilitory and inhibitory central and peripheral influences constantly bombard the final common pathway. Which of these influences may predominate in a given set of circumstances for different individuals with varying conditions is unclear. Therefore, the rationales presented in this chapter are by no means indisputable. Certainly much more clinically related research is needed to either verify or refute these hypotheses.

AUTONOMIC NERVOUS SYSTEM

The autonomic nervous system (ANS) can affect somatic functioning. Increases in the output of the sympathetic division of the ANS have been linked to abnormalities in the sensory–motor system.[2,3] It is therefore important for the therapist to recognize signs of an enhanced sympathetic output so that ap-

propriate techniques can be applied to restore homeostasis while promoting the stages of control. The following may be indicators of increased sympathetic output:

▶ lowered pain threshold;

▶ decreased or abnormal peripheral circulation;

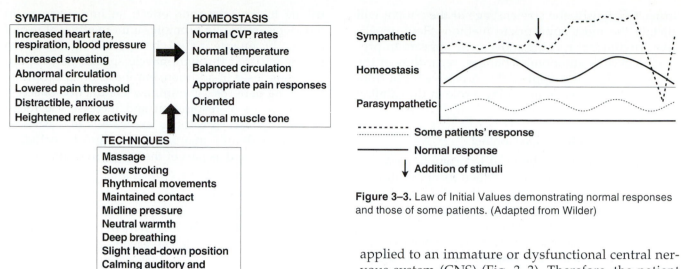

SYMPATHETIC	HOMEOSTASIS
Increased heart rate, respiration, blood pressure	Normal CVP rates
Increased sweating	Normal temperature
Abnormal circulation	Balanced circulation
Lowered pain threshold	Appropriate pain responses
Distractible, anxious	Oriented
Heightened reflex activity	Normal muscle tone

TECHNIQUES

Massage
Slow stroking
Rhythmical movements
Maintained contact
Midline pressure
Neutral warmth
Deep breathing
Slight head-down position
Calming auditory and visual stimuli

Figure 3–2. ANS values related to sympathetic and homeostatic behavior and techniques to promote homeostasis.

Sympathetic

Homeostasis

Parasympathetic

- - - - - - Some patients' response

———— Normal response

↓ Addition of stimuli

Figure 3–3. Law of Initial Values demonstrating normal responses and those of some patients. (Adapted from Wilder)

▶ mottled, cold, or shiny skin;

▶ hyperhidrosis;

▶ hypersensitivity to touch;

▶ accelerated heart rate;

▶ rapid, shallow breathing;

▶ dilated pupils;

▶ anxiety or distractibility;

▶ increased muscle tension or tone.

The therapist can expect a lowered threshold to stimuli, anxiety, and increased muscle tone or tension to adversely affect the amount and quality of movement. While controversy may exist regarding the exact mechanisms involved, literature and empirical evidence support the concept that dampening of sympathetic output aids in calming the patient and raising the threshold of pain.[4,5] In addition, balancing the ANS will help to stabilize the patient's response to stimuli so that results will be more predictable and rebound phenomena avoided. For example, a patient who is not in homeostasis may experience immediate pain relief with the use of either heat or cold, with a subsequent worsening of symptoms hours later. When homeostasis is achieved, this rebound exacerbation of symptoms may be avoided.

Several techniques can be applied either individually or in combination to decrease sympathetic activity (Fig. 3–2). These can be used as a precursor to more specific techniques aimed at increasing passive or active movement of individual segments. Many of the techniques designed to balance the ANS may produce an enhanced or unpredictable response when applied to an immature or dysfunctional central nervous system (CNS) (Fig. 3–3). Therefore, the patient should always be closely monitored and input altered if unwanted responses become evident. Many of these techniques promote general relaxation and incorporate slow, repetitive, rhythmical input and maintained skin contact. All are used in conjunction with calming verbal commands and should be applied whenever possible in a quiet environment conducive to the goal of relaxation.

Techniques to Balance the Autonomic Nervous System

Massage

Various types of massage or stroking have been used to influence muscle tension via circulatory and autonomic reflex pathways, including effleurage,[6] connective tissue massage,[7] and slow stroking down posterior primary rami.[4,8] The effects of these techniques may be local[9] or generalized, with changes noted in vital signs and muscle tone.

Slow stroking can be applied with the patient sidelying or prone. The therapist strokes over the paravertebral musculature extending from the cervical region to the buttocks, using the index and middle fingers of one hand on either side of the spine. As one hand approaches the buttocks, the other begins in the lower cervical region. Pressure is firm but not heavy and the motion continuous for approximately 3 to 5 minutes. Although slow stroking can have a calming effect, its effectiveness is not as well documented as the other massage techniques.

Rolling or Rocking

Rhythmical movements can be performed passively or actively in various ways, such as rolling repetitively from supine toward prone, rotating the lower trunk in hooklying, or rocking in a chair, a hammock, over a large ball, or even rocking in the therapist's arms. Obviously, the size and age of the patient will dictate the most appropriate method. Slow, repetitive, rhythmical rocking movement appears to produce reflexive autonomic changes, regardless of the plane in which it is applied.[10,11] Adaptive input from the vestibular system may play a role in the calming response.

Maintained Touch or Skin Contact

Maintained touch can be used to promote parasympathetic responses. Rood described its application to the distal extremities and to the abdomen.[8] Any mother knows that a fussy or hyperactive child may be calmed by being placed prone on a supporting surface, or by application of gentle but firm manual pressure to the abdomen. Lying prone over a ball or bolster will promote the same effect, especially when combined with rhythmical rocking.

Maintained contact to the entire body can be accomplished by wrapping the body in a blanket. Many cultures wrap or swaddle infants, which appears to have a calming effect as well as making it easier for the child to be carried. A neutral warmth effect is produced whenever maintained contact is applied, which has also been cited as contributing to a decrease in sympathetic output.[8,12]

The effectiveness of maintained touch can be attributed to the stimulation of slowly adapting tonic sensory receptors and C fiber firing or to the rapid adaptation of cutaneous receptors, which dampens the entering stimuli into the system.[9,12,13]

Breathing

Slow, deep breathing has been incorporated into several therapeutic regimens, including Jacobson's relaxation exercises,[14,15] yoga,[16] and transcendental meditation,[17] for purposes of decreasing muscle tension and anxiety. Various physiological events contribute to the relaxation effect: an improvement in blood gas exchange promotes a more efficient use of oxygen by muscle; reflex changes in muscle tension can be initiated through muscle spindles in respiratory muscles.[18] In addition, emphasis on appropriate breathing patterns can minimize contraction of accessory muscles of respiration and increase the relaxation response. Breathing exercises can easily be incorporated into treatment procedures, including those performed as part of the home program.

Carotid Sinus Reflex

Lowering the head in relation to the trunk can produce a decrease in muscle activity by activation of the carotid sinus reflex.[19,20] The carotid sinus is a slight enlargement located in the arterial wall at the beginning of the internal carotid artery. Increased pressure on the sinus magnifies the depressor effect on medullary centers and causes a decrease in blood pressure. The reflex can be elicited with the head tilted down in quadruped, by bending forward in sitting, or by lying over a large bolster or ball. An inverted or complete head-down position should not be performed, to avoid a marked drop in blood pressure or an increase in intracranial pressure.

Many of these techniques can be easily combined. For example, effleurage to the trunk can incorporate slow stroking down posterior primary rami; slow, rhythmical rolling can be performed in conjunction with breathing exercises, abdominal pressure, and a head-down position (Fig. 3–4). Calming auditory and visual stimuli should be incorporated, to the extent possible, into all procedures to establish homeostasis. Any of these general relaxation techniques can be repeated at various intervals within a treatment session and can be combined with the following techniques, which focus on increasing mobility of specific segments and tissues.

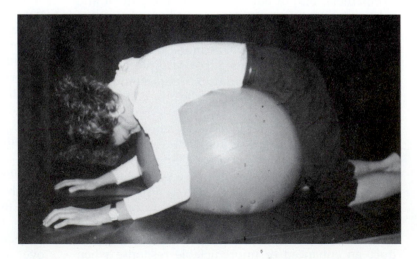

Figure 3–4. Rhythmical rocking, pressure, head down.

MOBILITY

Mobility is defined both as the presence of a functional range of motion through which to move and the ability to initiate and sustain active movement through range.

Patients with musculoskeletal or neurological dysfunction can experience difficulty with either parameter of mobility but for different reasons. For example, an individual who has had a cast removed because of a fractured olecranon may experience passive range of motion (ROM) restrictions caused by pain, swelling, and tissue tightness and decreased ability to initiate active contractions resulting from muscle disuse and weakness. An individual with multiple sclerosis may be unable to initiate movement as a result of muscle weakness and tissue tightness caused by alterations in muscle physiology or abnormal tone. Restrictions in mobility may also be compounded by an increase in sedentary behavior. Mobility techniques should not be used indiscriminately, regardless of the cause of restriction. The therapist should attempt to identify the cause of the immobility to determine the most effective choice of techniques. Indications for the various mobility techniques will be discussed in this section and appropriate modifications for musculoskeletal and neurological problems will be included.

Passive and Adjunctive Techniques

A variety of thermal and electrical modalities can be used as adjunctive or preparatory measures to decrease pain and swelling or to promote soft-tissue healing and extensibility. Such measures may be followed by any of the passive or active exercise techniques aimed at increasing tissue length, which will be discussed in this chapter (Fig. 3–5).

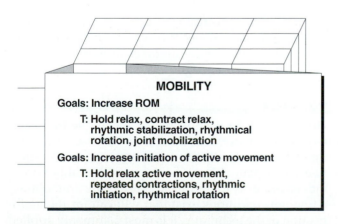

MOBILITY

Goals: Increase ROM

T: Hold relax, contract relax, rhythmic stabilization, rhythmical rotation, joint mobilization

Goals: Increase initiation of active movement

T: Hold relax active movement, repeated contractions, rhythmic initiation, rhythmical rotation

Figure 3–5. The treatment goals to be achieved at the mobility stage and suggested techniques.

Joint Mobilization

This is a passive technique that is indicated when joint capsule, connective tissue, or ligamentous tightness limits motion, regardless of whether the limitation is of musculoskeletal or neurological origin. For example, a patient 1 year post cerebral vascular accident (CVA) may be experiencing limitation in shoulder motion and impingement of soft tissue associated with a decrease in motor control. The decreased ROM and impingement may be similar to that found in an individual with a rotator cuff dysfunction resulting from overuse or trauma. Joint mobilization preceded by deep heating modalities may be indicated in both instances to gain mobility of the capsule. What may differ between these two groups, however, is the decision on the choice of active exercise techniques to promote the stages of control. Discussion of appropriate choices will be undertaken later in this chapter. The reader is referred to other texts for a detailed description of mobilization techniques and modalities and their indications for use.[21–23]

Prolonged Stretching

Stretching of contractile and non-contractile tissues can be applied manually in combination with joint distraction or by mechanical means, including pulleys or continuous passive motion machines. Regardless of the method, passive stretch must always be applied slowly and cautiously to avoid tissue tearing or pain while allowing for adaptation of tissue elements. Most passive stretch techniques are used to increase the number of sarcomeres in muscles as well as to increase the length of noncontractile components of muscle, including tendon and fascia.[24–26] Serial or inhibitory casting, a form of passive stretch, is often applied to individual joints of patients with hypertonia for purposes of normalizing tone as well as increasing mobility in the involved joint.[27–29]

Joint Distraction

Joint surfaces can be distracted to enhance the effect of passive stretching techniques, or can be applied for the sole purpose of relieving joint pain. However, when applied in combination with quick, external stretch, joint traction can enhance the initiation of active movement.

Rhythmical Rotation

Passive rhythmical rotation of an extremity performed slowly around a longitudinal axis may increase relaxation of a segment in a manner similar to that previously described for total body relaxation

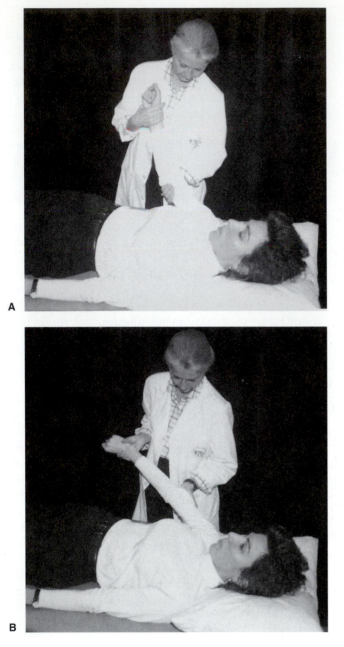

Figure 3–6. Rhythmical rotation of the upper extremity: **(A)** external rotation; **(B)** internal rotation.

with rolling (Fig. 3–6). This technique is effective when either pain, contractile or noncontractile tissue tightness, or hypertonia limit movement. Consequently, it is appropriate for use with a wide variety of patients. While the technique is thought to be completely passive, active movement often occurs automatically through the shortening response.[30] Efficacy of this technique may be due to inhibition from joint mechanoreceptors or from receptors such as the Golgi tendon organ.[31,32] Supraspinal inhibition will also contribute to a response whenever the patient is instructed to relax.[33]

Maintained Pressure

Maintained pressure on a muscle belly or tendon can be used to achieve local muscle relaxation. Manual pressure applied to a long tendon either manually or by a supporting surface can produce an increase in ROM.[8,34] For example, the application of deep manual pressure over the insertion of the biceps tendon can promote muscle relaxation in a patient who has been immobilized in a position of elbow flexion; maintenance of the quadruped position on a firm surface will place pressure on the patellar tendon and flexor tendons of the hand to promote inhibition of spastic quadriceps and finger flexors; holding a firm object in the hand can have a dampening effect on wrist and finger spasticity; air splints placed on limbs provide maintained manual contact and pressure and have been shown to decrease motor unit activity (Fig. 3–7). The effects of all types of pressure appear to be immediate, with little evidence of carry-over effects.[35-38]

Additional Adjunctive Techniques

Other adjunctive inputs can be used to more directly promote movement or mobility of a segment and include mechanical vibration or manual tapping over a muscle tendon or muscle belly.[34] Although the pathways differ, both are transmitted proprioceptively by the Ia ending of the muscle spindle. Stimuli such as phasically applied light touch or ice will facilitate movement through stimulation of cutaneous receptors.[34] Once any movement is elicited, the response must be reinforced with appropriate resistance. Choice of techniques is dependent on the integrity of the conducting systems and precautions.

Active Exercise Techniques to Increase ROM

Three specific active exercise techniques can be used to increase ROM: **Hold Relax, Contract Relax,** and **Rhythmic Stabilization.** All three involve active muscle contractions and therefore may be used when the cause of immobility involves muscle rather than noncontractile tissue tightness.

Hold Relax

Hold relax (HR) is an isometric technique that is effective when ROM is decreased because of muscle tightness on one side of a joint. It is particularly effective when pain either accompanies the limitation of movement or is the primary cause of the immobility. Although conditions exist that will call for the modification of the technique, it is most commonly applied in the following manner: The patient actively moves the segment or is assisted to the point of limitation of

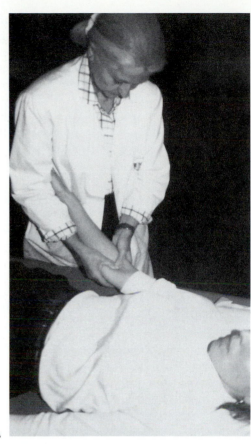

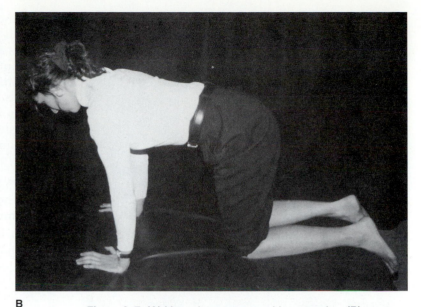

Figure 3–7. (A) Manual pressure over biceps tendon; **(B)** pressure on patellar tendon, wrist and finger flexors; **(C)** firm object in hand; **(D)** air splint.

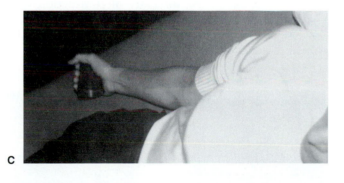

the available ROM; an isometric contraction of all the components of the agonistic muscles is elicited at this point in the range. If the patient is experiencing pain at the end point, the technique can be effectively applied 5 to 10 degrees short of the point of limitation in a more comfortable range. The isometric contraction is gradually increased and maintained for approximately 7 to 9 seconds, followed by a command to relax slowly. The intensity is kept in the minimal-to-moderate range below the pain threshold to avoid muscle splinting. Slow relaxation is important to avoid the pain that an abrupt relaxation response can

produce. Once relaxation occurs, the patient actively moves or is assisted into the gained range to the new point of limitation. If the agonistic muscles are too weak to move the part into the gained range, active assisted or passive movement is an alternative. Active movement is always preferred, however, to activate agonistic musculature and to provide reciprocal inhibition to antagonistic muscles during the movement phase. The technique is reapplied and the cycle continued approximately three to four times until no further increase in range can be accomplished during that treatment period.

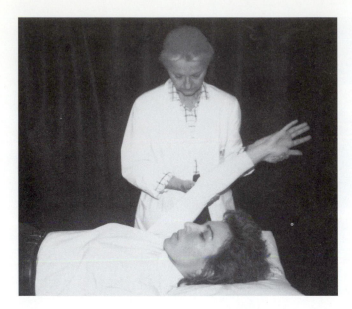

Figure 3–8. Hold relax to agonist.

HR can also be applied to the antagonistic, range-limiting pattern and is primarily used when the agonistic muscle group is too weak to be effective.

The application of the technique both to the agonist and to the antagonist is illustrated by the following examples: A middle-aged woman has idiopathic adhesive capsulitis of the shoulder with resulting pain and decreased movement into flexion, abduction, and external rotation (D2F). The **agonistic** shoulder muscles are the weakened middle deltoid, supraspinatus, and infraspinatus and the **antagonistic** muscles are the tight pectoralis major and minor, subscapularis, teres major, and latissimus dorsi (D2E). When applying HR to the **agonist,** or D2F, pattern, manual contacts (MC) are placed on the flexor, abductor surface, and the command is "Hold and don't let me push your arm down" as the therapist elicits an isometric contraction of the D2F muscle groups (Fig. 3–8). After contraction of the D2F muscles and reciprocal relaxation of the antagonistic groups, the limb moves, or is moved, into the newly gained range. When applying HR to the **antagonist,** or D2E, pattern, MC are placed on the extensor, adductor surface of the arm, and the command is "Hold and don't let me lift your arm" as the therapist elicits an isometric contraction of the D2E muscle groups (Fig. 3–9). After relaxation of the tight D2E muscles, the therapist changes MC to the opposite surface of the limb and the limb moves into flexion, abduction, and external rotation.

Both methods of application can produce gains in ROM. However, HR to the agonist appears to be especially effective during initial sessions when

avoidance of pain and gaining the patient's confidence is so important. Because the therapist's resistance is applied to nonpainful tissues, patient anxiety is minimized and greater relaxation can be attained. In addition, isometric contractions applied to weak agonists, particularly to postural muscles that have undergone adaptive lengthening, will help to facilitate restoration of spindle bias and improve stability of proximal muscle groups.

Summary

▶ The limb moves or is moved toward the point of limitation.

▶ A gradually applied isometric contraction of the agonistic or antagonistic muscle groups is elicited.

▶ The patient relaxes.

▶ Active assisted or resisted movement into the new range is promoted.

▶ The technique is applied until no further gains can be achieved

Contract Relax

Contract relax (CR) is another technique used to gain range when contractile tissue is limiting the motion required for functional activities. Unlike HR, CR is most effectively applied to tight antagonistic muscle groups. Because of the intensity of contraction with CR, attempts to apply this technique to the agonistic pattern result in unwanted cocontraction around

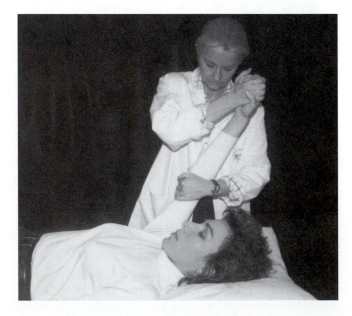

Figure 3–9. Hold relax to antagonist.

the joint rather than the desired reciprocal inhibition and relaxation of the antagonist. As in hold relax, the limb first moves toward the range of limitation. The contraction of the antagonist combines a maximal **isometric** contraction of the diagonal component (flexion, extension, abduction, or adduction) with an **isotonic** contraction of the rotational component (internal or external rotation) into its shortened range. The patient is asked, not "to hold," but to "turn and push" or "turn and pull" as much as possible for approximately 7 to 9 seconds. After relaxation, the limb actively moves or is moved into the shortened range, where the technique is reapplied. Because the technique incorporates a much more forceful contraction than hold relax and because rotational movement occurs, it is not appropriate if pain is a major complaint, if movement of the joint is contraindicated, or if rotation is contraindicated as in healing fractures or anterior cruciate ligament (ACL) repairs.

However, CR can be quite an effective technique and has been shown to yield greater increases in range than HR on two-joint muscles of normal subjects.[39]

Continuing with the previous example of the patient with adhesive capsulitis will help to illustrate the appropriate use of CR. When pain is no longer a factor but ROM remains limited, CR may be the technique of choice. With the patient supine or sitting, the upper extremity moves to the point of limitation (flexion, abduction, external rotation); the therapist's hands are positioned on the limb so as to resist the antagonistic motions (extension, adduction, internal rotation). The dynamic and forceful verbal commands are "turn your thumb down and pull your arm toward your opposite hip." The therapist allows full rotation to occur but prevents, as much as possible, movement into extension and adduction. After the maximal contraction of 7 to 9 seconds, the patient relaxes and the therapist changes MC to the opposite surface of the limb to resist or assist movement into the newly gained range of flexion, abduction, and external rotation. As with HR, the technique is repeated until no further range can be achieved during that treatment session.

Summary

- ► The limb moves or is moved close to the point of limitation.
- ► A maximal and rapid contraction of the antagonistic musculature is elicited: isometric of the diagonal component and isotonic of the rotational component.
- ► The patient relaxes.

- ► Active assisted or resisted movement into new range is promoted.
- ► The technique is applied until no further gains are achieved.

Traditionally, both HR and CR are applied at or near the point of limitation of the available range of movement. Studies have demonstrated, however, that the techniques can be applied at other points in the available range with equivalent gains in motion.[40,41] There has been very little investigation of the optimal time of application of one contraction or the number of contractions necessary to gain or maintain ROM. One study of normal subjects has indicated a positive relationship between the length of time of application of HR and immediate increases in motion.[42] Another study showed that the effects of CR lasted up to 1 hour when applied for two 15-second intervals.[43] Empirical evidence indicates that following the active contraction, the therapist should allow adequate time for muscle relaxation to occur before movement into the newly gained range is attempted. Research investigating the relationship between the H reflex and motoneuron activity following muscle contraction suggests that the relaxation period should not exceed 5 seconds to take advantage of the effects of postcontraction reflex depression.[44] Continued research is needed to further establish time and force parameters and their relationship to the efficacy of relaxation techniques.

Rhythmic Stabilization

Rhythmic stabilization (RS) is most often used to promote stability but can also promote mobility by decreasing muscle splinting around a joint, as occurs commonly with burn patients, with uncasted fractures such as those of the radial head, or with muscles of patients who have recently had a cast removed. The technique involves simultaneous isometric contractions of agonist and antagonistic muscles without allowing relaxation to occur between contractions (Fig. 3–10). Resistance is gradually increased. Because pain is usually a factor, relaxation, as with HR, should be gradual. If the part is very painful or the patient is apprehensive, RS can be simply and effectively applied in a similar manner, but away from the injured segment, termed an **indirect approach.** For example, to increase muscle relaxation around the right shoulder girdle, RS can be applied with graduated amounts of resistance to the right hand with the arm supported in supine, resulting in contraction of the muscles in the entire limb (Fig. 3–11). The same goal can be accomplished by applying RS to an up-

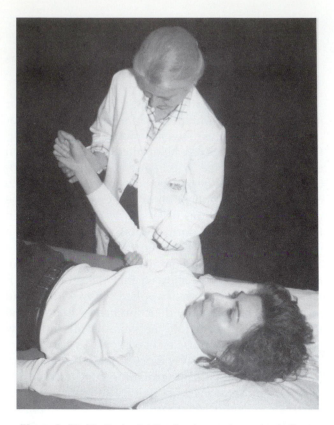

Figure 3–10. Rhythmic stabilization to muscles around elbow.

per-extremity trunk pattern, with the resistance applied primarily to the uninvolved left limb (Fig. 3–12). In addition to eliciting muscle relaxation around a joint, the intermittent muscle contractions produced by the contraction may increase local circulation via muscle pumping action and thus contribute to healing of tissue. Because RS requires more coordination than either HR or CR, it may not be the choice of techniques for some patients in early stages of treatment.

Rationale. The following is the rationale for all mobility exercise techniques used to gain ROM of contractile tissue. Many complex peripheral and supraspinal mechanisms may contribute to the relaxation or muscle inhibition, including:

▶ Resistance to agonistic muscles can produce reciprocal inhibition to tight antagonistic musculature.[45]

▶ Low-threshold, slowly adapting joint receptors may be stimulated by changes in isometric or isotonic muscle tension, as well as by rotational

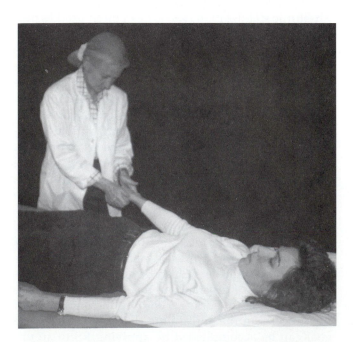

Figure 3–11. Rhythmic stabilization to hand—indirect approach.

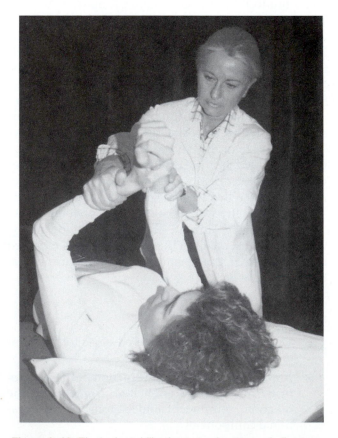

Figure 3–12. Rhythmic stabilization to trunk pattern—indirect approach.

movements, thereby contributing to muscle inhibition.[31]

▶ Verbal commands to relax can influence supraspinal inhibition of the final common pathway.[46]

▶ Fatigue of motor units may play a greater role in CR than in HR when applied to the antagonist. The maximal effort elicited throughout the application of CR, particularly when it is repeated, may recruit increasingly more phasic or fast-twitch motor units, which are quicker to fatigue than tonic or slow-twitch units.[47,48]

▶ Recurrent inhibition to the final common pathway (FCP) is produced by discharge of Renshaw cells, which receive synaptic input from supraspinal and segmental pathways. This inhibition appears to primarily affect low-threshold tonic motor neurons and may therefore have more of an inhibitory effect on those muscles with a predominance of tonic or slow-twitch motor units.[49]

▶ Motoneuron hyperpolarization and presynaptic inhibition of motoneurons both occur during muscle contraction and can contribute to the decrease in muscle responsiveness immediately following contraction.[44]

▶ Golgi tendon organs (GTOs) are extremely sensitive to active muscle tension and when activated result in autogenic inhibitory impulses of the FCP.[50] However, GTO firing is depressed immediately following a contraction—creating, in fact, disinhibition. Therefore, gains in ROM with these techniques are unlikely to be augmented by GTO stimulation.

The hold relax, contract relax, and rhythmic stabilization techniques were designed to increase muscle extensibility primarily in those patients with musculoskeletal involvement. The gains in range that occur have been postulated to be due, in part, to inhibitory mechanisms mediated at the spinal and cortical levels. Therefore, these techniques, although not contraindicated, may not be as effective in patients with neurological dysfunction, who may have abnormal functioning of inhibitory mechanisms. If applied to patients with hypertonia, the level of muscle contraction should be kept low to avoid associated reactions.

All ROM techniques, both active and passive, have one important common denominator that deserves repetition and emphasis. As stated, *relaxation or passive ROM once achieved, is followed by active movement with resistance into the newly gained range, whenever such active movement is possible.* There are two ba-

sic reasons for this principle: First, active movement of the agonistic pattern may perpetuate the inhibition to the tight antagonist via the afferents of the agonistic muscle spindles. Secondly, slight resistance, be it gravitational or manual, will serve to strengthen the agonistic pattern, a most important treatment goal. If this goal is not achieved, the antagonistic muscle may quickly return to its contracted or tight position and the active lag of the agonist will be perpetuated. For example, a patient who has had his elbow flexed at a 90-degree angle for a period of weeks has two major problems: adaptive shortening of elbow flexors and adaptive lengthening of elbow extensors. The extensors have not functioned in the shortened range for a period of time and have thus become weak in this range. Neurophysiologically, this means that extensor muscle spindles have become biased at a new resting length of 90 degrees of elbow flexion. Consequently, when the elbow is extended after relaxation of flexors has occurred, the extensor spindles are unloaded, that is, on slack, and gamma bias of the extensors then must be restored with the muscle at this new resting length. If gamma bias is not restored, the primary spindle afferents of the extensors will lack stretch sensitivity and be unresponsive to stretch in shortened ranges. This means that the extensors will not respond appropriately to resistive forces of gravity, weight bearing, or external loads; such readiness to respond is necessary to accomplish functional tasks. Resistance, particularly isometric resistance, facilitates static gamma motoneurons, which enhances the response of spindle afferents.[51,52] The application of HR to the agonist, therefore, is usually the technique of choice because it achieves the goal of relaxation of the tight antagonistic muscle groups and simultaneous isometric strengthening of agonists.

In summary, resistance to the agonist should follow the relaxation techniques, whether the agonist to be strengthened is a flexor or an extensor. Strengthening extensor muscles in the shortened range is particularly important, as this is the range in which these muscles most commonly function.

Active Exercise Techniques to Initiate Movement

Movement can be initiated by the application of **Hold Relax Active Movement, Repeated Contractions,** or **Rhythmic Initiation.** The use of each technique is determined by the patient's disability and muscle tone.

Hold Relax Active Movement

Hold relax active movement (HRAM) is appropriate when a muscle is 2/5 or weaker as determined by manual muscle testing and responds poorly to stretch. Although the technique can be modified to accommodate a variety of conditions, it is most appropriate when the weakness is not accompanied by pain, decreased ROM, or increased tone. The treatment goal is to improve the muscle's ability to initiate movement from the lengthened range and to sustain movement throughout the range. The technique is applied in the following manner: the muscle is passively placed near the shortened range, where a maintained isometric contraction is facilitated. Because the spindle intrafusal muscle fibers are on slack or in an unloaded position, this isometric contraction may need to be augmented by overflow from stronger segments. Muscle tapping, vibration, joint approximation, and dynamic verbal commands are types of sensory input that can be added to enhance the muscle's response. Once elicited, the isometric response is held for up to 10 seconds to allow optimal alpha and gamma coactivation to occur.[52] Fatigue of the weakened muscles should be avoided by keeping the intensity low and promoting overflow from stronger segments. Following the isometric contraction, the patient relaxes and the muscle is quickly and passively returned to the lengthened range, where a quick stretch is applied. The weak muscle should now be better able to respond to the stimulus. The therapist then assists or resists the response throughout the range depending on the amount of activation elicited. If too much assistance is provided, alpha gamma coactivation will be decreased. However, too much resistance will inhibit the muscle contraction. Thus, a balance of assistance and resistance must be achieved by the therapist to optimize the contraction. The result anticipated is an increase in the active range or a stronger contraction through the same excursion. The technique is repeated within one treatment session and over time until an adequate contraction throughout the range can be accomplished. The following example will illustrate the appropriate use of HRAM.

Your patient has a form of muscular dystrophy and presents with poor hip abductors and extensors. With the patient supine, the therapist places one of the lower extremities in extension and elicits an isometric contraction of the weak musculature with the aid of gravity, joint approximation, and overflow from the stronger knee and ankle musculature. The patient is then instructed to relax, and the leg is quickly moved into a mass flexor–adductor pattern to stretch the extensors and abductors (Fig. 3–13). The response to the stretch is manually resisted and augmented by verbal commands as the patient pushes the limb back into extension and abduction.

Rationale

▶ A maintained isometric contraction in shortened ranges will facilitate gamma bias or increase the stretch sensitivity of the intrafusal muscle fibers and thus improve the muscle's response to stretch.[50,51]

▶ Passive movement into the lengthened range from the shortened range is preferable to an active contraction of antagonists to prevent reciprocal inhibition of the weak agonistic muscles.

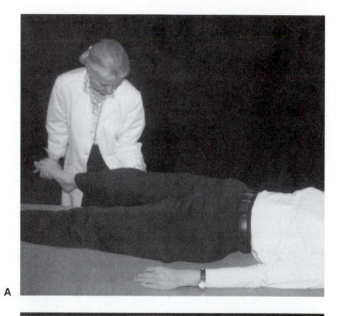

A

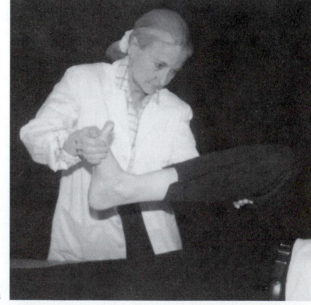

B

Figure 3–13. (A) Isometric contraction in shortened range of extensor pattern. **(B)** Quick stretch in lengthened range of extensor pattern.

▶ Quick stretch in the lengthened range places both the extrafusal and intrafusal muscle fibers on stretch.[45] If the stretch sensitivity of the intrafusal fibers has been appropriately increased, the spindle afferents will fire to increase motor unit activation.

▶ Dynamic verbal commands will arouse the reticular activating system and increase motoneuron firing.[53]

Repeated Contractions

As with HRAM, repeated contractions (RC) is appropriately applied when the muscle is very weak and cannot sustain the contraction throughout the range. With RC, however, repeated stretches are applied in the lengthened range of the muscle without first contracting isometrically in shortened ranges. Because the lengthened range is the range emphasized, the technique is most appropriate for flexor muscles that are not easily inhibited by quick stretch in lengthened ranges as are the one-joint extensors. For this reason, isometric contractions in a shortened range before stretching in the lengthened range are not necessary for flexor muscles, which always respond well to stretch.

To apply RC, the weak, below 3/5, phasic or flexor muscle is brought to the lengthened range, where a quick stretch or multiple stretches are provided along with verbal encouragement to promote an active contraction. Once the muscles respond, they must be resisted to perpetuate the isotonic contraction. The intensity of resistance must be kept at a level that will reinforce and not dampen the muscle contraction. An isometric contraction at the end of the active range will reinforce spindle bias at the part of

the range where spindle firing begins to diminish (Fig. 3–14).

Rationale. If the internal stretch of intrafusal fibers of muscle spindles by gamma motor neurons is deficient, the primary afferents of the spindles can be directly activated by the application of quick, moderately rapid external stretch of the muscle.[45]

However, resistance of even a very slight amount is then necessary to facilitate alpha-gamma coactivation; such resistance keeps the spindles loaded or taut and thus responsive to stimulation. Stretch without subsequent resistance can result in unloaded or slack intrafusal fibers of the muscle spindle and a subsequent decrease in spindle afferent firing and decreased extrafusal fiber contraction.[54] Strong verbal commands can enhance the response through the reticular activating system.

Rhythmic Initiation

Rhythmic initiation (RI) is indicated when a patient is unable to initiate movement, is limited in range because of hypertonia, or exhibits difficulty learning motor skills. With RI, movement of a limb or a body part progresses from completely passive to active assisted to slightly resisted as the patient relaxes and is capable of actively moving. The verbal commands are "Relax and let me move you," followed by "Now you do it with me." It is important that the verbal commands be soothing and the movements repetitive, slow, and rhythmic to initially decrease abnormal tone. Quick stretch to any muscle groups that need to be relaxed should be avoided. The technique can be made more difficult by increasing the range through which the movement occurs and by increasing the speed of movement as it progresses from passive to active contractions. If the patient has an intact CNS, active contractions will automatically occur as the technique is repetitively applied.[30] The goal achieved is increased active ROM.

RI is an effective technique for many patients who have difficulty initiating movement. Rolling, a total body pattern that is important both developmentally and functionally, may be one of the first activities included in a treatment program. RI can be applied in the following manner to promote active rolling. The patient is positioned on one side and MC are placed on scapula and pelvis. The patient is then instructed to relax while being passively moved toward prone and then supine. This passive stage is repeated until the therapist feels that the patient has relaxed and can thereby be moved more easily through increments of range. The patient is encouraged to exert some active control through the range. When this

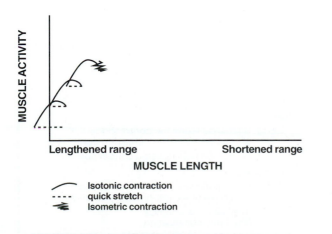

Figure 3–14. Repeated contractions in lengthened ranges.

occurs, slight resistance is added so that in effect RI becomes a slow reversal technique (see Controlled Mobility). In the case of a patient with parkinsonism with increased flexor tone, the resistance is applied primarily to the movement of rolling toward supine to emphasize extensor musculature. Conversely, resistance toward prone emphasizes flexor tone and is appropriate for patients with exaggerated extensor tone.

As stated earlier, RI also is of benefit when a motor learning or communications problem exists. Allowing the patient both to feel and look at the movement as the pattern is passively performed helps to facilitate subsequent active or resisted contractions, thus minimizing the frustration on the part of both patient and therapist. Enhancement or kinesthetic awareness is an important goal that can be achieved even if the patient cannot fully participate. If no increased tone is present, application of stretch may be applied in lengthened ranges to improve peripheral feedback and enhance muscle contraction.

Rationale

▶ The vestibular system may accommodate to the repetitive rhythmic movements and the calming verbal commands associated with RI. Decreased input to the reticular formation may result and thereby may minimize an arousal effect.[10,11]

▶ The calming effects of rocking may be due to reflexive autonomic changes and input from joint receptors.[11]

▶ Suprasegmental inhibition may occur with verbal commands to relax.[46]

▶ Muscles will actively assist with the passive movement if corticospinal pathways are intact.[30]

In summary, mobility passive ROM is promoted with HR, CR, and RS and the initiation of active ROM is facilitated by HRAM, RC, and RI (Fig. 3–15).

STABILITY

The ability of both proximal and distal muscle groups to stabilize joints is an inherent component of movement control (Fig. 3–16). Proximal postural muscles, in particular, need to provide a stable foundation upon which distal segments can function. This proximal stability can be established step-by-step by first eliciting an isometric contraction of muscles on one side of a joint in the shortened range, progressing to isometric contractions on all sides of the joint in preparation for postural demands. Attainment of postural stability is considered in this text as one of

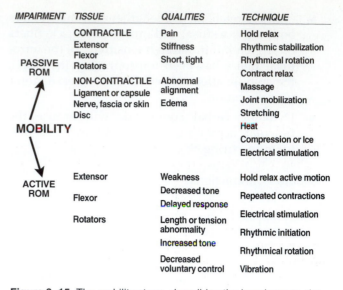

Figure 3–15. The mobility stage, describing the impairments, the tissues involved, the qualities of the involvement, and the treatment techniques.

the precursors to a higher level of control termed *dynamic stability.* Proximal dynamic stability is the ability of trunk and proximal segments to provide sufficient support during the performance of functional activities. The term indicates the presence of appropriate sequencing and timing of muscle contractions within and between segments to allow for coordinated movements. Attainment of dynamic stability begins with techniques to improve stability and is further enhanced as the patient moves through the controlled mobility, static dynamic, and skill levels of control.

Treatment goals that can be achieved at the stability stages include improved quality and duration of isometric holding of postural extensors, and improved ability to maintain postures with proper alignment. Stability is assessed by observing bilateral

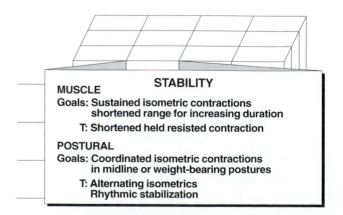

Figure 3–16. The treatment goals that can be achieved at the stability stage and the appropriate techniques.

equality of contraction and fluctuations or oscillations in muscles, which may indicate fatigue.

The following three techniques can be applied to develop stability: **Shortened held resisted contraction, alternating isometrics,** and **rhythmic stabilization.**

Shortened Held Resisted Contraction

Performance of graded isometric contractions in shortened ranges promotes muscle stability in non-weight–bearing postures prior to the stability needed in weight bearing. To accomplish a shortened held resisted contraction (SHRC), the postural extensor muscles are either passively positioned or actively moved into shortened ranges, where they most commonly function and where inhibitory factors are minimized. In this shortened range, a low-intensity, isometric contraction against gravitational, manual, or mechanical resistance is maintained for at least 10 seconds. The duration of 10 seconds seems to optimally increase gamma motor activation of intrafusal muscle fibers, which starts to decline after this 10-second interval. To compensate for this decline, however, and to maintain the force of the contraction, more motor units of participating muscles are recruited as the contraction is maintained.[52] A purpose, therefore, of SHRC is to improve muscle spindle stretch sensitivity and thus the muscle response when the stretch of body weight resistance is later applied in weight-bearing postures. An additional goal is to improve the recruitment of slow-twitch motor units and the control and endurance of the postural extensors in the range in which they most commonly function. To increase endurance, contractions of longer durations may be needed.

Resistance must be graded by the therapist to elicit a response that is limited to approximately 40% of a maximal voluntary contraction (MVC). This level of effort delays the decline of gamma or fusimotoneuron activity and limits the response primarily to slow-twitch, type I muscle fibers, which are responsible for aerobic activity, muscle stability, and endurance.[52,55,56] If the contraction is more forceful or performed too quickly, fast-twitch, type II fibers are increasingly recruited, resulting in an anaerobic response that is more likely to fatigue.

Keeping the response within the 40% range of a MVC is important to develop stability in patients with abnormal tone, weakness, or muscle imbalance. Patients with hypertonia may require stability training to the same degree as those patients with disuse weakness or low tone. Increasing evidence indicates that the decrease in function that occurs with hypertonia is not so much due to the increase in tone but is more likely the result of a problem with motor unit recruitment.[57,58] An abnormal number of motor units, altered rate of firing, or inappropriate recruitment order may result in inefficient movement, instability, and fatigue. Grading resistance will help promote a more normal recruitment order of slow-twitch fibers before fast-twitch and help limit recruitment to those motor units needed to accomplish most activities of daily living (ADL). An unwanted movement response, such as a sustained associated reaction that interferes with function, is a sign that either too much resistance is being applied or that the posture or activity is too difficult for the patient to perform. When this is evident, the therapist may either decrease the amount of resistance, the speed with which it is applied, or revert to a posture with a lower center of gravity (CoG) and larger bases of support (BoS).

SHRC can be performed in various postures against manual, gravitational, or mechanical resistance. For example, gluteal and quadriceps contractions can be actively elicited in supine with a pillow under the knees; manual resistance can be applied to the shortened range of a trunk extensor pattern with the patient supine; scapular adductors can be easily resisted in shortened ranges in any posture with use of Theraband* or pulleys (Fig. 3–17).

When the cardiopulmonary system is involved, the therapist must be extremely careful to monitor resistance so that isometric contractions do not excessively increase peripheral resistance to blood flow, thereby raising blood pressure.

Rationale

The range in which the postural extensors contract and the intensity and duration of the contractions are all important components of stability development.

▶ Slowly performed isometric contractions in shortened ranges promote the development of muscle spindle stretch sensitivity and feedback to higher centers in preparation for demands made on the muscle in a weight-bearing or a stretched position.

▶ Low-level contractions maintained for 10 seconds at approximately 40% of MVC will help to sustain gamma motoneuron activity and recruit primarily slow-twitch motor units needed for endurance, stability, and accuracy of movement.[56]

Alternating Isometrics

The alternating isometrics (AI) technique is a progression from a SHRC. Once the sensitivity of the

---

* Theraband, Hygienic Corporation, Akron, Ohio.

Figure 3–17. Shortened held resisted contraction of: **(A)** gluteals and quadriceps; **(B)** rotator cuff, lower trapezius; **(C)** middle trapezius, rhomboids.

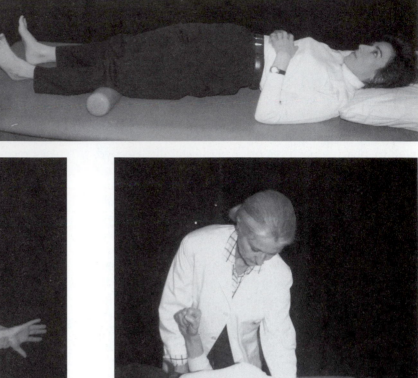

A

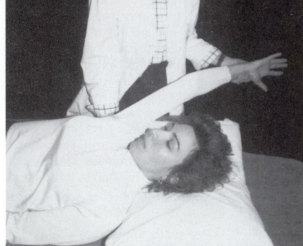

B

C

postural muscles has been improved, the body segment can be brought either into a midline or weight-bearing position. With the therapist's MC on either side of the segment, isometric contractions are rhythmically alternated from one side of the joint to the other, with no relaxation occurring between contractions. If the goal is to increase endurance, the level of patient effort is kept low; if the goal is isometric strengthening, the level of effort can be increased. The direction of resistance can be applied in one or more planes. In bridging, for example, AI applied to the pelvis in an anterior–posterior plane will activate the trunk abdominals and back extensors; resistance applied in a medial–lateral plane will enhance the trunk lateral flexors and the hip abductors and adductors; resistance applied in a horizontal plane will

facilitate rotators; AI applied in a diagonal direction will promote a combination of flexors and extensors with abductors and adductors (Fig. 3–18).

Rhythmic Stabilization

RS is a progression from AI, since it facilitates a smooth performance of isometric contractions in all three planes simultaneously around the segment, rather than alternately. The placement of MC may be similar to AI, but the forces applied differ (Fig. 3–19). The following examples will illustrate the appropriate use of both techniques. With the patient sidelying and MC placed posteriorly on the pelvis and shoulder, verbal commands (VC) for AI are "hold and don't let me push you forward" followed by sliding the hands anteriorly and stating "hold and don't let

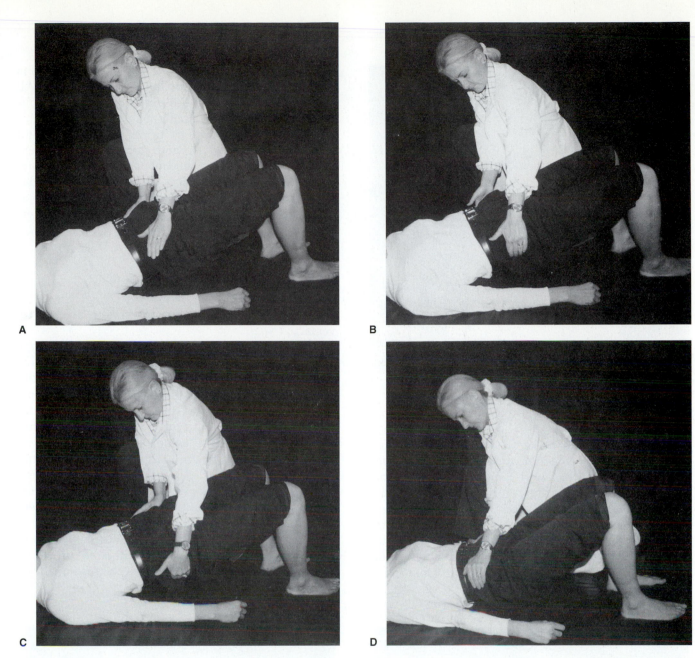

Figure 3–18. Alternating isometrics in bridging: **(A)** anterior–posterior resistance; **(B)** medial–lateral resistance; **(C)** horizontal direction for rotation; **(D)** diagonal direction.

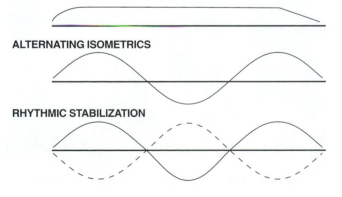

Figure 3–19. A depiction of the application of resistance during the stability techniques.

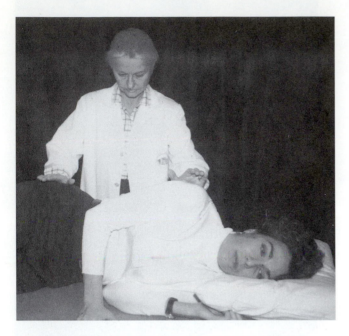

Figure 3–20. Alternating isometrics to trunk in sidelying.

me pull you backward" (Fig. 3–20). With RS, contacts are placed on opposite joint surfaces simultaneously. With one hand on the anterior shoulder and the other placed posteriorly on the pelvis, VC are "hold and don't let me move you" as both trunk flexion and extension and rotation are resisted simultaneously; the therapist's pressure is then gradually altered to the opposite surfaces without allowing relaxation to occur (Fig. 3–21). Because the patient must hold all of

the muscles around the trunk simultaneously, RS is considered to be a more advanced technique than AI. RS may be applied in all postures following the application of AI to enhance postural stability.

RS can also be applied to bilateral or unilateral extremity patterns to promote stability of a weak extremity or to indirectly promote stability of the trunk (Fig. 3–22). Bilateral application of RS is of particular benefit when one or both of the extremities is of good to normal strength and can be used to produce overflow effects.

Slow Reversal Hold Through Decrements of Range

(see Controlled Mobility for description of slow reversal)

Slow reversal hold through decrements of range (SRH ↓ Range) is used as a stepping-stone to promote stability in those patients with excessive mobility, such as occurs with athetosis or ataxia. Such patients usually have difficulty responding to AI or RS with appropriate holding patterns. As a precursor to either technique, SRH ↓ range can be applied. The purpose of the technique is to gradually introduce isometric contractions into the patient's movement pattern while slowly decreasing the arc of movement. For example, to promote stability in quadruped, the patient is allowed to rock forward and backward through wide ranges while the therapist introduces an isometric contraction at the end of range in either direction. The range of movement is gradually reduced, termed

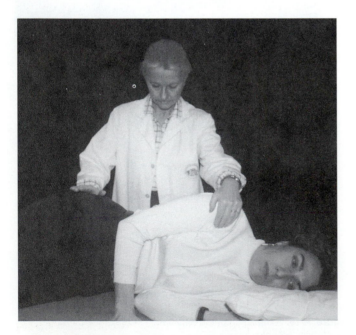

Figure 3–21. Rhythmic stabilization to trunk.

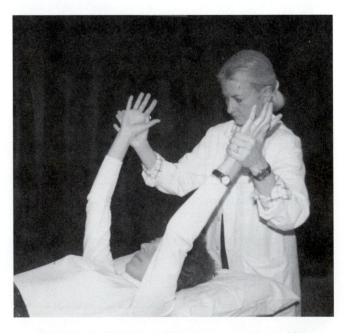

Figure 3–22. Rhythmic stabilization to upper extremities.

moving through decrements of range, until holding at mid range (AI) can be achieved. In quadruped, weight bearing enhances stability through approximation of the joints.

If a patient is capable of responding initially to RS in any weight-bearing posture, the therapist may not need to apply SRH ↓ range or AI.

Various adjunctive measures can precede or be combined with exercise techniques to further increase stability: Vibration with a mechanical vibrator can be applied to a muscle belly or over a tendon to enhance the isometric or tonic response; manual approximation of joint surfaces can be added to the approximation that occurs in weight bearing to further increase holding; MC should be firm and maintained to avoid stimulation of a phasic response.

Rationale

▶ Isometric contractions applied on either side of a joint as occurs with SRH ↓ range, AI, and RS result in coactivation of alpha and gamma motoneurons and motor-unit recruitment.

▶ The simultaneous muscle contractions that occur around a joint when resistance is applied or that occur during weight bearing when stretch-sensitive postural muscles are lengthened may be a result of various factors: motor-unit recruitment through muscle-spindle afferent firing or supraspinal mechanisms, reciprocal facilitatory effects of GTOs that occur from tonic to phasic muscle groups, and Renshaw cell firing, which results in inhibition of inhibitory interneurons (disinhibition) from more tonic to phasic muscle groups.

▶ Although the neural pathways are unclear, joint receptors responding to the approximation of joint surfaces can contribute to stability in weight-bearing postures.[59]

Figure 3–23 summarizes the impairments in stability and the techniques used to promote improvements.

CONTROLLED MOBILITY

Controlled mobility (Fig. 3–24) is weight shifting or movement in weight-bearing postures such as rocking or arching in quadruped. Rotation around the longitudinal axis, as occurs with segmental or total trunk rolling, is also controlled mobility.

Movement in weight-bearing postures, closed-chain activities, can be used to achieve proximal dynamic stability, promote postural control, and strengthen muscles concentrically and eccentrically within the available ROM. Enhancing controlled mobility within various postures will enable the patient to more easily assume and move between postures independently. The patient's ability within this stage can be measured by the amount of movement the patient can control compared to what is available. For example, a patient may only be able to bridge through approximately 50% of range even though passive movement into extension is not restricted.

The techniques that are most effective in promoting this level of control are slow reversal (SR), slow reversal hold (SRH), and agonistic reversal (AR).

Slow Reversal and Slow Reversal Hold Through Increments of Range

Both techniques can be used in all weight-bearing postures to promote controlled movement throughout range. SR involves slow, resisted rhythmical concentric contractions alternating between agonistic and antagonistic muscle groups without relaxation occurring between reversals. Quick stretch may be applied in the lengthened range to initiate movement as needed.

SRH varies from SR in that an isometric contraction is introduced at the end of range in either direction to enhance holding of weakened muscles in that range or to emphasize weight bearing on a limb.

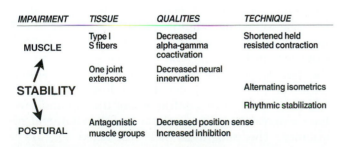

Figure 3–23. The stability stage, describing the impairments, tissues involved, the quality of the involvement, and the techniques.

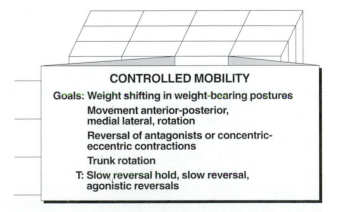

Figure 3–24. Controlled mobility, with the treatment goals that can be achieved and techniques.

If the goal is increased muscle activation, sufficient manual or other means of external resistance is applied. In cases of muscle imbalance, resistance may be applied first to the stronger pattern of movement to facilitate subsequent movement of the weaker pattern.

If the goal is to increase postural control, minimal resistance or guidance by the therapist may be needed. In addition, the range through which the patient moves from the mid position progresses from minimal to maximal, termed moving through increments of range (SRH ↑ range). The excursion gradually increases as the patient learns to control movements that shift the CoG further away from the midpoint of BoS. For patients with tonal abnormalities, increasing the speed of reversal as well as the excursion is an important goal (see Chapter 10).

Rationale

▶ The effects of SR may be explained by Sherrington's law of successive induction, which maintains that a pattern of movement is facilitated by the immediate preceding contraction of its antagonist.[60] The rationale underlying this phenomenon is unclear. One explanation could be that as the stronger pattern actively approaches the shortened range and as the external stretch of the muscles in this pattern diminishes, the unloading of the muscle spindle reduces the spindle afferent input from these receptors to higher centers. Unless resistance, particularly isometric resistance, is emphasized in the shortened range to facilitate the gamma system and subsequent spindle afferent firing, the inhibitory influences of GTOs and Renshaw cells on agonistic anterior horn cells could predominate. The result, therefore, could be one of inhibition of the contracting pattern and reciprocal facilitation to the antagonist.

▶ An isometric contraction applied at the end of range will recruit static gamma motoneurons and increase motor unit activation in the shortened range of the movement.

▶ The simultaneous stretching of the antagonistic muscles at the end of the range can result in facilitation to those muscles via the primary afferents of the muscle spindles.

▶ Electromyographic studies have shown that the onset of antagonistic activity occurs prior to the time when these muscle groups are stretched. This evidence strongly suggests that facilitation to the antagonistic pattern may be a result of central programming rather than influences from peripheral mechanisms.[61]

Agonistic Reversals

Research in the past several years has suggested several beneficial effects of eccentric exercise including muscle hypertrophy, modification of connective tissue, decreasing spasticity, and improvement of tendonitis and patellar tracking.[62–64] From a practical standpoint, muscles need to be able to contract eccentrically for performance of functional activities. For example, hip and knee extensors contract eccentrically to control the body as it is lowered into a chair or descends stairs; trunk extensors exert eccentric control whenever the trunk flexes from an upright position, as occurs during dressing or brushing teeth; rotator cuff muscles contract eccentrically to decelerate the shoulder during throwing movements. Inability of a muscle group to contract eccentrically to adequately decelerate a limb may subject ligaments, cartilage, and bone to abnormal stresses, since they are required to absorb the forces normally absorbed by muscle.[62]

AR is a technique used to promote eccentric control of any muscle group and should be incorporated into treatment programs to attain optimal function of trunk and extremity musculature. Although it can be used to promote skill level activities in non–weight-bearing postures, it is commonly used to promote controlled mobility activities and thus will be described in this section.

Unlike SR, AR emphasizes muscle groups on one side of a joint at a time. The technique is applied by having the patient first concentrically contract the muscle or pattern through the range against manual or gravitational resistance or both. At the end of the range the patient is instructed to "lower slowly." The lowering must counteract either the force of gravity, externally applied resistance, or both. "Make me work at pushing your (arm, leg) down" or "make me work at pulling it up" is the command. If the patient has difficulty controlling the eccentric movement, it can be preceded by an isometric contraction in the shortened range to enhance the muscle's response.

The following example illustrates the use of AR to promote eccentric control of the hip and low-back extensors in bridging. The therapist's hands are on the pelvis near the anterior superior iliac spines (ASIS) and the patient elevates the lower trunk, performing a concentric contraction of the hip and low-back extensors against manual and gravitational resistance. The patient is then instructed to "lower

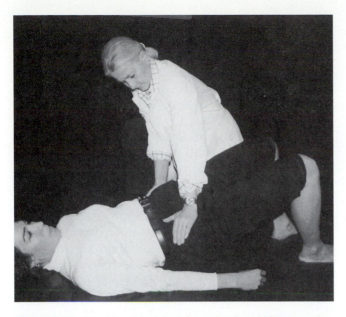

Figure 3–25. Agonistic reversals to lower trunk and hip extensors.

IMPAIRMENT	TISSUE	QUALITIES	TECHNIQUE
WEIGHT SHIFTING	Antagonistic muscle groups	Decreased reciprocal facilitation	
↑	Postural extensors	Decreased coordinated eccentric ability	Agonistic reversals / Slow reversal hold
CONTROLLED MOBILITY	Deep intrinsic	Decreased muscle interaction same and opposite sides of segment	Slow reversal
↓ ROTATION	Superficial multijoint muscles		

Figure 3–26. Controlled mobility, describing the impairments, tissues involved, the quality of the involvement, and the techniques.

slowly" as gravity and the therapist resist the eccentric contraction (Fig. 3–25). Before the patient reaches the mat and relaxes, the sequence of concentric, then eccentric contractions is repeated. Eccentric control, particularly in postural muscles, becomes increasingly more difficult as lengthened ranges are approached, but control throughout the range is important for accomplishment of many functional goals.

Patients with hypertonia often have difficulty performing controlled eccentric contractions throughout the range. Empirical evidence indicates that emphasis on slow eccentric movement has a dampening effect on spasticity and thus should be emphasized during treatment to improve control.

AR can be easily incorporated into a home program using Theraband weights or gravity as the resistive force.

Rationale

▶ The combination of both external and internal stretch of the intrafusal fibers of the spindles that occurs during an eccentric contraction should enhance firing of the spindle afferents.[65]

Figure 3–26 summarizes the impairments in controlled mobility and the techniques used to promote improvements.

STATIC–DYNAMIC

The **static–dynamic** level of control is a transitional stage between controlled mobility and skill. In weight-bearing postures it includes the ability of the trunk and proximal segments to control the body as one or two limbs are lifted from the supporting surface (Fig. 3–27). Static–dynamic activities can be performed in any weight-bearing posture and are indicated for patients with orthopaedic or neurological dysfunction who need enhancement of trunk stabilization or an increase in dynamic stability or postural control.

There are no techniques particular to the static–dynamic level. AI and RS can be performed to improve the patient's ability to stabilize in the posture with the reduced BoS and SR, and SRH or AR can be performed on the dynamic or moving limb to further increase the demands on supporting segments and to enhance development of dynamic stability.

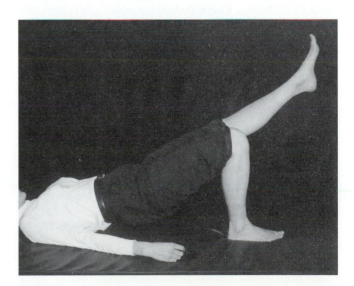

Figure 3–27. Static dynamic control.

SKILL

Skill implies consistency in performing functional tasks with economy of effort (Fig. 3–28).[66] The upper limbs must be able to move freely in space (open chain) to perform all ADL including occupational and recreational activities; the lower limbs must be able to combine and coordinate non–weight-bearing (open-chain) and weight-bearing (closed-chain) movements for functional ambulation on varied surfaces.

For limbs to perform in a skilled manner, there must be dynamic stability of the trunk and proximal limb musculature, which has been gradually developed during the attainment of the previous levels of control.

Unfortunately, patients are often asked to perform skill-level activities for which they do not possess the appropriate neuromuscular control. The result is frustration on the part of the patient but, more importantly, the development of inefficient and ineffective movement patterns, causing undue stress on the supporting structures. A common example is requiring a patient with shoulder disability, with accompanying pain and weakness, to climb a wall with his fingers. Successful performance of such an overhead movement requires dynamic stability of all scapulohumeral musculature, particularly the rotator cuff. Inability of these muscles to adequately stabilize the shoulder results in shoulder shrugging and impingement during attempts to move the arm above shoulder level (see Chapter 5).

The independent performances of occupational and recreational activities are associated with the skill level of control and are usually stated as functional outcomes. These outcomes will differ, depending on the patient's age, disability, and life-style:

▶ Outcome for elderly individuals with a hip fracture: the patient shall ambulate independently on all surfaces and stairs with a cane.

▶ Outcome for the recreational athlete with an ankle sprain: the patient shall run 5 miles three times a week.

The skill level of control focuses on the proper timing, sequencing, speed, and coordination of body and limb segments during the performance of a functional task. The techniques of resisted progression (RP) and normal timing (NT) can promote these aspects of skilled movement and can be easily adapted to enhance the patient's abilities and to promote functional goals. The previously described SR, SRH, and AR can also be used to promote concentric or eccentric control of extremity movements at the skill level.

Normal Timing

NT promotes the distal-to-proximal timing integral to the performance of functional movement. A segment may have sufficient strength to move through range, but the timing of the movement in relation to the other segments may be faulty. A commonly seen abnormality for patients at advanced levels is for movement to occur proximally while the distal segment lags behind. During the application of NT, the proximal segments are manually prevented from moving through the range as the distal segments are simultaneously facilitated by quick stretch and appropriate resistance. Once the distal component is activated the other components of the pattern are allowed to move through the range (Fig. 3–29). Repetition of this distal-to-proximal sequencing will reinforce a coordinated movement pattern.

NT is usually applied with the limb in an elongated position to simulate functional use. If, however, the patient is unable to initiate distal movement with proximal segments elongated, the technique can be made easier by beginning in more shortened ranges and progressing to lengthened. For example, hemiplegic patients can usually initiate wrist and finger extensors with the shoulder elevated beyond 90° (Souques' phenomenon).[67] In such cases NT would begin with shoulder elevation and progress to initiation of distal extension with the arm in more neutral ranges. Distal-to-proximal sequencing of muscle activity occurs during postural control strategies. For example, during an ankle strategy, the distal ankle musculature is active prior to the more proximal musculature.[68] Following the facilitation of NT in non–weight-bearing activities, this sequence is promoted in standing (Fig. 3–30).

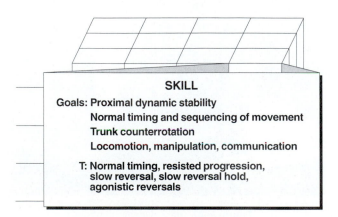

SKILL

Goals: Proximal dynamic stability
Normal timing and sequencing of movement
Trunk counterrotation
Locomotion, manipulation, communication

T: Normal timing, resisted progression,
slow reversal, slow reversal hold,
agonistic reversals

Figure 3–28. Skill, with the treatment goals and techniques.

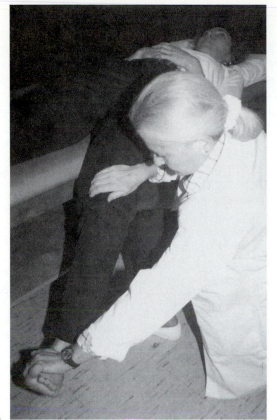

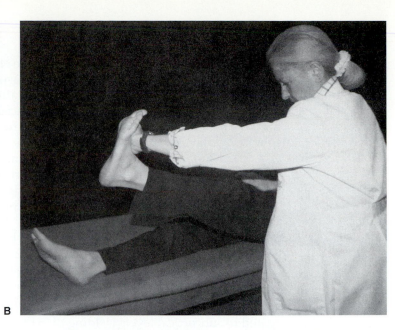

Figure 3–29. Normal timing for ankle dorsiflexion: **(A)** lengthened range; **(B)** midrange.

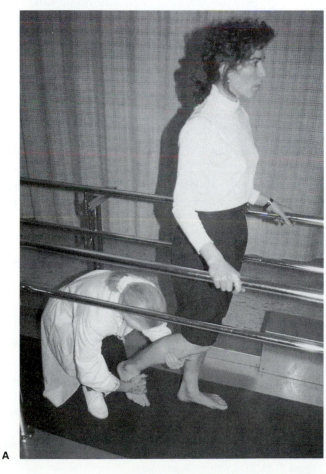

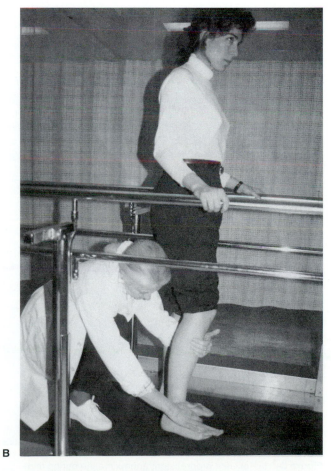

Figure 3–30. Normal timing in standing: **(A)** dorsiflexion lengthened range; **(B)** mid swing.

Biofeedback can be used to enhance any of the stages of control, including the normal timing of distal musculature during the actual performance of the functional activity. For example, electrodes can be placed on the anterolateral surface of the leg of a patient with hemiplegia to facilitate balanced dorsiflexion during the swing phase of gait. Patients with weakness or tonal abnormalities may benefit from this additional or alternative input.[69]

Rationale

Repetition and practice is an important principle in motor learning.[66] If impulses constantly travel over the same pathways, transmission of those impulses will become easier. A movement may first be initiated cortically, but with repetition and sensory feedback it may be relegated to subcortical levels yielding more automatic responses. Repetition of faulty movement patterns should therefore be avoided.

Resisted Progression

RP is applied during the gait cycle to facilitate and reinforce the sequencing of proximal components. Unlike NT, which focuses on the distal segments, RP emphasizes coordination of pelvic, hip, and knee musculature during ambulation. MC are commonly placed on the pelvis to control lateral shifting and forward progression as well as pelvic rotation during the swing phase and to increase stability during stance. If the therapist must provide maximal support to prevent the patient from falling, lower-level procedures to develop proximal control need to be emphasized before this technique can be effective.

Initially, the patient may be positioned in parallel bars or with other ambulatory aids as needed to increase the BoS. The feet are positioned in stride and the therapist's contacts are on the pelvis (Fig. 3–31). A minimal stretch to facilitate pelvic rotation and lateral shifting is followed by tracking resistance applied to the ipsilateral pelvis as the leg swings through. The pelvis is guided forward as the foot begins heelstrike. Approximation is applied and maintained through the pelvis as the foot moves into midstance to enhance extension of the limb. The sequence is then repeated on the contralateral side.

This deliberate, resisted walking pattern may enhance and reinforce the gait pattern of some patients. However, because walking is an automatic function, emphasis on and attention to component parts may not produce the desired effect. For many patients the total activity needs to be promoted at a subcortical level to achieve a coordinated gait pattern.

Rationale

▶ Sensory input provided by the manual contacts, stretch, resistance, and verbal commands will help the patient to use pelvic and hip musculature in proper sequence.

▶ If the prerequisite motor control abilities are present guided practice may promote learning of the functional task. Figure 3–32 summarizes the impairments at the skill stage and the techniques used to promote improvements.

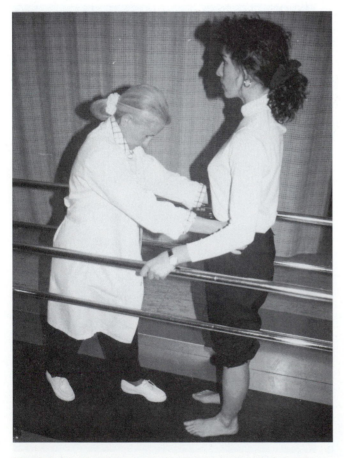

Figure 3–31. Resisted progression: approximation during midstance.

IMPAIRMENT	TISSUE	QUALITIES	TECHNIQUE
DISTAL FUNCTIONAL MOVEMENT	Limb muscles	Decreased timing, sequencing	Normal timing
			Slow reversal
↑			
SKILL			Slow reversal hold
↓			Agonistic reversals
PROXIMAL DYNAMIC STABILITY	Trunk and proximal muscles	Decreased postural control	
			Resisted progression

Figure 3–32. Skill, with the impairments, involved tissues, the quality of involvement, and techniques.

STRENGTH

Strength is an integral component of movement at all levels of control and is influenced by several factors, including the cross-sectional size of the muscle and its myofibrils and the motivation of the patient.[70,71] In this text, *strength* is defined as a sufficient amount and appropriate type and timing of motor unit recruitment to perform goals related to the tasks. Strengthening, according to this definition, can be acquired with several of the aforementioned techniques and is a goal to be achieved at all levels of control. Timing for emphases (TE) and repeated contractions (RC) are two particularly effective techniques that can be applied to increase motor unit recruitment for a wide variety of patients at any stage of their program (Fig. 3–33).

Repeated Contraction

RC was previously discussed under mobility as a technique to initiate movement of a very weak muscle. However, RC also can be used to promote strength throughout range when the muscle grade is above 2/5. At the point in the range that a decline in muscle contraction is felt, a quick stretch is superimposed on the contracting musculature, followed immediately by an appropriate amount of resistance to augment and reinforce the contraction. This stretch and resistance can be applied at any point or points in the range and can be repeated until a smooth, continuous contraction throughout range can be achieved by the patient. The therapist must be sure that the stretch and resistance are not of such magnitude as to prevent or overwhelm the muscle response. The amount of stretch needed to strengthen a response of a contracting muscle is not as great as that needed to

initiate a response of poor musculature. To further enhance the response, an isometric contraction can be elicited prior to the application of the stretch.

If the weakness is unidirectional, the application of RC can be enhanced by a preceding contraction of the stronger antagonistic muscle or movement pattern. For example, if the anterior and middle deltoid and supra- and infraspinatus are 3/5, the technique can begin by applying resistance to the antagonistic muscle groups or movement pattern (extension, adduction, internal rotation). Quick stretch is added to the agonistic muscles at any point in the range that the response begins to weaken (Fig. 3–34).

Rationale

▶ Quick stretches superimposed on an isotonic contraction will increase spindle afferent firing and motor unit recruitment.[72]

▶ An isometric contraction at the point of weakness will increase gamma motoneuron activity and thus increase spindle stretch sensitivity.[50–52]

▶ Resistance to the antagonistic or stronger movement prior to the contraction of the agonistic or weaker movement will enhance the response of the agonist through successive induction (see rationale for slow reversal).

Timing for Emphasis

TE combines the physiological principle of overflow with the technique of RC to strengthen either one component of a movement or an entire movement pattern. The term implies that one or more strong segments are contracting isometrically to create irradiation or overflow effects while weaker segments are being stretched and isotonically resisted through

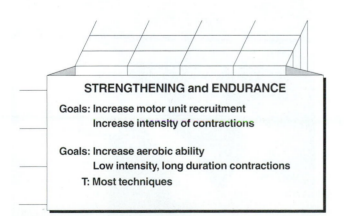

Figure 3–33. The performance characteristics of strength and endurance with the treatment goals and techniques.

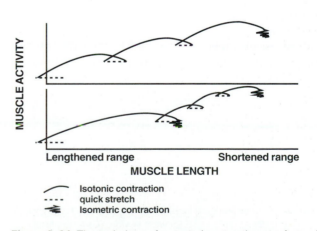

Figure 3–34. The technique of repeated contractions performed throughout the range and near the shortened range.

range, that is, they're performing a repeated contraction. Overflow is maximized by holding flexor muscles in mid ranges and extensor muscles in shortened ranges. The following examples illustrate the use of TE:

▶ PROBLEM: WEAK LEFT BICEPS (2+/5)

The patient is supine. The movement combination is flexion, adduction, and external rotation of the shoulder, which provides optimal facilitation of biceps. Resistance is applied to an isometric contraction of all three shoulder components in conjunction with wrist flexion in midrange, where maximal resistance is usually best elicited. While the shoulder and wrist segments are being resisted isometrically, stretch and resistance are applied to an isotonic contraction of the biceps with the goal of completing elbow flexion through the range (Fig. 3–35A).

▶ PROBLEM: WEAK RADIAL WRIST FLEXOR (2/5)

The patient position and movement pattern remain the same as the above example. Resistance is again applied to an isometric contraction of shoulder flexion, adduction, and external rotation, and elbow flexion in midrange while stretch and resistance are applied to the distal components, wrist flexion with radial deviation (Fig. 3–35B).

▶ PROBLEM: GENERALIZED WEAKNESS OF RIGHT UPPER EXTREMITY MOVING INTO FLEXION, ADDUCTION, AND EXTERNAL ROTATION

With the patient supine, a bilateral symmetrical D1 thrust can be performed. An isometric contraction of the stronger left upper extremity is maintained in middle ranges of the thrust, while stretch and resistance are simultaneously applied to the same muscle pattern on the weaker right extremity throughout the range (Fig. 3–35C).

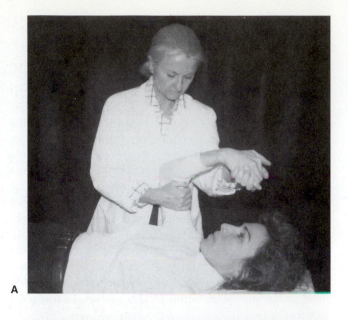

A

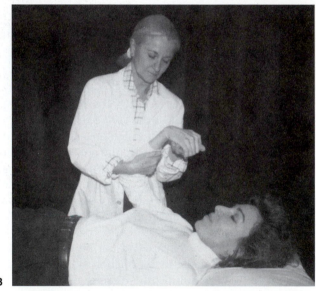

B

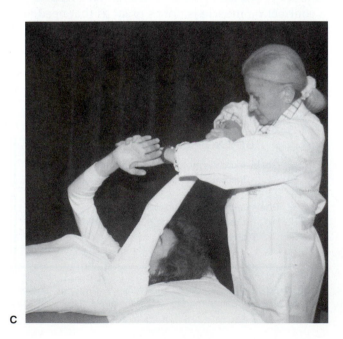

C

Figure 3–35. Strengthening techniques: **(A)** A: D1F; T: TE for elbow flexion; **(B)** A: D1F; T: TE for wrist flexion; **(C)** A: Bilateral thrust; T: TE R shoulder; **(D)** A: BS knee extension; T: TE for R knee extension; **(E)** A: Bilateral reciprocal LE motion; T: TE R knee extension; **(F)** A: Lower trunk flexion; T: TE trunk flexion.

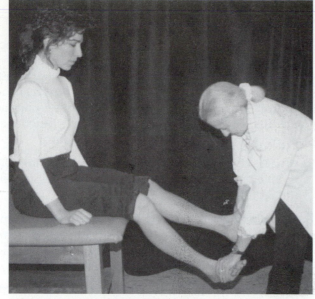

D

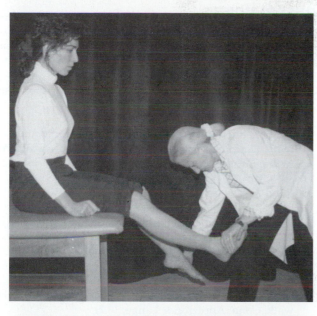

E

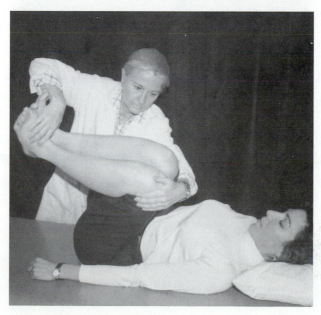

F

TE can be applied to weak segments of the lower extremity following the same procedure. For example, a weak quadriceps can be strengthened in sitting by manually resisting a bilateral symmetrical pattern and eliciting overflow from the contralateral quadriceps (Fig. 3–35D); the quadriceps may also be strengthened by resistance to a bilateral reciprocal pattern, which elicits overflow from the contralateral hamstrings (Fig. 3–35E). In addition, upper or lower extremities can be resisted together to obtain overflow effects into trunk musculature (Fig. 3–35F).

Many muscles and segments can be activated simultaneously with TE. For many conditions, strengthening in this manner is preferable to the use of machines, which usually emphasize only one segment at a time.

TE is a very effective technique to facilitate and reinforce muscle contraction but requires coordination of verbal commands and manual skills of the therapist who must resist isometric and isotonic contractions simultaneously.

Rationale

▶ Maintained isometric contraction of strong muscle groups is capable of producing overflow effects to weaker musculature.[73]

▶ Quick stretch superimposed on a contracting muscle will enhance firing of spindle afferent and increase alpha motoneuron response.

ENDURANCE

Endurance training, as well as strength, is needed if a skill level of functioning is to be maintained. Essential to the performance of functional activities is the presence of sufficient aerobic capacity to sustain controlled movement.[54,70] Duration, frequency, and intensity are parameters of all movements that can be manipulated to improve endurance training of specific muscle groups or of the cardiovascular system. Use of mechanical equipment such as pulleys, treadmills, stationary bicycles, or progression of a home program with Theraband or free weights are ways in which endurance can be accomplished. Holding of a muscle against low-intensity resistance for an increased duration will increase the circulatory bed of the muscle and improve muscular aerobic capacity.[74] For example, a SHRC of scapula adductors in sitting can be performed against the resistance of lightweight Theraband. As stated throughout this text, isometric contractions are particularly important for postural muscles, which must be able to sustain contractions during performance of functional activities.

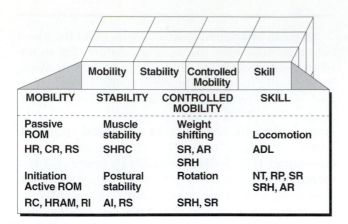

Mobility	Stability	Controlled Mobility	Skill
MOBILITY	**STABILITY**	**CONTROLLED MOBILITY**	**SKILL**
Passive ROM	Muscle stability	Weight shifting	Locomotion
HR, CR, RS	SHRC	SR, AR SRH	ADL
Initiation Active ROM	Postural stability	Rotation	NT, RP, SR SRH, AR
RC, HRAM, RI	AI, RS	SRH, SR	

Figure 3–36. A summary of the techniques to achieve the stages of control.

▶ SUMMARY

Techniques are used in conjunction with activities to achieve the stages of control (Fig. 3–36). Balancing of the ANS is a precursor to the development of the stages of control and can be achieved with certain techniques geared to the dampening of sympathetic function. In conjunction with promoting homeostasis, the treatment goals encompassed within the mobility, stability, controlled mobility, static–dynamic, and skill stages can be achieved with a variety of techniques. An understanding of the mechanisms responsible for the efficacy of each technique will aid the therapist in choosing the most appropriate techniques for a patient with a particular disorder.

▶ REVIEW QUESTIONS

1. What is the purpose of a technique?

2. You have a patient with pain and limited ROM in the knee, as well as other impairments leading to decreased function. The impairment of decreased ROM is what stage of control? Which techniques are appropriate to promote the goal of increasing ROM? Which tissues are affected by each technique?

3. Why is active movement of the agonist important in maintaining gains in ROM?

4. Why are isometric contractions indicated for the treatment of postural extensor muscles? What techniques incorporate this type of contraction? What is the importance of intensity and duration of the contractions?

5. Why should eccentric contractions be empha-

sized? What technique will achieve control of eccentric contractions? Why is an eccentric contraction of a postural muscle difficult in lengthened ranges? If a patient has difficulty with eccentric contractions of the gluteus maximus, gluteus medius, or quadriceps, during which functional activities might you observe abnormalities?

6. What is dynamic stability? During which stages is it developed? Why is dynamic stability critical for the performance of functional activities?

7. Describe how all the levels of control are encompassed in a functional task such as stepping up onto or off a curb, throwing a ball, or getting dressed.

REFERENCES

1. Knott M, Voss D. *Proprioceptive Neuromuscular Facilitation.* 2nd ed. New York: Harper & Row Publishers Inc; 1968.
2. Koizumi K, Brooks CM. The integration of autonomic reflexes, their control and their association with somatic reactions. *Ergeb Physiol.* 1972;67:1–68.
3. Lanting P, Faes TJ, Ijff GA, et al. Autonomic and somatic peripheral nerve function and the correlation with neuropathic pain in diabetic patients. *J Neurol Sci.* 1989;94:507–17.
4. Rood M. The use of sensory receptors to activate, facilitate and inhibit motor response, autonomic and somatic, in developmental sequence. In: Sattely C, ed. *Approaches to the Treatment of Patients with Neuromuscular Dysfunction.* Dubuque, Iowa: William C. Brown; 1962.
5. Selye H. *The Stress of Life,* rev ed. New York, NY: McGraw-Hill Book Co; 1976.
6. Tappan FM. *Healing Massage Techniques,* 2nd ed. Norwalk, Conn: Appleton & Lange; 1988.
7. Ebner M. *Connective Tissue Massage: Theory and Clinical Application.* New York, NY: Robert E. Krieger Publishing Co; 1962.
8. Stockmeyer SA. *Procedures for Improvement of Motor Control.* Unpublished notes from Boston University, Sargent College of Allied Health Professions; 1978.
9. Sullivan J, Williams LRT, Seaborne DE, et al. Effects of massage on alpha motoneuron excitability. *Phys Ther.* 1991;71:555–560.
10. Pederson DR. The soothing effect of rocking as determined by the direction and frequency of movement. *Can J Behav Sci.* 1975;7:237–243.
11. Ter Vrugt D, Pederson DR. The effects of vertical rocking frequencies on the arousal level of two-month old infants. *Child Dev.* 1973;44:205–209.
12. Umphred DA, McCormick GL. Classification of common facilitory and inhibitory treatment techniques. In: Umphred DA, ed. *Neurological Rehabilitation.* St. Louis, Mo: CV Mosby Co; 1985.
13. Heiniger MC, Randolph SL. *Neurophysiological Concepts*

in Human Behavior—The Tree of Learning. St. Louis, Mo: CV Mosby Co; 1981.

14. Jacobson E. *Progressive Relaxation.* Chicago, Ill: University Press; 1939.

15. Jacobsen E. *Anxiety and Tension Control.* Philadelphia, Pa: J.B. Lippincott Co; 1964.

16. Telles S, Desiraju T. Heart rate and respiratory changes accompanying yogic conditions of single thought and thoughtless states. *Indian J Physiol Pharmacol.* 1992;36: 293–4.

17. Blackwell B, Bloomfield S, Gartside P, et al. Transcendental meditation in hypertension. Individual response patterns. *Lancet.* 1976;1:223–226.

18. Bouhuys A. *Physiology of Breathing.* New York, NY: Grune & Stratton Inc; 1977.

19. Stockmeyer SA. An interpretation of the approach of Rood to the treatment of neuromuscular dysfunction. *Am J Phys Med.* 1967;46:950–56.

20. Gellhorn EL. *Principles of Autonomic-Somatic Integration.* Minneapolis, Minn: University of Minnesota Press; 1967.

21. Kaltenborn FM, Evjenth O. *Manual Mobilization of the Extremity Joints: Examination and Basic Treatment Techniques.* Oslo, Norway: Olaf Norlis Borhandel; 1989.

22. Maitland GD. *Peripheral Manipulation.* 3rd ed. Boston, Mass: Butterworth-Heinemann Ltd, 1991.

23. Michlevitz SL. *Thermal Agents in Rehabilitation.* Philadelphia, Pa: FA Davis Co; 1986.

24. Williams PE, Goldspink G. Changes in sarcomere length and physiological properties in immobilized muscle. *J Anat.* 1978;127:459–468.

25. Gossman MR, Rose SJ, Sahrmann SA, et al. Length and circumference measurements in one joint and multi joint muscles in rabbits after immobilization. *Phys Ther.* 1986;66:516–520.

26. Ada L, Canning C. Anticipating and avoiding muscle shortening. In: Ada L, Canning C, eds. *Key Issues in Neurological Physiotherapy.* London, England: Butterworth-Heinemann Ltd. 1990:219–236.

27. Zablotny C, Andric MF, Gowland C. Serial casting: clinical applications for the adult head injured patient. *J Head Trauma Rehabil.* 1987;2:46–52.

28. Mills V. Electromyographic results of inhibitory splinting. *Phys Ther.* 1984;64:190–193.

29. Zachazewski J, Eberle ED, Jefferies M. Effect of tone-inhibiting casts and orthoses on gait: a case report. *Phys Ther.* 1982;62:543–545.

30. Sahrmann S, Norton BJ, Bomze HA, et al. Influence of the site of the lesion and muscle length on spasticity in man. *Phys Ther.* 1974;54:1290–1297.

31. Zimny ML. Mechanoreceptors in articular tissues. *Am J Anat.* 1988;182:16.

32. Houk J, Singer J, Henneman E. Adequate stimulus for tendon organs with observation on mechanics of the ankle joint. *J Neurophysiol.* 1971;34:1051–1065.

33. Basmajian JV. Neuromuscular control of voluntary movement. In: Buerger AA, Tobis JS, eds. *Neurophysiologic Aspects of Rehabilitation Medicine.* Springfield, Ill: Charles C Thomas Publisher; 1976.

34. Sullivan PE, Markos PD, Minor MAD. *An Integrated Approach to Therapeutic Exercise: Theory and Clinical Application.* Reston, Va: Reston Publishing Co; 1982.

35. Kukulka CG, Beckman SM, Holte JB, et al. Effects of intermittent tendon pressure of alpha motoneuron excitability. *Phys Ther.* 1986;66:1091–1101.

36. Leone JA, Kukulka CG: Effects of tendon pressure on alpha motoneuron excitability in patients with stroke. *Phys Ther.* 1988;68:475–480.

37. Belanger AY, Morin S, Pepin P, et al. Manual muscle tapping decreases soleus H-reflex amplitude in control subjects. *Physiotherapy (Canada).* 1989;41:192–196.

38. Robichaud JA, Agostinucci J, Vander Linden DW. Effect of air-splint application on soleus muscle motoneuron reflex excitability in nondisabled subjects and subjects with cerebrovascular accidents. *Phys Ther.* 1992;72: 176–183.

39. Markos PD. Ipsilateral and contralateral effects of proprioceptive neuromuscular technique on hip motion and electromyographic activity. *Phys Ther.* 1979;59: 1366–1373.

40. Shapiro CH. *Effects of Hold Relax at Different Muscle Lengths.* Boston, Mass: Boston University, Sargent College of Allied Health Professions; 1978. Thesis.

41. Bernier S. *Effects of Contract Relax at Different Muscle Lengths.* Boston, Mass: Boston University, Sargent College of Allied Health Professions; 1980. Thesis.

42. Cole D, Cooper L, Murphy M, et al. Hold relax effects over time. Boston, Mass: Boston University, Sargent College of Allied Health Professions; 1978. Unpublished study.

43. West A. *Duration Effects of Contract Relax.* Boston, Mass: Boston University, Sargent College of Allied Health Professions; 1983. Thesis.

44. Moore MA, Kukulka CG. Depression of Hoffman reflexes following voluntary contraction and implications for proprioceptive neuromuscular facilitation therapy. *Phys Ther.* 1991;71:270–363.

45. Gordon J, Ghez C. Muscle receptors and spinal reflexes: the stretch reflex. In: Kandel E, Schwartz JH, Jessell TM, eds. *Principles of Neural Science,* 3rd ed. New York, NY: Elsevier Publishing Co; 1991.

46. McCandless CA, Rose DE: Evoked cortical response to stimulus change. *J Speech Hear Res.* 1970;13:624–634.

47. Burke RE, Rymer WZ, Walsh JV. Functional specialization in the motor unit population of cat medial gastrocnemius muscle. In: Stein RB, Pearson KA, Smith RS, et al, eds. *Control of Posture and Locomotion.* New York, NY: Plenum Press; 1973.

48. Structure and function of skeletal muscle. A discussion. *Physician and Sports Medicine,* May 1977;34–48.

49. Gordon J. Spinal mechanisms of motor coordination. In: Kandel E, Schwartz JH, Jessel TM, eds. *Principles of Neural Science.* 3rd ed. New York, NY: Elsevier Publishing Co; 1991.

50. Brooks VB. *The Neural Basis of Motor Control.* New York, NY: Oxford University Press; 1986.

51. Ribot-Ciscar E, Tardy-Gervet MF, Vedel JP, et al. Postcontraction changes in human muscle spindle resting discharge and stretch sensitivity. *Exp Brain Res.* 1991; 86:673–679.

52. Macefield G, Hagbarth KE, Gorman R, et al. Decline in spindle support to alpha motoneurons during sustained voluntary contractions. *J Physiol.* 1991;440:497–512.

53. Buchwald JS. Exteroceptive reflexes and movement. *Am J Phys Med.* 1967;46:127.

54. Crutchfield CA, Barnes MR. *The Neurophysiological Basis of Patient Treatment.* 2nd ed. Atlanta, Ga: Stokesville Publishing Co; 1975;1.

55. Henneman E. Peripheral mechanisms involved in the control of muscle. In: Mountcastle VB, ed. *Medical Physiology.* 13th ed. St. Louis, Mo: CV Mosby Co; 1974;1.

56. Astrand PO, Rodahl K. Neuromuscular function. In: *Textbook of Work Physiology.* New York, NY: McGraw-Hill Book Co; 1986.

57. Petajan JH. Motor unit control in movement disorders. *Adv Neurol.* 1983;39:897–905.

58. Grimby L, Hannerz J. Tonic and phasic recruitment order of motor units in man under normal and pathological conditions. In: Desmedt JE, ed. *New Developments in Electromyography and Clinical Neurophysiology.* Basel, Switzerland: Karger; 1973.

59. Johansson H, Sjolander P, Sojka P. A sensory role for the cruciate ligaments. *Clin Orthop.* 1990;288:161–178.

60. Kabat H. Proprioceptive facilitation in therapeutic exercise. In: Licht S, ed. *Therapeutic Exercise.* 2nd ed. New Haven, Conn: Elizabeth Licht Publisher; 1961.

61. Angel RW. Antagonistic muscle activity during rapid arm movements: central versus proprioceptive influences. *J Neurol Neurosurg Psychiatry.* 1977;40:683–686.

62. Stauber WT. Eccentric action of muscles: physiology, injury and adaptation. In: Pandolf KB ed. *Exercise and Sports Sciences Reviews.* Baltimore, Md: Williams & Wilkins; 1989.

63. Stanish WD, Rubinovich RM, Curwin S. Eccentric exercise in chronic tendonitis. *Clin Orthop.* 1986;208:65–68.

64. Hughston JC, Walsh WM, Puddu G. *Patellar Subluxation and Dislocation.* Philadelphia, Pa: WB Saunders Co; 1984;5.

65. Burke D, Hagbarth K, Lofstedt L. Muscle spindle activity in man during shortening and lengthening contractions. *J Physiol.* 1978;277:131–142.

66. Gentile AM. Skill acquisition: action, movement, and neuromotor processes. In: Carr JH, Shepherd RB, eds. *Foundations of Physical Therapy Rehabilitation.* 1988.

67. Brunnstrom S. *Movement Therapy in Hemiplegia.* New York, NY: Harper & Row Publishers Inc; 1970.

68. Nashner LM, McCollum G. The organization of human postural movement: a formal basis and experimental synthesis. *Behav Brain Sci.* 1985;8:135–172.

69. Basmajian JV. *Biofeedback—Principles and Practice for Clinicians.* 2nd ed. Baltimore, Md: Williams & Wilkins; 1983.

70. McArdle WD, Katch FI, Katch VL. *Exercise Physiology.* 2nd ed. Philadelphia, Pa: Lea and Febiger; 1986.

71. Kisner C, Colby LA. *Therapeutic Exercise–Foundations and Techniques.* Philadelphia, Pa: FA Davis Co; 1985.

72. Ashworth B, Grimby L, Kugelberlg E. Comparison of voluntary and reflex activation of motor units. *J Neurol Neurosurg Psychiatry.* 1967;30:91–98.

73. Portney LG, Sullivan PE. *EMG Analysis of Ipsilateral and Contralateral Shoulder and Elbow Muscles During the Performance of PNF Patterns.* Presented at the Annual Conference of the Society for Behavioral Kinesiology. 1980; Boston, Mass.

74. Smith JL, Hutton RS, Eldred E. Postcontraction changes in sensitivity of muscle afferents to static and dynamic stretch. *Brain Res.* 1974;78:193–202.

Evaluation

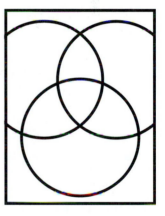

The purpose of the evaluation is to determine the patient's physical functional capability. This determination is made by ascertaining: the etiology of the dysfunction, the environmental constraints or physical impairments contributing to the functional limitations, and the extent to which the impairments and constraints can be rectified by physical therapy intervention to achieve the functional outcome (Fig. 4–1).[1] The following information is included for the purpose of relating evaluative findings to the interventions, with the primary focus on determination of appropriate therapeutic exercise procedures. The clinical chapters that follow will relate the general discussion presented in this chapter to each particular situation. This chapter is not intended to provide an in-depth description or analysis of measurement procedures. The reader is referred to the bibliography in the appendix for more detailed information on evaluative methods.

The functions that are assessed include: locomotion, which encompasses ambulation, transfers, and the use of the lower body to perform daily, occupational, or recreational tasks; manipulation of environment, comprising the activities of daily living (ADL), including the use of the upper body in vocational and recreational activities; communication, encompassing temporomandibular joint

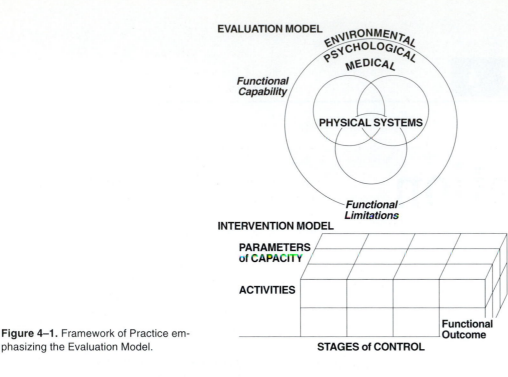

Figure 4–1. Framework of Practice emphasizing the Evaluation Model.

(TMJ) function and other oral motor activities, such as feeding and the motor prerequisites for speech and nonverbal communication.

The evaluation process includes:

▶ an overview of patient's complaint;

▶ a subjective analysis of past and current physical problems;

▶ an assessment of the contribution of environmental, psychological, and medical factors to functional limitations;

▶ an in-depth analysis of the physical systems to determine physical impairments, tissue involvement, and the potential to change.

After the data has been gathered, the therapist determines the extent to which a change in the physical impairments, an augmentation of attributes, and modification of environmental constraints can improve function. Functional outcomes and treatment goals and the frequency and duration of therapy can then be established. Referrals are made to other practitioners for information or treatment and the findings documented and communicated.

The **overview** of the patient's complaint includes date of onset of symptoms and, when possible, the patient's description of the problem and his or her goals.

The **subjective analysis** includes gathering of information pertaining to previous injury to the area, the response to previous interventions, and results of special diagnostic and laboratory tests including roentgenogram, computerized tomographic (CT) scan, magnetic resonance imaging (MRI), electromyogram (EMG), and pulmonary function tests. Reading a surgical report, when appropriate, may provide useful information. Various portions of the history will influence judgments regarding intervention. The following examples will illustrate this point: the time elapsed since injury will help determine the acuteness or chronicity of the condition and the projected healing time; the tissue reactivity will influence the treatment's duration, frequency, and intensity; a history of repeated injury with the addition of an acute trauma may suggest long-standing subclinical tissue strain that may follow a different course from an initial trauma to healthy tissue; the variability of the symptoms will help determine whether subsequent changes in patient's response should be attributed to the condition or to the intervention; reports of cardiac involvement or elevated blood pressure will influence the choice of postures and intensity of exercise. In general, if symptoms cannot be related to a particular trauma or incident or if a biomechanical cause of disability cannot be identified, referral to a physician should be considered.

ENVIRONMENTAL, SOCIAL, CULTURAL, AND PSYCHOLOGICAL AND MEDICAL FACTORS

Environmental, social, and cultural factors need to be considered, including family support, living conditions, nutrition, education, occupation, and recreation (Fig. 4–2).[2–4] For example, a truck driver who has a back injury and who has limited education may have difficulty finding alternative employment. His financial situation may not allow environmental modifications, such as changing the driver's seat or adding a lift on the truck. Thus his inability to work may be as limited by external factors as by physical impairments. A referral to vocational counseling may be appropriate. Environmental, occupational, and recreational strains may be the immediate cause of the injury or, in the case of many patients, may have resulted in repetitive trauma weakening tissues to the extent that they become prone to injury. Therefore, discussing the home or occupational environment may reveal conditions that require modification.

Relevant **psychological** factors may include the individual's self-esteem, the sense of mastery and control, life satisfaction, depression, and anxiety.[5–7] These factors may influence health either positively, with the development of appropriate coping mechanisms, or negatively, with resultant strain or stress re-

sponses. For example, the increased strain of unemployment or of an unhappy home situation may lead to depression or anxiety. These factors have been shown to contribute to increased pain behavior and chronic pain syndromes.[4,8]

From the patient or medical record the patient's **medical history** needs to be ascertained. Dysfunction in many internal organs can refer symptoms to other regions such as to the shoulder and back. The patient should be questioned regarding possible cardiac, pulmonary, gallbladder, and breast involvement. Certain disease processes such as osteoporosis, osteopenia, or diabetes can alter tissue density or compliance, requiring that caution be taken in the application of some treatment procedures. Medications, both those prescribed by a physician and those self-prescribed, should be ascertained as well as their influence on physical performance. If the patient is referred by a medical practitioner, the diagnosis that guides the medical intervention is noted.

Any of these factors, which cannot be changed by physical therapy, may account for the lack of improvement in functional status. In some cases, referral to other health professionals may be warranted to provide medical care or to modify environmental and psychological strains and help the patient develop more effective coping mechanisms. With such help the patient will often respond more favorably to physical therapy intervention.

Environmental limitations, including architectural barriers, may restrict the individual's independence.[8] The home environment needs to be addressed. For example, the height of stairs and toilet seats may limit ambulation and ADL for those with hip arthritis, those receiving postsurgical lower-extremity care, or any patient who has lower-extremity ROM, strength, or postural control impairments.

The patient should be questioned regarding the functional gains that are anticipated with therapy. For example, the patient's goals may be to regain pain-free use of the trunk or limbs, to perform ADL and occupational tasks, or to resume recreational activities such as golf or tennis. Certain goals may not be realistic because of permanent physical impairment. As the evaluation continues, the appropriateness of these goals can be more clearly determined.

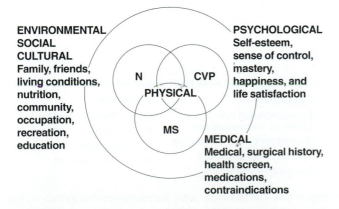

Figure 4–2. The environmental, social, cultural, psychological, and medical factors that need to be considered.

EVALUATION OF THE PHYSICAL SYSTEMS

The foci of the physical therapy evaluation are the structures of the **musculoskeletal (MS), nervous,** and **cardiovascular–pulmonary (CVP) systems** and the functions of **movement control** and **capacity** (Fig. 4–3). The evaluative strategies used to assess the physical impairments and tissue involvement may vary for each area; the influence of each system on functional capability differs and each responds to direct and indirect injury or disease differently.

Despite these variations, the evaluation includes assessment of certain common denominators: ROM and the ability to initiate active movement, to sustain muscle contractions and maintain postures, to move within and between postures, and to perform functional activities with the appropriate timing and sequencing of movement with varying intensities, durations, and frequencies. These characteristics of movement control and capacity comprise the primary components of physical functional capability. The assessment attempts to determine the structures or physiological functions that limit or cause the impairments and the extent to which they can be changed. The findings are considered with respect to normal variability, which is influenced by age,[9] sex,[10] and body structure.[11]

From the history and description of the complaint, the therapist should be able to hypothesize which physical system is most involved.[12] An in-depth assessment of the structures of this particular system and the functions of the overlapping areas will probably yield the most pertinent information linking the physical impairments to the functional limitations. Additional measures to screen the other systems may be performed if more than one system seems involved. Such screening reduces the possibility of omitting important data. The sequence of the assessment begins with the autonomic nervous system (ANS), progressing to the other systems. For example, if gait is limited as a result of pain and apparent MS involvement of the knee, the assessment begins with the ANS, followed by the MS structures and the areas of movement control and capacity. The initial assessment of a patient with acute hemiplegia may include the ANS, neurological, and CVP systems as well as movement control. However, another hemiplegic patient, with a chronic problem, may present with MS system and movement capacity deficits that also need to be assessed.

The evaluative measures are chosen according to the structures and functions of the system. For example, goniometry, palpation, and observation may be appropriate measures to assess ROM in the MS system. Muscle tone may be assessed by deep tendon reflex (DTRs), resistance to passive stretch, and the adequacy of postural tone while maintaining postures. Recognition of the reliability and validity of the measures improves decision making by establishing the degree of confidence that can be placed on the findings.[13,14]

Autonomic Nervous System

The ANS deserves special consideration during both the evaluation and intervention, for it is affected by environmental and psychological strains and, in turn, influences the functioning of the other systems (Fig. 4–4). Patients may demonstrate heightened sympa-

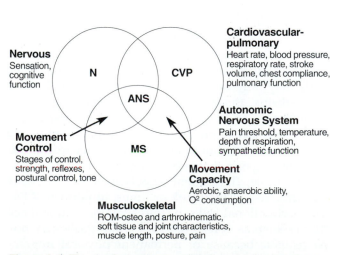

Nervous
Sensation, cognitive function

Movement Control
Stages of control, strength, reflexes, postural control, tone

Musculoskeletal
ROM-osteo and arthrokinematic, soft tissue and joint characteristics, muscle length, posture, pain

Cardiovascular-pulmonary
Heart rate, blood pressure, respiratory rate, stroke volume, chest compliance, pulmonary function

Autonomic Nervous System
Pain threshold, temperature, depth of respiration, sympathetic function

Movement Capacity
Aerobic, anaerobic ability, O² consumption

Figure 4–3. The physical systems and their evaluative measures.

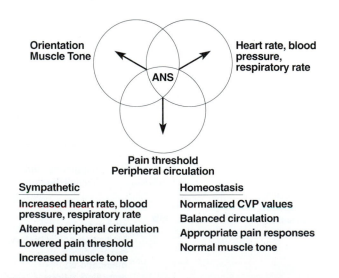

Orientation
Muscle Tone

Heart rate, blood pressure, respiratory rate

Pain threshold
Peripheral circulation

Sympathetic

Increased heart rate, blood pressure, respiratory rate

Altered peripheral circulation

Lowered pain threshold

Increased muscle tone

Homeostasis

Normalized CVP values

Balanced circulation

Appropriate pain responses

Normal muscle tone

Figure 4–4. The influence of the autonomic nervous system on the other systems.

thetic function[15] identified by increased heart rate, blood pressure, and respiration rate, altered peripheral circulation and skin temperature, lowered pain threshold with increased pain behavior, and increased muscular tension, muscle tone, and general sensory awareness and orientation.[16] All these findings may influence the interpretation of other evaluative findings. For example, the amount of pain reported by a patient with low back dysfunction may be heightened by anxiety about beginning physical therapy; the altered temperature in the involved area and the report of increased pain following the application of a hot pack may be a manifestation of sympathetic activity; the distractibility of a patient with brain injury may be accentuated by ANS fluctuations. A goal is to normalize the state of the ANS and maintain a level of homeostasis[17] that will enhance the effectiveness of other interventions (see Chapter 3).

The Structures of the Musculoskeletal System

The assessment of the MS system will help determine if abnormalities in these tissues are related to the functional limitation (Fig. 4–5). The anatomical structures to be assessed include the muscles, tendons, fascia, ligaments, capsules, joints including menisci or discs, and bone. These structures are examined for integrity, alignment, and length. The assessments used include history, observation, palpation, and measures of range, girth, length and accessory motion. The results of other tests including roentgenography and MRI are reviewed. Because skin can limit range, it needs to be assessed for extensibility. Muscle strength, which is a composite of control and capacity

functions, will be included in those discussions later in the chapter. As previously stated, an understanding of the healing process and healing times needs to be considered when assessing the tissues. For example, immediately after joint surgery, swelling, tenderness, and limited range are expected; however, they should not be excessive or prolonged. Although differences between the limbs exist, bilateral comparison provides norms for the individual patient.

If **pain or discomfort** are present, the patient should be questioned regarding various parameters to help determine type and extent of tissue involvement. Because pain is such an individual experience, the therapist needs to gather both subjective and objective base-line information and repeat the measures at intervals to assess change. The patient can indicate on a body chart many of the descriptors that follow. The parameters that should be ascertained include:

- ▶ **location:** is pain focused, diffuse, or radiating?
- ▶ **type:** is pain dull or sharp, burning, or catching?
- ▶ **frequency:** is pain constant or intermittent?
- ▶ **duration:** does pain last for minutes or hours?
- ▶ **intensity:** how severe is the pain when rated on a 1-to-10 scale or on a visual analogue scale?[18,19]

Activities or movements that aggravate or relieve the symptoms may help determine which movements reduce abnormal forces and how successful the patient is at relieving the pain. Constant pain that is not relieved by positional or movement changes may reflect non-mechanical causes of pain necessitating referral to a physician. Throughout the evaluation, the therapist observes the patient to determine if behavior is consistent with reports of pain. An example of inconsistency may be a patient who calmly remains seated while reporting pain as 8/10.

To help differentiate whether the pain is in contractile or noncontractile tissues, isometric contractions are contrasted with passive movement. Active tension should affect only muscle, tendon, and its bony attachment; passive movement can influence all involved tissues.[20]

Alignment—Posture. Malalignment may result from congenital or acquired conditions and may be associated with bony structures, such as a hemivertebra, or occur as a result of laxity or tightness in ligaments, capsule, and muscle. Standing and sitting posture may also indicate the individual's ability to sustain low-intensity, long-duration contractions. Abnormal alignment of segments may increase strain on shortened tissues and reduce the effectiveness of

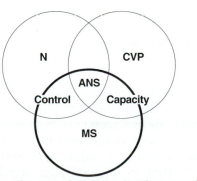

- PAIN: Location, type, frequency, duration, associated factors
- Soft tissue characteristics
- ROM: Osteokinematic, arthrokinematic
- POSTURE: Structural alignment, bony landmarks, muscle length

Figure 4–5. The measures of the musculoskeletal system.

lengthened tissue to provide adequate support. Alignment may be clinically assessed by observation and palpation; viewing roentgenograms may be helpful. Common areas of involvement include: the humerus, which may sit anteriorly in the glenoid; the vertebra on the lumbar spine, which may be shifted laterally or rotated; or the foot, which may excessively pronate in weight bearing. These abnormalities may adversely affect both the area primarily involved and the surrounding joints and structures.

Palpation. The structures and tissues of the involved segment(s) are systematically palpated to examine for alignment, density, pliability, swelling, sensitivity, and differences in temperature. Increased density coupled with tenderness may indicate local muscle "spasm." Decreased tissue length may limit both passive and active range. Areas of elevated temperature may indicate inflammation that may require medical referral. Ligaments and joint lines are assessed for tenderness and smoothness.

Active Range of Motion. The patient is asked to move the segment through the available range. In addition to assessing the muscle's ability to move against gravity and noting the patient's reports of pain, the therapist observes for abnormal movements that may indicate imbalances of tissue length. For example, during active trunk movement, tight hamstrings may limit forward bending before tightness in the lumbar extensors is noted. During active shoulder flexion, excessive trunk lateral flexion or scapula elevation may occur (see section on Movement Control below).

Passive Range of Motion. The segment is passively moved through osteokinematic range. If the tissues are limited in length or are stiff, edematous, or painful, range may be decreased. A slight over pressure at the limit of range may be added to help determine the range-limiting tissue and the extent of reactivity. Depending on the tissue, the feeling at the end of the range will vary: the feel of capsular, ligamentous, and fascial limitation resembles stiff elastic, whereas the contractile portion of muscle is more pliant; a bony end feel is hard.[21] Arthrokinematic movements will assess the extent of joint play, and stress tests will determine ligamentous integrity. Limitations in range resulting from muscle length need to be differentiated, whenever possible, from limitations in the joint capsule and ligament. Muscle tissue is implicated if range can be gained by application of a hold relax technique at the point of limitation (see Chapter 3).

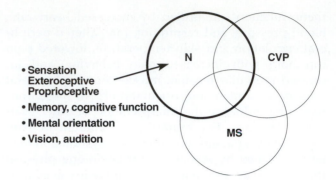

Figure 4–6. The measures of the nervous system.

The Nervous System

Evaluation of the nervous system includes assessment of sensation, space cognition, orientation, and memory (Fig. 4–6). Assessment of movement ability, reflexes, tone, and postural control is deferred to the section on movement control, since these functions are measured by motor responses and reflect the overlap of nervous and MS systems.

Sensation. This includes the measures of light touch, pressure, temperature, vibration, and position sense and may be rated as intact, diminished, or absent depending on the number of correct responses with 10 trials. Sensation may be limited by peripheral compression or obstruction or may reflect deficits more centrally. The therapist uses the information gained from these assessments to choose the most effective treatment procedures. For example, if sensation is lacking, techniques that rely on touch may not be effective. If the patient has a peripheral proprioceptive deficit, procedures designed to improve proprioception are indicated; at the same time, the patient may need to be encouraged to compensate with vision for improvement of safety and function.

Cognition, Orientation, and Memory. The involvement of these mental functions can be assessed by the Glasgow coma scale or Rancho Los Amigos cognitive scale, which measures orientation to person, place, and time, and the ability to follow two- or three-step commands.[22,23] This information is critical in determining the individual's safety and potential for independence. The patient's ability to relearn or learn motor tasks is dependent on many factors including the integrity of perception, cognitive functioning, and efferent processing.

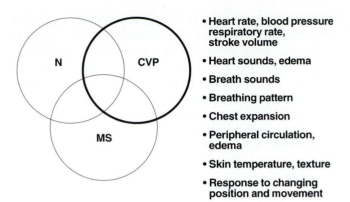

- Heart rate, blood pressure respiratory rate, stroke volume
- Heart sounds, edema
- Breath sounds
- Breathing pattern
- Chest expansion
- Peripheral circulation, edema
- Skin temperature, texture
- Response to changing position and movement

Figure 4–7. The measures of the cardiovascular–pulmonary system.

The Cardiovascular–Pulmonary System

Measures of this system include: heart rate, blood pressure, respiratory rate, breath sounds, breathing pattern, chest expansion, peripheral circulation, and skin temperature and texture (Fig. 4–7). Results of other tests, including pulmonary function studies, electrocardiogram (ECG), and measures of stroke volume need to be taken into consideration. In relation to the performance of therapeutic exercise, this system is assessed for the ability to sustain sufficient heart rate and blood pressure when different postures are assumed and during exercise procedures. For example, when moving between supine, sitting, and standing, does the patient experience lightheadedness or in such horizontal postures as supine or prone, does the patient have difficulty with breathing or with the increased return of blood volume? Also assessed is the change in cardiac and pulmonary signs when the intensity, duration, or frequency of exercise procedures increase.[24]

EVALUATION OF MOVEMENT CONTROL ___

As stated, the assessment of movement control measures the functions that occur as a result of the interaction of the MS and nervous systems (Fig. 4–8). Movement control encompasses the stages of control, various aspects of muscle performance, reflexes, reactions, and postural control, and muscle tone. Movement control is emphasized in this discussion, for it provides information integral to the development of a therapeutic exercise intervention program.

Stages of Control

Mobility—Passive ROM. Range may be limited by many factors including abnormal tissue length, pain,

and abnormal tone. Measurement of the passive extensibility of the MS tissues has been previously described. Neural tissue also may be restricted or compressed in the spinal foramen or along the course of the tissue, resulting in limited range or reports of pain.[25,26]

Mobility—Initiation of Active Movement. This is assessed by measuring the amount of active ROM. If it is diminished compared to the available passive range, the particular tissue involvement needs to be determined so that appropriate treatment techniques can be applied (see Chapter 3). For example, muscle activation may be inhibited by pain from a tendinitis or joint effusion, or voluntary movement may be restricted by the anticipation of pain; weakness may be a result of insufficient actin-myosin bonding that occurs with disuse atrophy or may be secondary to diminished neural innervation, such as occurs with a peripheral nerve injury; voluntary, reflexive, and automatic movement may be affected by central nervous system (CNS) lesions resulting in hemiplegia or multiple sclerosis. The agonist's ability to contract through a range may be limited because of stiffness or abnormal tone in the antagonist. The cause of the dysfunction will determine the choice of procedures.

Stability—Muscle Holding. Stability of the postural muscles is assessed by the ability to sustain an isometric contraction in the shortened range, for example a quadriceps or gluteal set. Both the quantity and quality of the contraction are considered. The contraction should be sustained for approximately 10 seconds and the intensity of the contraction should be no more than about 40% of a maximum effort. This combination minimizes the decline in gamma motoneuron firing,[27] recruits primarily slow-twitch, aerobic fibers,[28] and allows a normal breathing pattern to be maintained. Fatigue may be noted by muscle

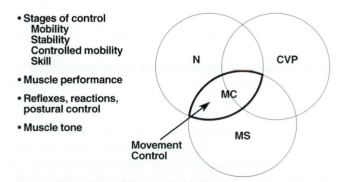

- Stages of control
  Mobility
  Stability
  Controlled mobility
  Skill
- Muscle performance
- Reflexes, reactions, postural control
- Muscle tone

Figure 4–8. The measures of movement control.

"flickering." Deficits in muscle stability may be observed as an active lag, which may be due to decreased ability to activate a sufficient number of motor units to sustain the contraction in the shortened range. Patients with CNS lesions may demonstrate abnormalities in the type and number of motor units recruited, as well as in the firing pattern.[29] For example, some patients may activate more motor units within a muscle than required for the actual task and may have difficulty restricting effort to specific muscles.

Stability—Maintaining Postures. Postural stability can be assessed by the ability to maintain joint alignment during weight-bearing activities such as sitting, standing, bridging, or quadruped. The time the posture is maintained with good alignment may be the measure; for example, the patient can maintain standing with equal weight bearing for 20 seconds. Both the duration and the quality of the postural alignment is assessed. For example, some patients may have difficulty maintaining an erect sitting posture; others may excessively sway in a posture. To help determine the reason for the impairment the previous stages also are assessed: is there sufficient muscle stability in the abdominals and back extensors and sufficient range in the spine and hips? Any increase in pain or tone with weight bearing should be noted. Patients who have difficulty contracting antagonistic muscles may hyperextend the weight-bearing joints to produce an abnormal compensatory stabilization with capsular and ligamentous structures. Both muscle and joint receptors provide feedback regarding body position and thus play a major role in postural stability.[30]

The sensory–motor component to postural stability may be measured in a variety of ways. The sensory component can be assessed by position sense and the ability to detect motion. To assess the interaction of the sensory–motor response, the technique of alternating isometrics can be applied to the antagonistic muscles and the delay from the time of application of resistance to the time the muscle responds is noted. The test is performed to determine if the patient can sense and respond to the change in joint movement or manual pressure. The technique is applied so as to elicit a low-intensity contraction in non–weight-bearing postures, progressing to weight bearing in a range that simulates function of the segment(s). For example, to test the knee, the postures chosen may be sitting, then standing with the knee near full extension. The patient is instructed to maintain the limb position while minimal resistance is provided to the quadriceps, then rhythmically altered to the hamstrings. The muscles should respond to maintain the position. Some patients may require a few learning repetitions with tactile, visual, and verbal input such as "don't let me bend or straighten your knee," or "just keep your leg where it is and match my pressure, but don't try to beat me." Minimal or no lag between the force application and the muscle's response is normal. Terms used to describe the response may be a *minimal lag of the quadriceps*, or the *hamstrings' response is delayed with 5-to-10 degrees of joint movement occurring before the muscles contract.*

Controlled Mobility. Movements within the base of support (BoS) are assessed in weight-bearing postures, for example, weight shifting in sitting, rocking in quadruped, and weight shifting and small-range squats in standing. If these activities can be performed pain free and slowly with control, speed is increased. Fatigue may be noted as "flickering" or reduced smoothness of the movement. Depending on the movement, muscles can contract in different combinations: a reversal of antagonists promotes concentric–concentric movements; movement of the agonist against body weight resistance promotes concentric–eccentric contractions. Both eccentric and concentric ability is essential to control weight shifting in various postures. For example, in standing, a posterior weight shift and resumption of upright are controlled by an eccentric, then concentric contraction of the anterior muscles, whereas an anterior shift is controlled by the same contraction pattern of the posterior muscles;[31] short-range squats require eccentric quadriceps contraction to lower the body and a concentric quadriceps contraction balanced by an eccentric hamstring contraction to raise the body while the knees extend. An imbalance of antagonists may be noted as uneven reciprocal movement or a tendency to hyperextend the weight-bearing segment. Controlling the eccentric contraction of the lengthening extensor becomes more difficult as greater ranges are attempted.

The amount of movement excursion that can be controlled can be the measure. For example, in bridging, the patient can control lowering the pelvis though 50% of the range; in quadruped the patient can weight-shift over the involved right arm 25% of the full range before the scapula elevates from the thorax as compared to the intact upper extremity.

Controlling trunk rotation while rolling or during weight shifting in postures also is assessed in this stage and can be measured in a manner similar to that described above.

Static–Dynamic. Sustaining a posture with a reduced BoS or moving between postures assumes sufficient range through which to move (mobility), postural stability, and the ability to weight-shift in the posture (controlled mobility). Both the quantity and quality are assessed during static and dynamic postural adjustments. Measures of the static posture may include the number of seconds the position can be maintained, along with observation of any abnormal limb or trunk movement. For example, unilateral standing can be maintained for 5 seconds; however, excessive upper extremity movement occurs. The measure of dynamic function is observed as the patient intentionally moves the trunk or non–weight-bearing upper or lower extremity or performs weight shifting.[32] For example, the therapist observes the control with which weight can be shifted forward onto the ball of the foot or backward toward the heel while in unilateral standing; in quadruped, the ability to maintain trunk alignment is observed as one limb or contralateral limbs are flexed and extended. Moving between postures, such as between sitting and standing, may be assessed according to: time required to perform the transition, bilateral equality of limb weight bearing, ability to maintain midline during the movement, and the amount of assistance needed.

Skill. Functional daily, occupational, and recreational activities are assessed for safety, the level of independence, and control of the timing and sequencing of movement. Numerous scales exist to measure functional independence and assess gait.[33] Defects may be due to abnormalities occurring in any of the previous stages, as well as with the more advanced aspects of control. For many patients, performing daily activities safely with the minimum amount of assistance is the goal. For others, with fewer permanent impairments, the quality and coordination of the activity is measured by observing the timing, sequencing, and smoothness of the limbs during both slow and quick movements, and the proximal dynamic stability of the trunk and proximal segments. When functional outcomes include a return to sports, the sequencing of movement may become more critical. For example, the timing of hip, knee, and ankle movements should be observed while jogging on a treadmill or during the practice of "cutting" movements performed actively or against the resistance of a Sports Cord.

Muscle performance can also be assessed by an isokinetic measure of torque, work, power, and endurance.[34] Devices can provide a detailed between-limb comparison and relate the individual's response to an age- and sex-matched standard. Specific variables on sequential trials can be measured to assess progress although the correlation between isokinetic values and function have not been shown to be clini-

cally significant.[14] Other measures of muscle performance include the ability to hold or move weights. The ability to resist one maximum effort or repetitions of various intensities can be assessed.

Reflexes, Reactions, Postural Control

Reflexes and reactions are assessed to determine the extent to which they interfere with the ability to assume and move in various postures.[35] For example, rolling from supine toward prone may be difficult if the tonic reflexes are dominant; maintaining quadruped and bridging may be problematic for those with a grasp reflex or an extensor thrust; maintaining sitting or standing may be difficult for those with abnormal righting reactions or postural responses. The therapist observes for increases in tone or changes in limb position consistent with phasic or tonic reflexes, or for a lack of head, trunk, and extremity movements in response to changes in the body's orientation in space. This lack of movement may indicate diminished righting or postural responses.

Many aspects of **postural control** are assessed during the measures of postural stability, weight shifting, and static–dynamic movements. In these stages the amount of movement and the segment where movement occurs is noted. For example, a common response while standing is minimal movement at the ankle. However, when requested to maintain standing, the patient may sway excessively at the ankle, hip, or trunk or use the upper limbs to help maintain the posture.[36] Abnormal responses may be related to deficits in sensory or motor areas. The challenge of postural tests is increased as the sensory stimuli are varied. For example, visual input can be obscured; standing on foam, a balance board, or uneven surfaces also alters peripheral input. To focus on automatic responses, the patient can be distracted from the motor task by reciting a familiar phrase or being questioned about the home environment while performing the task. The assessment of the vestibular ocular system is described in depth in other texts.[37]

Muscle Tone

Altered muscle tone may result from pain, anxiety, stress, tension, peripheral nerve injury, or CNS lesions. Decreased tone related to diminished neural innervation may be accompanied by a decreased ability to initiate an active contraction. Increases in tone or muscle density as a result of pain, tension, or stress is commonly localized and transient and not accompanied by increases in reflex responses, in contrast to the increased tone that occurs with CNS lesions. Passive tone, while the muscle is not voluntarily active, may be assessed by DTRs and the resistance to passive stretch. Active tone is more difficult to quantify. However, adaptability of muscle responses in the trunk can be observed as the upper extremities are lifted at different angles from the BoS[38]. Although not always clinically feasible more objective measures can be obtained with EMG.[39]

ASSESSMENT OF THE CAPACITY FOR MOVEMENT

Included in this assessment are both general exercise capacity as well as the ability of a specific muscle group to perform low-intensity, long-duration, repetitive movements (Fig. 4–9).

Patients who have been immobilized or sedentary for any length of time may have decreased exercise capacity. The measures of heart rate, blood pressure, respiratory rate, and the rating of perceived exertion during sustained aerobic activity provide an indication of the patient's capacity for movement.[39] Deficits may be assessed as fatigue, chest pain, abnormal heart rate, irregular heartbeat, dyspnea, or leg cramps.

Assessing a muscle or group of muscles during the performance of repetitive activity at less than maximum effort will measure aerobic ability. When these tests are performed in positions in which the segments normally function, the effort required during most functional activities can be simulated. For example, a functional test of the knee musculature is to time the quadriceps and hamstrings while maintaining a neutral knee position in unilateral weight bearing and while performing a short-range squat. The length of time, number of repetitions or intensity included in this test is gradually increased. More blood needs to be supplied to the working muscles as the duration and number of repetitions of the activity increases.

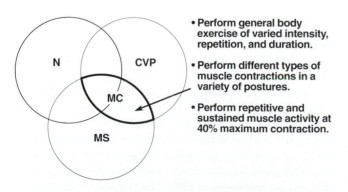

- **Perform general body exercise of varied intensity, repetition, and duration.**
- **Perform different types of muscle contractions in a variety of postures.**
- **Perform repetitive and sustained muscle activity at 40% maximum contraction.**

Figure 4–9. The measures of movement capacity.

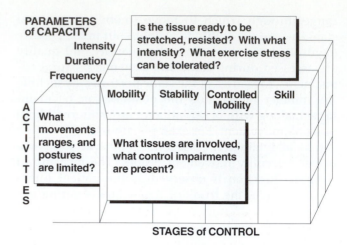

Figure 4–10. Translating evaluative findings into the Intervention Model.

SUMMARY

At this juncture in the evaluation process, most of the information has been collected. The therapist compiles the data regarding the physical impairments that seem to be related to the functional limitations, the extent of tissue involvement, and the potential to change, as well as the constraints imposed by the environment and the ability to make appropriate modifications. The therapist determines the most effective and efficient means of achieving the maximum functional outcome by considering the intervention strategies of changing the individual, providing compensatory aids, and modifying the environment. The length of time required to achieve the functional outcome and the cost of implementing each of the possible strategies must be taken into account. The treatment goals are developed by transposing the impairments into the control and capacity movement characteristics delineated in the intervention model. Referrals to other practitioners are initiated as is communication of the evaluation results (Fig. 4–10).

REVIEW QUESTIONS

1. Why are the environmental, social, medical, and psychological factors considered in addition to the specific analysis of the physical systems?

2. What physical signs or symptoms might a patient demonstrate if the ANS is more sympathetic than normal?

3. Why might different evaluative sequences be used when assessing the three physical systems?

4. Translate the following evaluative findings into the classifications of the intervention model: decreased ROM in the elbow, decreased stability of the ankle following sprain, a list to the right while attempting to maintain sitting, hyperextension of the knee during unilateral standing, delayed finger extension while reaching for a cup.

5. What are ways that the environment may be modified to decrease strain and what compensatory strategies or aids may be appropriate for a patient with low-back involvement, for a patient with hemiplegia experiencing difficulty walking, or for a patient with chronic obstructive pulmonary disease?

REFERENCES

1. Guccione AA. Physical therapy diagnosis and the relationship between impairments and function. *Phys Ther.* 1991;71:499–504.
2. Tech SN. *Hidden Arguments: Political Ideology and Disease Prevention Policy.* New Brunswick, NJ: Rutgers University Press; 1988.
3. Dohrenwend BP, Dohrenwend BS. Socioenvironmental factors, stress and psychopathology. *Am J Community Psychol.* 1981;9:128–164.
4. Campbell A, Converse PE, Rogers WL. *The Quality of American Life—Perceptions, Evaluations, and Satisfactions.* New York, NY: Russell Sage Foundation; 1976.
5. Frankenhaeuser MP. Coping with Stresses at Work. *Int J Health Serv.* 1981;11:491–510.
6. Antonovsky A. *Unraveling the Mystery of Health: How People Manage Stress and Stay Well.* San Francisco, Calif: Jossey-Bass Inc, Publishers; 1987.
7. Kobasa SC, Massi SR, Courington S. Personality and constitution as mediators in the stress-illness relationship. *J Health Soc Behav.* 1981;22:368–378.
8. Kutner NG. Social ties, social support and perceived health status among chronically disabled people. *Soc Sci Med.* 1987;25.
9. Murry MP, et al. Age-related differences in knee muscle strength in normal women. *J Gerontol.* 1985;40:275–280.
10. Bendall MJ, Bassey EJ, Pearson MB. (Sex) gender factors affecting walking speed of elderly people. *Age Ageing.* 1989;18:327–332.
11. Klein-Vogelbach S. *Functional Kinetics.* New York, NY: Springer-Verlag; 1990.
12. Echternach J, Rothstein J. Hypothesis-oriented algorithms. *Phys Ther.* 1989;69:559–564.
13. Portney LP, Watkins MP. Foundations of Clinical Research: Applications to Practice. Norwalk, Conn: Appleton & Lange; 1993.
14. Rothstein JM, ed. *Measurement in Physical Therapy.* New York, NY: Churchill Livingstone, Inc; 1985.
15. Hoskins TM, Troy L, Dossa A. Effects of slow stroking on the autonomic nervous system. Unpublished research conducted at Physical Therapy Dept., New England Medical Center, 1984.
16. McClelland DC, Floor E, Davidson RJ, et al. Stress, power, motivation, sympathetic activation, immune function and illness. *J of Human Stress.* 6(2) 1980.
17. Wilder J. Basimetric approach (law of initial value) to biological rhythms. *Ann NY Acad Sci.* 1962;98:1211–1220.
18. Pain scale, Huskisson EC: Measurement of pain. *J Rheumatol.* 1982;9:768–769.
19. Waddell G. How patients react to low back pain. *Acta Orthop Scand.* 1993;64(suppl 251):21–24.
20. Cyriax J. Textbook of Orthopedic Medicine. 8th ed. London, England: Baillière Tindal Ltd; 1982.
21. Kaltenborn FM, Evjenth O. *Manual Mobilization of the Extremity Joints: Basic Examination and Treatment Techniques.* 4th ed. Oslo, Norway: Olaf Norlis Bokhandel; 1989.
22. Jennett B, Bond M: Assessment of outcome after severe brain damage—a practical scale. *Lancet,* March 1:480–484; 1975.
23. Hagen C, Malkus D, Dorham P. Levels of cognitive functioning. In: Rehabilitation of the Head Injured Adult: Comprehensive Physical Management. Downey CA: Professional Staff Association of the Ranchos Los Amigos Hospital Inc; 1980.
24. Cohen M, Hoskins TM: Cardiopulmonary Symptoms in Physical Therapy Practice, New York, NY: Churchill Livingstone, 1988.
25. Elvey RL. Treatment of arm pain associated with abnormal brachial plexus tension. *Aust J Physiother.* 1986;32:226–230.
26. Butler DS. *Mobilisation of the Nervous System.* Melbourne, Australia: Churchill Livingstone; 1991.
27. Macefield G, Hagbarth KE, Gorman R, et al. Decline in spindle support to alpha motoneurons during sustained voluntary contractions. *J Physiol.* 1991;440:497–512.
28. Henneman E. Peripheral mechanisms involved in control of muscles. In: Mountcastle VB, ed. *Medical Physiology.* St. Louis, Mo: CV Mosby Co; 1974; 1.
29. Brooks VB. *The Neural Basis of Motor Control.* New York, NY: Oxford University Press; 1986.
30. Johansson H, Sjolander P, Sojka P. A sensory role for the cruciate ligaments. *Clin Orthop.* 1990;288:161–178.
31. Nashner LM, McCollum G: The organization of human postural movement: a formal basis and experimental synthesis. *Behav Brain Sci.* 1985;8:135–172.
32. Duncan PW, Studenski SA, Chandler JM. Functional reach: predictive validity. *J Gerontol.* 1992;47:M93–M98.
33. Jette AM, Davies AR, Cleary PD, et al. The Functional Status Questionnaire: reliability and validity when used in primary care. *J Gen Intern Med.* 1984;1:143–149.

34. Davies GJ. Use of isokinetics in rehabilitation of selected surgical knees. In: Davies GJ, ed. *Rehabilitation of the Surgical Knee.* Ronkonkoma, NY: Cypress; 1984.

35. Barns MR, Crutchfield CA, Heriza CB, et al. *Reflex and Vestibular Aspects of Motor Control.* Atlanta, Ga: Stokesville Publishing Co; 1990.

36. Woolacott H, Shumway-Cook A, Nashner L. Aging and posture control: changes in sensory organs and muscular coordination. *Int J Aging Hum Dev.* 1986;23:97–114.

37. Herdman SJ. Assessment and treatment of balance disorders in the vestibular deficient patient. In: Duncan P, ed. *Balance Proceedings of the American Physical Therapy Association Forum.* Alexandria, Va: APTA Publications; 1990; 87–94.

38. Shenkman M, Butler RB: A forum on assessment and management of tone. APTA Conference. Boston, Ma: 1991.

39. Austrand PO, Rodahl K. *Textbook of Work Physiology, Physiological Basis of Exercise.* 3rd ed. New York, NY: McGraw-Hill Book Co; 1986.

CHAPTER 5

Shoulder

EVALUATION
ENVIRONMENTAL, SOCIAL AND CULTURAL FACTORS
MEDICAL AND PSYCHOLOGICAL FACTORS
PHYSICAL SYSTEMS
CLINICAL IMPRESSIONS
INTERVENTION
SPECIAL TREATMENT CONSIDERATIONS
TREATMENT PLAN
SUMMARY
PATIENT CASE
REVIEW QUESTIONS

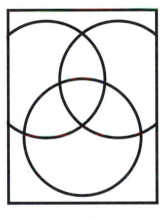

A wide variety of causes, both direct and indirect, can lead to shoulder dysfunction, thereby challenging the therapist's skill in determining a diagnosis and developing an appropriate intervention plan.[1] Some of the most common causes of disability include sprains, strains, soft-tissue and skeletal trauma, overuse and maluse syndromes, instability secondary to capsular or muscular laxity, postural deficits, neurological impairment, surgical repairs, and chest wall procedures such as mastectomy or thoracotomy. The exercise and total intervention program needs to be developed according to an individual's diagnosis, age, pain, tissue integrity, and functional goals. The program for a 20-year-old baseball pitcher with a rotator cuff strain varies considerably from that of a 70-year-old with the same diagnosis but who has a sedentary life-style. Age-related variations may include range-of-motion (ROM) and movement-control requirements, the speed of progression through the treatment program, and the ability to tolerate stress in any of the parameters of exercise.[2] Greater emphasis might be placed on the normal timing and sequencing of movement during advanced-level activities for some athletic patients to provide the strength, speed, control, and variety of movement patterns needed, whereas a more sedentary person might require emphasis on movements that simulate functional needs. Regardless of these multiple variables, certain treatment principles can be applied, although the manner and timing of application and emphasis may differ.

The procedures in this chapter are sequenced according to the treatment principles emphasized throughout this text. They are meant to serve as a guide in helping the therapist formulate appropriate programs for each patient. Indications for modifications of the procedures will be addressed according to patient needs. Home and independent programs that complement therapy sessions are included for each phase of treatment.

EVALUATION

The evaluation is sequenced to assess the environmental, medical, and psychological factors that may influence the patient's symptoms and is followed by an in-depth assessment of the involved physical and physiological systems to determine the etiology of the dysfunction and the structures that may be involved. These include: bone, cartilage, capsule, ligament, nerve, tendon, and muscle. During the initial interview the therapist gathers information regarding the history and symptoms of the present complaint to differentiate a dysfunction of a biomechanical origin from other causes. When the external and internal strains are determined, an appropriate intervention can be implemented. This may include modifying the environment as well as altering the individual's physical abilities.

Environmental, Social, and Cultural Factors

Occupational and vocational activities need to be assessed to determine the particular strains placed on the upper extremity (Fig. 5–1); repetitive activities that may lead to tissue injury are noted. For example, activities requiring maintained abduction near 90° may lead to stress of the lateral structures; frequent traction forces such as occur with lifting heavy objects can lead to stress of the capsule, especially if the surrounding musculature is not of sufficient strength to counteract such forces.

The patient's age and activity level will influence the integrity of the tissues. For example, the elderly have reduced vascular supply, increased tissue stiffness, and may have calcium deposits in particular tissues of the shoulder.[2] Postural changes such as increased kyphosis may alter the position of the scapula and biomechanics of the shoulder. A sedentary life-style may reduce muscle endurance, resulting in increased complaints of discomfort with repetitive movement.

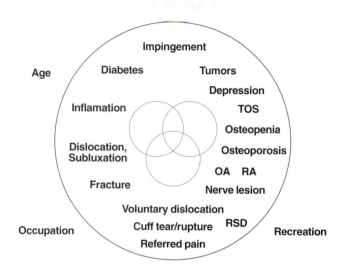

Figure 5–1. Environmental, medical, and psychological factors influencing patients with shoulder involvement. OA, osteoarthritis; RA, rheumatoid arthritis; RSD reflex sympathetic dystrophy; TOS, thoracic outlet syndrome.

The combination of repetitive trauma with circulatory insufficiency may reduce the effectiveness of the rotator cuff in maintaining the alignment of the humeral head in the glenoid fossa.[3,4] To prevent further trauma and impingement and to rest the involved tissues, the patient should be taught to move in the sagittal plane and to avoid painful abduction motions. Educating the patient to alter body position relative to the task is one way to alter stress on the glenohumeral joint. For example, lifting an object and moving it to the side can be accomplished by turning the body rather than by shoulder abduction. Environmental modifications and education in compensatory movements are strategies to help achieve functional goals, especially if changing the individual's physical abilities is not possible. Altering the height and configuration of the work station or home cabinets and modifying the intensity of vibratory, rotational, or traction forces will reduce environmental stresses on the shoulder.

The patient should be questioned regarding the functional gains that are anticipated with therapy.

For example, the patient may wish to return to complete recreational activities, including playing golf or tennis, or the goal may simply be the use of the limb during normal activities of daily living (ADL). As the evaluation continues the probability of attaining these goals can be more clearly determined.

Medical and Psychological Factors

Dysfunction in many internal organs can refer symptoms to the shoulder region. The patient should be questioned regarding possible cardiac, pulmonary, gallbladder, and breast involvement. Certain disease processes, such as osteoporosis, osteopenia, or diabetes, indicate to the therapist that precautions must be taken in the application of some treatment procedures because of altered tissue density or compliance (see Fig. 5–1). Therefore, a medical screen should be included in the evaluation as part of the procedure to rule out medical origin of the dysfunction and to determine if pain is referred from internal organs. History should also include present and past trauma or other injury to the involved area. Previous dysfunction in the same area may decrease the anticipated functional outcome.

If the shoulder dysfunction has altered the patient's occupational status, the patient may show signs of depression. Some abnormal psychological states seem to be associated with voluntary shoulder dislocation, reducing the success of both surgical and physical therapy rehabilitation.[5]

Physical Systems

Autonomic Nervous System

An imbalance in the autonomic nervous system (ANS) will influence pain threshold, peripheral circulation, and potential for developing reflex sympathetic dystrophy or shoulder–hand syndrome.[6] Measures such as heart rate, blood pressure, skin temperature, texture, and moisture indicate the integrity of central and peripheral circulation. Balancing the ANS should be included in the treatment plan if the patient demonstrates abnormalities in these measures, seems to be excessively anxious, and seems to have a low threshold of pain (see Chapter 3). If abnormal heart rate and blood pressure are noted, referral to a medical practitioner is appropriate.

Musculoskeletal System

Screening of the cervical and upper thoracic spine is performed to rule out spinal causes for the shoulder dysfunction. Assessment measures include neck ROM, palpation, and sensory testing of the limb (Fig.

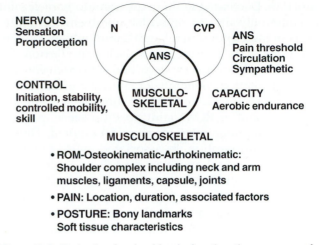

Figure 5–2. Evaluation for shoulder dysfunction: the measures of the physical systems that need to be considered.

5–2). Neural tension tests may reveal discomfort or ROM limitations when tension is placed on particular nerve roots by movements of the neck and upper extremity.[7] The patient may complain of altered sensation and muscle strength in the limb if pressure on the thoracic outlet compresses neural and vascular structures.[8] Although not common, specific injuries to portions of the brachial plexus, including the axillary nerve, may result in localized muscle weakness.

The muscles, ligaments, capsule, and joint structures of the shoulder girdle are palpated, observed, and measured to determine their contribution to ROM, tenderness or pain, and postural abnormalities. Assessment of the glenohumeral, acromioclavicular, sternoclavicular, and scapulothoracic articulations includes measurement of arthro- and osteokinematic movements, muscle length, strength, alignment, and posture. Various measures can be used to differentiate noncontractile from contractile restrictions: an end feel of noncontractile capsular and ligamentous tissue feels like stiff elastic, whereas the contractile tissue of muscles is more pliant; complaints of pain with isometric tension implicate muscle, tendon, and bony attachments; gains in range of motion following hold or contract relax indicate that muscle tightness contributes to the limitation.

Range. After immobilization or disuse, a reduction in passive movement into scapula adduction and diminished proximal stabilization may be evident. These problems may be attributed to tightness of the pectoralis minor and other anterior structures or weakness and abnormal timing of posterior muscles, or both. This combination of tightness on one side of the joint and weakness of opposing muscles is a common finding, and both must be treated to restore function. Decreased ROM in the scapulothoracic joint is commonly due to muscular involvement; limitations in the glenohumeral joint commonly include restrictions of the capsule and muscles into flexion, abduction, and external rotation, and into extension and internal rotation. Generalized splinting of surrounding musculature is a common finding. During the measurement of ROM, joint position sense, particularly of shoulder rotation, should be noted. Diminished proprioception is associated with abnormal movement control and may contribute to decreased automatic control of the rotator cuff and faulty shoulder mechanics.[9] During functional movements, excessive scapular elevation and "impingement" in the shoulder may be due to impaired automatic activity of the lower and middle trapezius and rotator cuff. Automatic muscle responses may be diminished if proprioceptive input from the muscle or capsule is dampened, as occurs when these structures are strained, stretched, or lax.[10]

Tenderness or Pain. When asked to indicate the area of pain with one finger, the patient may point specifically to the superior or anterior aspects of the shoulder or may state that pain is diffuse or that it courses down the arm. Although all parameters of an evaluation must be considered before a definitive diagnosis can be determined, indication of the area of pain will implicate certain tissues. For example, pain in the lateral shoulder may be indicative of impingement of the supraspinatus tendon between the greater tuberosity and acromion; anteriorly located pain may indicate involvement of the biceps or subscapularis tendons and diffuse shoulder pain may be caused by bursitis or an arthritic condition. Pain also may be the result of a torn labrum, a condition that may require surgical intervention. Although not as obvious as in other joint conditions, swelling in the shoulder may limit ROM and cause diffuse pain. Stress can be differentially applied to specific tissues to determine if the patient's pain can be reproduced. The amount of stress required and the patient response is indicative of the reactivity of the tissue.

Posture. Postural abnormalities may be due to muscle imbalances and bone or joint malalignment. For example, muscle tightness in the pectoralis major and minor, the teres major, subscapularis, and in the latissimus dorsi may result in an internally rotated shoulder and abducted or anteriorly tilted scapula. Bone and joint findings may include excessive laxity in the capsule or a shallow labrum, both associated with a tendency toward subluxation. This may result in an anteriorly or inferiorly placed humeral head.[11] Pa-

tients with instability resulting from capsular or labral abnormalities should be referred to an orthopaedic surgeon.

Movement Control

Movement Initiation. The ability to initiate and sustain active movement throughout full range can be assessed by having the patient attempt movement through the available range. The amounts of active and passive range are compared to determine if an active lag is present. A manual muscle test can be used to assess strength although pain may limit the amount of resistance that can be applied.

Stability. Stability of the scapula and shoulder joints is assessed by performing isometric contractions of surrounding musculature, particularly of the trapezius, rhomboids, serratus anterior,[12] and the rotator cuff[4] in both non-weight–bearing and weight-bearing postures. The patient's ability to maintain joint alignment in weight-bearing postures is an indication of the balance between the scapular abductors and adductors and the response to compressive forces. Flickering of the shoulder musculature during movement may be a sign of joint instability.

Controlled Mobility and Skill. Scapulohumeral rhythm is a kinesthetic term describing the coordinated movement of the scapula on the thorax in conjunction with the dynamic alignment of the humerus within the glenoid fossa. Normal scapulohumeral rhythm requires a coordinated dynamic stability within the scapular muscles, between the scapula and shoulder musculature, and within the shoulder. A common finding is abnormal deltoid and rotator cuff control or decreased glenohumeral ROM, leading to substitution of shoulder movement by scapular movement.

Scapulohumeral rhythm is observed as the patient shifts weight in closed-chain postures such as modified plantigrade and during attempts at arm elevation during open-chain activities. Common findings are excessive scapula elevation or abduction during the initiation of shoulder flexion and continued excessive scapular movement rather than the normal 2:1 glenohumeral to scapulothoracic movement ratio.[13]

Lateral flexion of the trunk away from the involved limb is often substituted for scapular and shoulder motion. Both abnormal scapulohumeral rhythm and lateral trunk flexion are associated with muscular and capsular tightness at the glenohumeral joint and with weakness of the scapula and rotator cuff musculature. Table 5–1 summarizes the stages of control.

TABLE 5–1. STAGES OF CONTROL

Mobility	Stability	Controlled Mobility	Static Dynamic	Skill
ROM or extensibility of muscle, nerve, capsule, and ligament.	Holding of scapula adductors, serratus anterior, and rotator cuff.	Controlling scapulohumeral rhythm in weight-bearing postures.	Proximal dynamic stability with increased weight-bearing and increased range.	Movement with normal timing, sequencing, and endurance.
Initiation of all movements.	Maintaining weight-bearing postures.			

Movement Capacity

Limited endurance in the scapular and shoulder muscles may be evident with repetitions of active movements. The patient may report fatigue and aching toward the end of the day, which may indicate an inability to sustain muscle contractions. Many individuals become generally deconditioned because of a decrease in overall activity levels. This is particularly evident in the elderly if the fractured arm or sprained rotator cuff was caused by a fall, resulting in fear of falling and a subsequent restriction of daily activities (see Chapter 9).

Clinical Impressions

At the conclusion of the evaluation, the functional limitations and the associated impairments are enumerated. Shoulder dysfunction, particularly of the dominant arm, may result in **functional limitations** including:

▶ reduced skills in activities of daily living (ADL), such as dressing, feeding, hygiene;

▶ decreased occupational or vocational abilities including a diminished ability to lift or hold objects; and

▶ curtailed recreational activities because of pain that may occur during a tennis serve, a golf swing, or even jogging. These limitations need to be documented as clearly as possible indicating the extent of involvement.

The specific **impairments** that seem to be causing these functional limitations can be categorized according to the control and capacity classifications.

The **functional outcomes** are determined by the therapist to be achievable changes in the functional limitations. Possible modification of both the individual and the environment are taken into account when these determinations are made. The **treatment goals** reflect the incremental changes in the amount of control and capacity and other impairments that are required to attain the functional outcomes.

To help sequence the treatment plan the impairments are classified according to the attributes of movement delineated in the intervention model.

INTERVENTION

The treatment procedures are developed to achieve treatment goals and functional outcomes. The initial treatment goal is to promote movement and control in the least painful ranges. To realize this goal, the activities consist of postures that provide the most support and movements that are the least difficult or painful. The techniques, combined with complementary sensory inputs, enhance the beginning stages of control: mobility, stability, and control of mobility. The parameters of frequency, intensity, and duration are adjusted according to the reactivity of the tissues, and to promote learning, strength, and endurance. Intervention progresses toward the functional outcomes by increasing the difficulty of the three units of the procedure: the **activity, technique,** and **parameter.**

The therapist initially determines the movements and the stages of control that need to be achieved. Because ROM often is limited, the first logical step in treatment is to increase mobility. The movements that are more limited, painful, and problematic are usually external rotation, abduction, and flexion,[14] the components of D2F as well as movement into extension and internal rotation. Flexion with adduction, or diagonal 1 flexion (D1F), and the anatomical motions of adduction and internal rotation are usually less painful. Reactivity is patient-specific and depends on factors such as the time since the injury or surgery and the integrity of the circulatory bed in the tissues.

Special Treatment Considerations

▶ During normal pain–free shoulder flexion, the humeral head is aligned within the glenoid fossa to allow sufficient space for the tendons and bursa. Altered muscular and capsular extensibility may change this relationship, and dysfunction of the rotator cuff may allow the humerus to abnormally elevate in relation to the glenoid and impinge on tissues.[15,16] These impairments make the combination of flexion, abduction, external rotation, D2F, a movement that may reproduce or aggravate the patient's pain. The D1F pattern requires movement into two of the usually limited motions, external rotation and flexion. However, the ranges of the movements that occur in D1F are less than those in D2F. Because the shoulder is adducting and moving through incomplete range, there is less tendency for the greater tubercle to abut the acromion and impinge on the supraspinatus tendon and its bursa. *With most shoulder conditions, activity of the rotator cuff is initiated in D1F before advancing to D2F.*

▶ Exceptions to this principle are made when the dysfunction and pain are not caused by rotator cuff insufficiency, common capsular restrictions, or the biomechanical abutment of the greater tubercle and the acromion. For example, biceps tendonitis or acromioclavicular joint pain may be aggravated with D1F movements. If such is the case, treatment begins with non-painful movements of flexion and abduction or in a straight plane before the difficult or painful motions are introduced.

▶ Full range into flexion, abduction, and external rotation is contraindicated for any condition which results in anterior displacement or anterior laxity of the humeral head such as conservative or surgical management of a shoulder dislocation.[17] For these patients, movement into D2F in early stages of treatment should not proceed beyond 90° so that the involved structures are not stressed. Conversely, if the posterior structures are lax, weight bearing with the shoulder in flexion, as occurs in quadruped, is avoided.

▶ Because the myotome corresponds with the dermatome of the shoulder, the use of various pain-relieving modalities such as transcutaneous nerve stimulation (TNS) may be effective.[18]

To increase the challenge of the intervention, the motor abilities described by each stage of control are progressed from:

▶ movement into D1F or within anatomical planes to the more limited D2F movement;

▶ postures are progressed by increasing range and weight bearing to increase the challenge to the scapular and shoulder musculature;

▶ parameters are altered to improve endurance and transfer the movement ability to functional tasks.

Treatment Plan

The intervention is designed to achieve **functional outcomes,** primarily: use of the limb for activities of daily living and occupational and recreational tasks.

To achieve the control and capacity needed for functional use of the upper extremity, a balance of joint and muscular mobility and dynamic stability are required. Initial treatment procedures will emphasize ROM and proximal stability; dynamic stability is gradually progressed for skilled function.

Treatment is divided into two phases. The *initial phase* emphasizes the first three levels of motor control: mobility, stability, and controlled mobility, whereas in the *advanced-skill phase* the normal timing and sequencing of movement is promoted. The treatment is described and progressed according to the stages of control.

Initial Phase

The goals of the initial phase are to:

▶ decrease pain;

▶ increase ROM, the mobility level of control;

▶ promote scapular and shoulder stability and controlled mobility in progressively more challenging postures.

Proximal dynamic stability is primarily developed during the stability and controlled mobility procedures in closed-chain activities.

Decrease Pain. The findings from the assessment will help the therapist determine the appropriate means to relieve pain.

▶ Pain may be caused by and also result in a generalized increase in tension and in localized splinting of the musculature around the shoulder. Massage, deep-breathing exercises, and neutral warmth or cold may promote generalized relaxation (see Chapter 3) and improve local tissue nutrition in preparation for exercise procedures.

▶ Tissue swelling and inflammation may be an acute reactive response to trauma. The beneficial physiological effects of thermal, electrical, sound modalities, and massage may be indicated.

► If swelling and inflammation are not symptoms, and if the patient has normal peripheral circulation, heat may be used to increase tissue extensibility before other interventions designed to increase ROM.

► If the individual has a decreased activity level, general conditioning exercises may improve tissue circulation and improve the balance within the ANS. Use of the treadmill and lower extremity ergometry may precede other aspects of treatment. This "warm up" will increase the patient's general exercise tolerance and may help to increase the pain threshold. In addition, the weight bearing that occurs through the upper extremities during these activities can be beneficial for most patients. This portion of the general treatment plan may be practiced with supervision and then included in the home program.

► Because abnormal alignment may cause tissue impingement and pain, the procedures designed to improve mobility–ROM may be appropriate to alleviate this possible cause of pain. TNS may be effective in decreasing pain and may be applied prior to or in conjunction with other therapeutic procedures.

If the pain and localized splinting reduce the ability to voluntarily activate musculature or if atten-tion directed to the shoulder results in an increased perception of pain, an indirect approach may prove effective. **Indirect procedures** include resistance to contralateral upper-extremity motions and resisted alternating isometric contractions (alternating isometrics [AI], rhythmic stabilization [RS]) with manual contacts positioned distally on the forearm or hand of the involved limb (Fig. 5–3). These procedures will facilitate isometric contractions of the involved shoulder muscles without focusing the patient's attention on those areas.[19] The alternating isometric contractions within the involved limb resulting from these indirect procedures may increase local circulation. The tendency toward painful scapular elevation can be reduced by techniques such as RS and hold relax (HR) applied to scapula patterns, which also indirectly promote isometric contractions of the shoulder musculature (Fig. 5–4).

Increase ROM–Mobility Stage. Following the reduction of generalized tension and local splinting, mobility, or improved extensibility of the contractile muscle tissues and noncontractile joint structures, can be initiated. Because patients commonly "posture" their arm at their side and avoid moving the scapula and shoulder, a typical limitation of ROM occurs, with shortening of the capsule and the pectoralis minor, subscapularis, pectoralis major, latissimus dorsi, and the teres major.

The **activities** include the **postures** of supine, sidelying, and sitting, and the **movements** that combine shoulder flexion with adduction and abduction

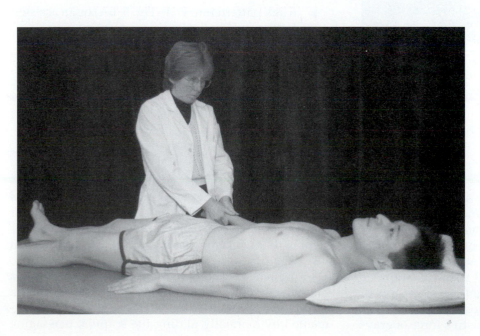

Figure 5–3. A. Supine, D1E involved limb. T. AI to shoulder, MC on forearm.

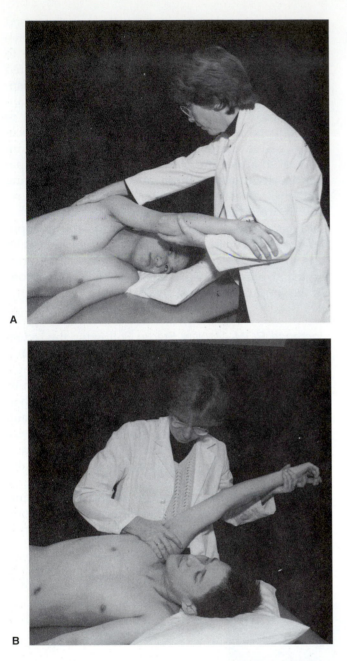

Figure 5–4. A. Supine or sidelying: **(A)** D1F; **(B)** D2F. T. Hold relax to shoulder.

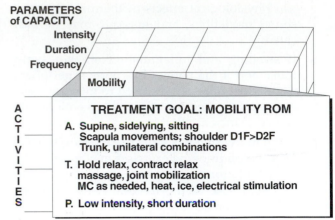

Figure 5–5. The treatment goal of increasing mobility–ROM with the treatment procedures.

and internal or external rotation (Fig. 5–5). Supine and sidelying have a large base of support (BoS) and low center of gravity (CoG), thus encouraging patient relaxation. In supine, shoulder movements can be the focus, whereas scapula movement can be emphasized in sidelying. In sitting, both scapula and shoulder movements can be performed with full scapular and clavicular movement. Although sitting is appropriate if the cardiovascular pulmonary (CVP) status limits horizontal positions, the resistive force of grav-

ity increases as the limb reaches 90° of forward flexion or abduction, making relaxation and active movement more difficult.

The scapula and shoulder movements progress from flexion, adduction D1F, to flexion, abduction, and external rotation, D2F. Later in treatment movement into shoulder extension and internal rotation, D1E, is included to promote reaching behind the back. A trunk pattern is initially used to provide support of the involved limb, followed by a unilateral movement. The elbow can be initially flexed in all of these combinations to decrease the length of the lever arm, to reduce the amount of resistance placed on proximal structures, and to emphasize the rotational component. The progression of movements is:

▶ trunk pattern into D1F (Fig. 5–6A) or an assisted D1 thrust (Fig. 5–6B),

▶ unilateral D1F pattern (Fig. 5–6C),

▶ trunk pattern into D2F (Fig. 5–6D),

▶ unilateral D2F pattern (Fig. 5–6E).

$$\text{trunk} \to \text{bilateral} \to \text{unilateral}$$
$$\text{D1} \to \text{D2}$$
$$\text{elbow flexion} \to \text{extension}$$

Trunk and unilateral patterns are usually performed when the goal is to increase ROM. Bilateral patterns are more commonly used to increase motor unit activity and overflow or to promote various combinations of movement and are not included at this stage.

Codman's exercises may be suggested by a physician after fracture of the proximal humerus. This passive, gravity-eliminated exercise can be augmented by manually gliding the scapula, massaging

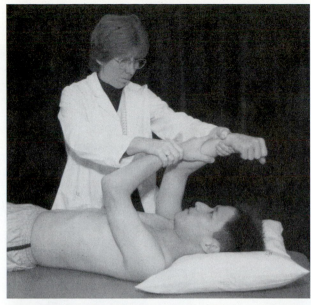
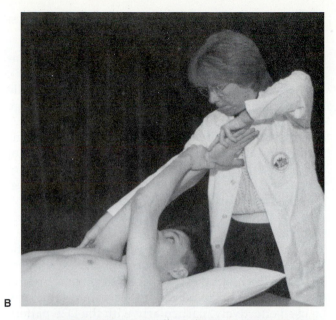

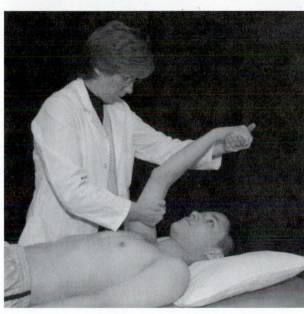

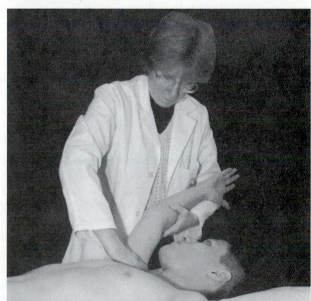

Figure 5–6. A. Supine: **(A)** D1 flexion assisted; **(B)** D1 thrust assisted; **(C)** D1 flexion unilateral; **(D)** D2 flexion assisted; **(E)** D2 flexion unilateral. T. Hold relax; MC on involved or uninvolved limb.

the medial axillary border, and performing HR to increase extensibility of the pectoral muscles (Fig. 5–7).

When indicated, mobilization of hypomobile noncontractile tissues is performed to increase range of the capsule and ligamentous tissues. To improve arthrokinematic movement, appropriate distractions and glides are performed to achieve pain-free joint range. A thorough description of the mobilization procedures are included in other texts. Caution must be taken and consultation should occur after recent fractures and surgical repairs or if bone is osteopenic.

To actively increase muscle extensibility the techniques of HR and contract relax (CR) are applied. HR is the technique of choice when pain is present (see Chapter 3). The relaxation technique of CR can be used effectively, particularly with the D2F pattern to increase ROM when increased muscle tension or rotational movements do not cause pain.

The following are examples of procedures which can be applied at the initial stages of treatment:

TREATMENT GOALS: DECREASING PAIN
AND INCREASING ROM

A. Supine, sidelying, sitting
    Trunk and unilateral movements into D1F
    and D2F;
T. HR progressing to CR, soft-tissue and joint mobilization; manual contacts (MC) on arm, forearm, or both limbs, ice, TNS, ultrasound, interferential current
P. Low-intensity active contractions and minimal passive forces. The duration, frequency, and intensity of these mobility procedures depends on the integrity and reactivity of the tissues and the patient tolerance.

Home and Independent Program

The reader is referred to the visuals for the home exercises at the end of the chapter (pp. 129–133). The home exercise program should be designed to follow the treatment sequence emphasized during the clinic visits. The primary goals of the home exercise program are to maintain the range gained during the clinic sessions and to improve general capacity, especially if the patient has been or will be sedentary following the trauma or surgical intervention. To maintain the scapular and shoulder ROM, the patient can perform active scapular movements with the arm maintained in a relaxed position or supported with the other arm or sling. Codman's exercises and other passive movements can, when appropriate, be modified to include active movement. Cane- or wand-assisted movement or assistance provided by the

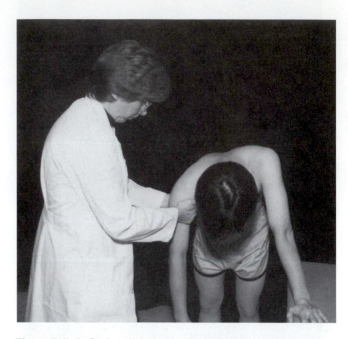

Figure 5–7. A. Codman's exercise. T. Hold relax and passive mobility; MC axilla.

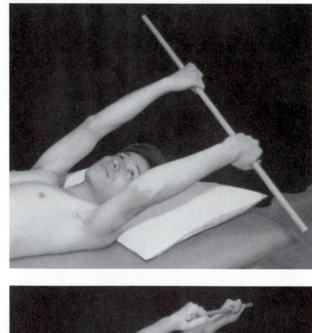

A

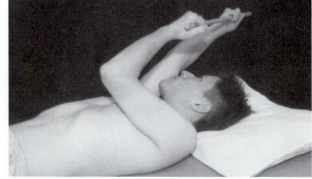

B

Figure 5–8. Home exercise: A. Supine or sitting, shoulder flexion: **(A)** D1F; **(B)** D2F. T. Active assisted with wand or uninvolved limb.

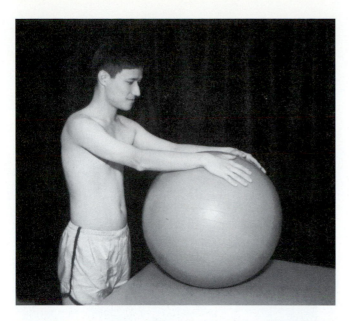

Figure 5–9. A. Standing or sitting, shoulder flexion. T. Active assisted movement with ball.

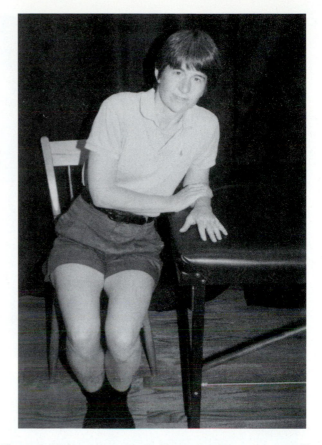

Figure 5–10. Home exercise: A. Sitting, shoulder movements. T. Self-mobilization.

uninvolved limb can be performed in a posture with a large BoS, such as supine and sitting (Fig. 5–8). A medium-size gym ball upon which the hands can be rested is useful to promote proximal relaxation and gentle motion (Fig. 5–9). Self-mobilization activities can be performed in various postures incorporating distraction and gliding movements (Fig. 5–10). If weight bearing is indicated the patient can perform weight shifting in sitting or modified plantigrade. Use of a finger ladder or finger-walking up the wall is not recommended at this stage. Such attempts at this early stage will only reinforce abnormal scapula elevation or lateral trunk flexion. These and similar home exercises therefore should be deferred until more advanced levels of control have been achieved.

To maintain or improve exercise capacity, essential to achieving full function, the patient should be encouraged to walk, ride a stationary bicycle, or perform resisted lower-extremity exercise. A program to improve balance and self-confidence during physical tasks may be indicated for the elderly (see Chapter 10). Maintaining aerobic ability is essential to achieving full function for all age groups.

Stability and Controlled Mobility in Progressively More Challenging Postures

Normal stability in the scapulothoracic and glenohumeral joints encompasses the ability to maintain proper alignment during open- and closed-chain activities in varying ranges with different biomechanical stresses against isometric resistive forces. Controlled mobility implies normal scapulohumeral rhythm during weight shifting in weight-bearing postures. Both stability and controlled mobility are components of proximal dynamic stability, a quality of movement control occurring during the normal timing and sequencing of skilled movement.

Scapular and rotator cuff stability is initially developed by performing low-intensity isometric contractions, first in shortened ranges and then in more lengthened ranges (Fig. 5–11). The isometric contractions may improve the muscles' automatic responses by enhancing the proprioceptive sensitivity of the muscle spindle.

TREATMENT GOAL: DYNAMIC STABILITY IN THE PROXIMAL MUSCLES IN NON-WEIGHT–BEARING POSTURES

A. Supine, sidelying, and sitting
   D1F → D2F with emphasis on scapula depression and adduction and shoulder internal and external rotation
T. Shortened Held Resisted Contraction (SHRC), AI → slow reversal hold (SRH) or slow reversal (SR) ↑ range and Agonistic Reversals (AR)
P. Intensity to about 40%, using body segment resistance or low poundage weights or Thera-

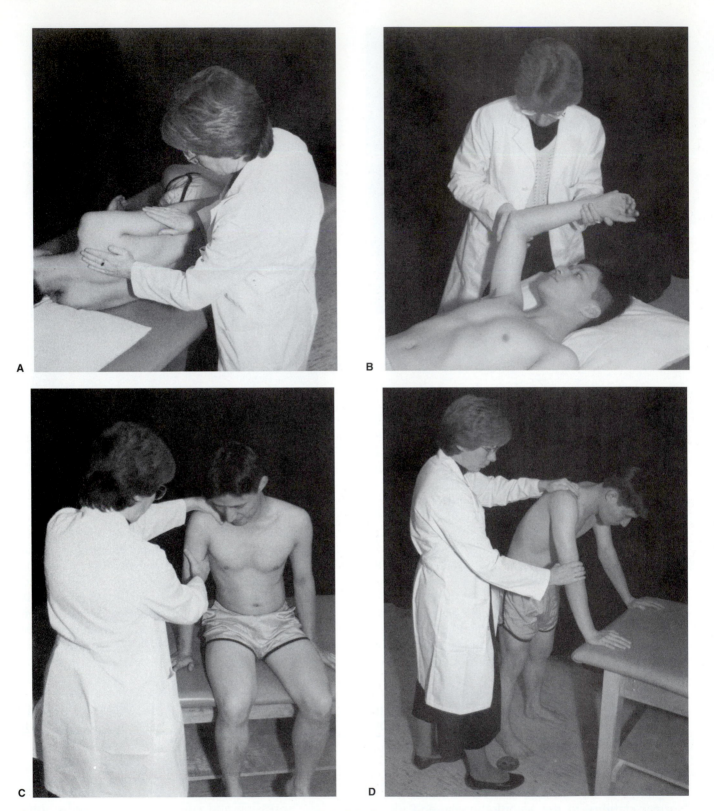

Figure 5–11. Procedures to promote stability: **(A)** A. Sidelying T. SHRC; **(B)** A. Supine; D2F T. AI; **(C)** A. Sitting T. AI RS; **(D)** A. Modified plantigrade. T. AI → RS; **(E)** A. Quadruped T. AI → RS A. Standing at stall bars; **(F)** Shoulders at 60°; **(G)** Shoulders at 120°.

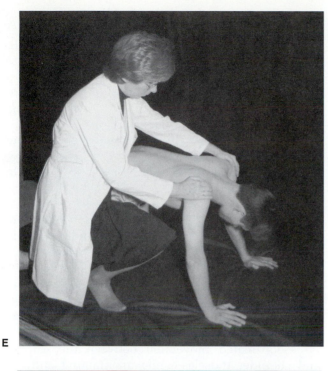

E

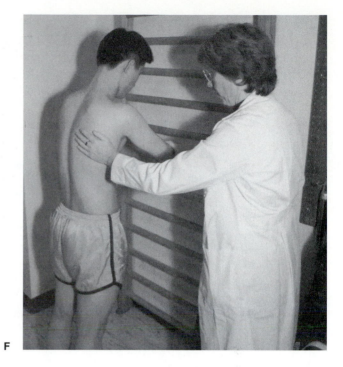

F

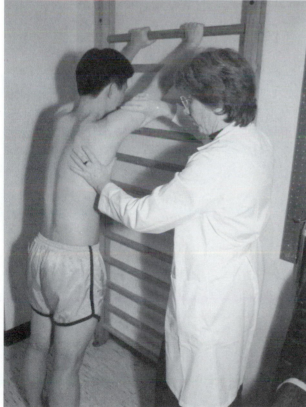

G

Maintaining the contraction at approximately 40% maximum will emphasize contraction of the type I, slow twitch muscle fibers needed for stability (see Chapter 3). Dynamic control of these muscles is enhanced with SRH or SR through increments of range; eccentric control is promoted with AR. As with the mobility sequence, each of these techniques is first performed in D1F (see Fig. 5–8A) progressing to D2F (see Fig. 5–8B) and straight plane abduction. The sequence of movements is chosen to gradually increase the challenge to the rotator cuff muscles, to maintain the proper relation of the humeral head in the glenoid, and initially to avoid the movements that are likely to cause impingement. To simulate the control needed during automatic muscle responses, the duration and rhythm of the contractions are varied and the verbal and visual cues removed as the patient's response improves.

TREATMENT GOAL: PROXIMAL STABILITY IN WEIGHT-BEARING POSTURES (Fig. 5–12)

A. Sitting, modified plantigrade, quadruped
T. AI, RS, approximation
P. Moderate intensity, longer duration, increased frequency

Proximal stability is further challenged in weight-bearing postures in which the amount of weight borne through the shoulder and the range of shoulder movements can be increased. The postures of sitting, modified plantigrade, and quadruped represent activities in which the range in the shoulder

band (Hygienic Corporation, Akron, Ohio). Length of contraction increasing in duration from 10 to 30 seconds. Frequency: 5 to 10 times throughout the day, incorporated into the home program.

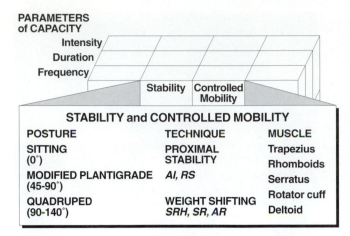

PARAMETERS of CAPACITY

Intensity
Duration
Frequency

| Stability | Controlled Mobility |

STABILITY and CONTROLLED MOBILITY

POSTURE	TECHNIQUE	MUSCLE
SITTING (0°)	PROXIMAL STABILITY	Trapezius
		Rhomboids
MODIFIED PLANTIGRADE (45-90°)	*AI, RS*	Serratus
		Rotator cuff
QUADRUPED (90-140°)	WEIGHT SHIFTING *SRH, SR, AR*	Deltoid

Figure 5–12. The stability and controlled-mobility treatment progressions.

progresses from 0° to 90° with increasing amounts of weight bearing:

▶ sitting with upper extremity support or standing in the parallel bars, 0° degrees of flexion (Fig. 5–11C);

▶ modified plantigrade (Fig. 5–11D) or prone on elbows, 45° to 60° of flexion; and,

▶ quadruped (Fig. 5–11E) or standing with the upper extremities flexed against the wall or holding the stall bars (Fig. 5–11F,G), 60° to 120°.

The therapist needs to observe scapular position and the quality of the contraction of the shoulder musculature. Abnormal responses include excessive scapular abduction, elevation off the thorax, or flickering of the muscles around the shoulder. These responses may indicate that the intensity of body weight or external resistance is too great or that the duration of maintaining the posture is too long. The techniques can be applied by placing MC directly on the involved segment or indirectly away from the involved part. For example, with the patient in modified plantigrade or quadruped, the MC can be on the scapula and pelvis or on both hips. Joint approximation may be applied to further facilitate proximal muscular activity.

When functional movements are performed in sitting or standing, gravitational resistance is greatest when the lever arm is the longest, at 90° of shoulder flexion or abduction. Resistance at this angle increases the challenge to the scapular and rotator cuff muscles. Although control throughout range needs to be promoted, the 90° arc, which seems to be the most difficult range to control, needs to be emphasized. This can be achieved in quadruped or with the arms weight-bearing on the wall or holding onto the stall bars.

TREATMENT GOAL: CONTROLLED MOBILITY OF THE SCAPULA AND SHOULDER

A. Sitting, modified plantigrade, quadruped, progressing the amount of weight bearing through the involved limb (Fig. 5–13)

T. SRH ↑ range, AR with manual resistance and equipment

P. Moderate intensity, increased duration, increased frequency

The range and direction of proximal motion and the amount of weight-bearing resistance at the involved shoulder can be varied. The direction of rocking can progress from D1F, to anterior-posterior, to D2F. To promote a reversal of antagonists, manual resistance is applied; a concentric-eccentric reversal can be promoted with manual and mechanical resistance, or with independent movement.

Coordinated movement between the scapular and shoulder muscles while maintaining and performing more biomechanically challenging activities is indicative of the presence of dynamic stability.

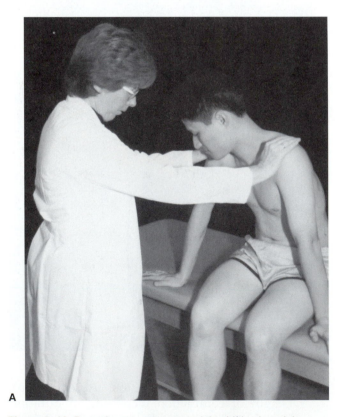

A

Figure 5–13. Procedures to promote weight shifting in weight-bearing postures: A. **(A)** Sitting; **(B)** Modified plantigrade; **(C)** Quadruped. T. SRH → SR → AR

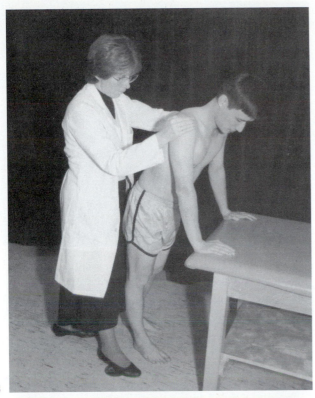

B

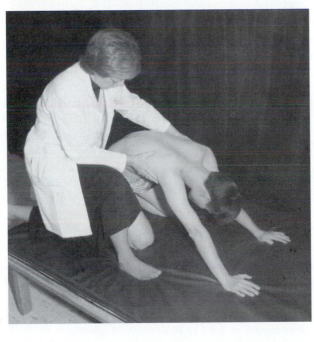

C

Static–dynamic activities further increase the dynamic stability around the involved weight-bearing segment. One manual contact can be positioned on the involved weight-bearing shoulder to apply approximation while the other arm is resisted through range. Increased proximal dynamic stability of the involved weight-bearing extremity is promoted as larger excursions of range against increased resistance are performed by the uninvolved limb. Resistance can be provided by a weight, Theraband (Fig. 5–14), or a pulley (see Chapter 2).

Dynamic stability of all the proximal muscles is essential for effective scapulohumeral rhythm and the normal timing of skilled movement. This control increasingly is developed as the stability, controlled mobility, and static–dynamic stages are performed in the sequence of weight-bearing postures.

In all of these procedures, the therapist is observing the quality of control and the endurance of the muscles around the scapula and shoulder. Smooth and equal control of the scapulae is desired as the muscles contract and the body moves through range. Abnormal scapular movements may include: lifting of the scapula off the thorax, usually indicative of serratus anterior weakness; upward tilt of the inferior

Within the scapula, this level of control requires a "balance" between the adductors and abductors and between the elevators and depressors to maintain a mid-range position as body weight resistance and stretch increases the challenge to stabilize. In the shoulder a balance of forces between the rotator cuff and the extrinsic muscles is required.

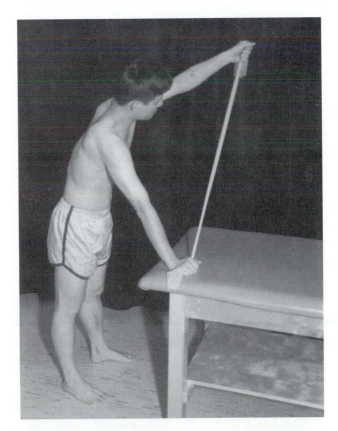

Figure 5–14. A. Modified plantigrade, lifting uninvolved limb. T. Resisted movement; elastic or hand-weight resistance.

angle, indicative of lower trapezius weakness;[12] excessive abduction into the axilla, indicative of either tightness of the joint capsule or teres major, or weakness of the middle trapezius or the rhomboids. Observation of any of these abnormal movements is an indication that the posture or the technique is too difficult. A less difficult weight-bearing procedure along with specific muscle strengthening or relaxation may need to be performed before control can be gained with more challenging procedures.

Overlapping of Treatment Goals

The procedures performed to achieve the goal of increased ROM–mobility are overlapped with those that focus on stability and controlled mobility. While range is being gained in supine, sidelying, or sitting with the mobility techniques, appropriate techniques can be performed in weight-bearing postures to increase the activity of the scapular and shoulder muscles needed for stabilization in the gained range.

The overlapping of treatment procedures can be clearly demonstrated during the progressions within the three postures of sitting, modified plantigrade, and quadruped. Within each posture, the techniques are sequenced to promote the stages of control (Fig. 5–15). When the patient is performing controlled mobility in modified plantigrade, for example, initial stability control also can be developed in quadruped, which incorporates more stressful weight bearing for the upper extremity. As more advanced control is

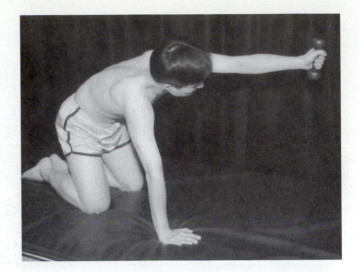

Figure 5–16. Home exercise: A. Quadruped, lifting uninvolved limb. T. Resisted movement; elastic or hand-weight resistance.

promoted in quadruped, such as controlled mobility and static–dynamic activities, the patient may be ready to begin procedures to develop the skill level of control in supine, sitting, and standing.

Home and Independent Program

Weight bearing through the limb and rocking in different directions can easily be performed in the same sequence of postures used during the clinic treatments. Because weight shifting and static–dynamic activities in modified plantigrade and in quadruped are easy to perform and control, they are excellent exercises to incorporate into a home program (Fig. 5–16). Resistance can be provided by body weight or additional force with a free weight or Theraband. As an independent program within the clinic setting, the patient can gradually push into a small trampoline to promote additional joint compression. When the patient is weight shifting in the parallel bars or on a balance board, automatic shoulder activity occurs.

In summary, the focus of the initial phase of treatment is to: (1) maintain or increase **mobility**— the extensibility of skin, fascial, muscle and capsular tissues of the shoulder girdle by appropriately applying specific and general soft-tissue and joint mobilizations and relaxation techniques; (2) promote dynamic stability by increasing the **stability, controlled mobility,** and **static–dynamic** levels of control in postures that incrementally increase weight bearing and the range of shoulder motion with the techniques of SHRC, AI, RS, SR(H), or AR.

PARAMETERS of CAPACITY

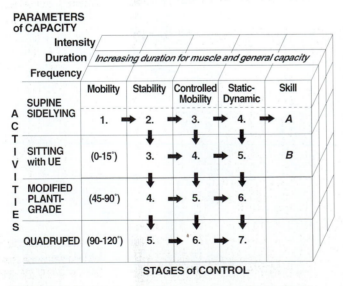

	Mobility	Stability	Controlled Mobility	Static-Dynamic	Skill
SUPINE SIDELYING	1. →	2. →	3. →	4. →	A
SITTING with UE	(0-15°)	3. →	4. →	5.	B
MODIFIED PLANTI-GRADE	(45-90°)	4. →	5. →	6.	
QUADRUPED	(90-120°)	5. →	6. →	7.	

STAGES of CONTROL

Figure 5–15. The Intervention Model sequencing the treatment procedures.

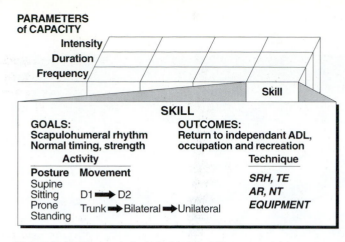

PARAMETERS of CAPACITY

Intensity
Duration
Frequency

Skill

SKILL

GOALS:
Scapulohumeral rhythm
Normal timing, strength

OUTCOMES:
Return to independant ADL,
occupation and recreation

Activity		Technique
Posture	**Movement**	
Supine		*SRH, TE*
Sitting	D1 ➡ D2	*AR, NT*
Prone		*EQUIPMENT*
Standing	Trunk ➡ Bilateral ➡ Unilateral	

Figure 5–17. The goals included at the skill stage and the treatment progressions.

Advanced Phase

At the advanced phase of treatment for a patient with shoulder dysfunction, the **treatment goals** (Fig. 5–17) include:

▶ the normal timing of movement emphasizing scapulohumeral rhythm in non-weight–bearing, open-chain activities; and,

▶ sufficient strength and endurance to perform required functional tasks.

Impairments that may persist at this phase may include weakness of the scapula abductors and adductors and decreased rotator cuff control as the limb moves into ranges greater than 90°. Some patients may have residual ROM limitations into full flexion, abduction, external rotation, and extension with internal rotation which may or may not interfere with the functional needs of the patient. For example, a sedentary individual may not need the full 180° of shoulder range to perform their functional tasks whereas a construction worker may require complete range.

Treatment Procedures

Although the activities at the skill stage are performed as open-chain movements, treatment may continue to include some of the procedures in weight bearing. For example, procedures performed in quadruped or while grasping onto the stall bars with the shoulders in more flexion may help to promote dynamic stability in these more difficult ranges.

A. Supine, prone, sitting
Bilateral and unilateral D1F, D2F, [and extension combined with internal rotation (Fig. 5–18)]

T. SR(H), timing for emphasis (TE) repeated contractions (RC), AR, Ice

P. Intensity, frequency, and duration as required by occupation and recreation

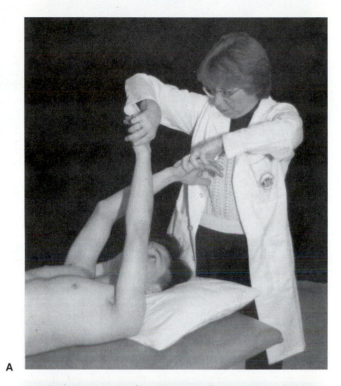

A

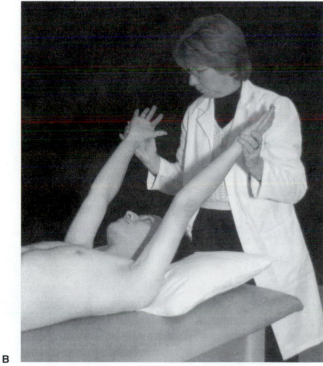

B

Figure 5–18. Procedures at the advanced phase: A. **(A)** Supine, BS D1 thrust; **(B)** Supine, BS D2 flexion; **(C)** Sitting, BS D2 flexion; **(D)** Supine, unilateral D2F; **(E)** Sitting, BS D1 withdrawal; **(F)** Standing, D1 thrust. T. SRH, SR, TE, AR; MC forearms or wrist and arm; manual elastic or mechanical resistance.

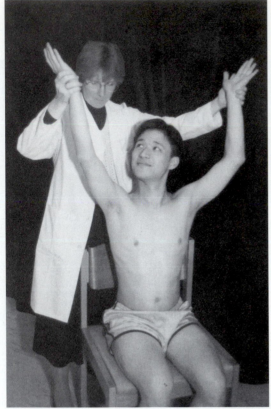

C

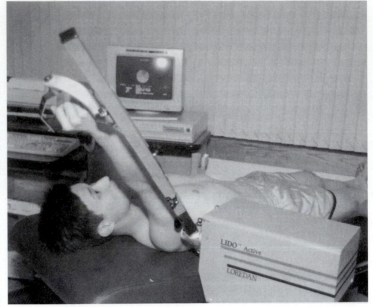

D

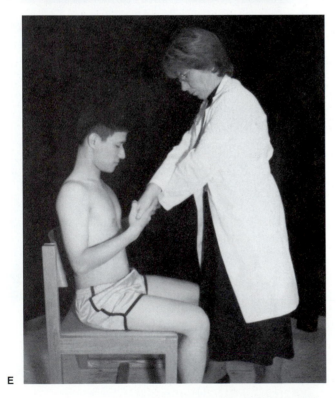

E

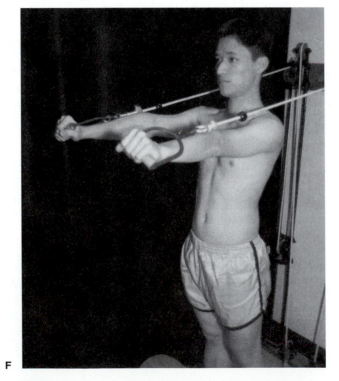

F

In this advanced phase the **activities,** or movements, of the involved limb are sequenced similarly to the preceding stages: flexion, adduction external rotation, D1F, proceeding to flexion, abduction exter-

nal rotation, D2F (Fig. 5–19). Resistance to bilateral combinations now are included in the treatment plan to promote overflow from the stronger limb and increase "strength" of the involved scapular and shoul-

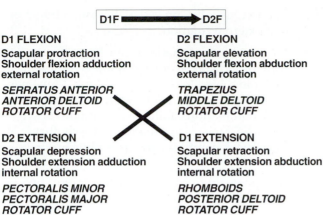

D1F ➡ D2F

D1 FLEXION	**D2 FLEXION**
Scapular protraction	Scapular elevation
Shoulder flexion adduction	Shoulder flexion abduction
external rotation	external rotation
SERRATUS ANTERIOR	*TRAPEZIUS*
ANTERIOR DELTOID	*MIDDLE DELTOID*
ROTATOR CUFF	*ROTATOR CUFF*
D2 EXTENSION	**D1 EXTENSION**
Scapular depression	Scapular retraction
Shoulder extension adduction	Shoulder extension abduction
internal rotation	internal rotation
PECTORALIS MINOR	*RHOMBOIDS*
PECTORALIS MAJOR	*POSTERIOR DELTOID*
ROTATOR CUFF	*ROTATOR CUFF*

Figure 5–19. The movements and muscles emphasized in the diagonal patterns.

der muscles.[20] Unilateral movements are incorporated to promote the normal timing and sequencing of scapula and shoulder movements.

$$\text{Trunk} \rightarrow \text{Bilateral} \rightarrow \text{Unilateral}$$
$$\text{D1F} \rightarrow \text{D2F}$$

Although the sequence of movements is similar to the mobility stage, the control expectations differ. At the mobility stage the goal is ROM, the *quantity* of movement; at the skill stage of control the goal is improved *quality* of timing and strength.

Bilateral D1 is performed most easily using the thrust pattern. The serratus anterior and the anterior deltoid are emphasized during the flexion movement and the rhomboids and posterior deltoid promoted as the shoulder moves into extension. During the D2F movement, control of the trapezius and middle deltoid are enhanced, whereas D2E activates the pectoralis minor and major. When these are performed in supine, the patient may be able to produce more motor unit activity because the BoS is large and the CoG is low; in sitting or standing, the timing and sequencing of the scapula and shoulder muscles can be emphasized; in prone, the scapular adductors can be resisted against gravity in combination with either shoulder flexion or extension.[21,22]

The techniques that accompany these activities include SR to promote a smooth reversal of antagonists, TE, or RC to enhance strengthening of specific muscle groups or movements, and AR to improve eccentric control. Facilitory inputs should be unnecessary at this stage because of increased voluntary control. Ice may be used after a vigorous exercise session to prevent swelling.

Home and Independent Program

Strengthening and endurance exercises can be emphasized with various types of equipment (Fig. 5–20).

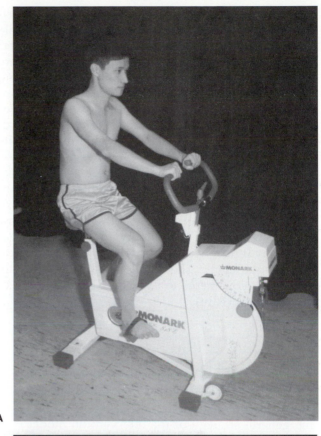

A

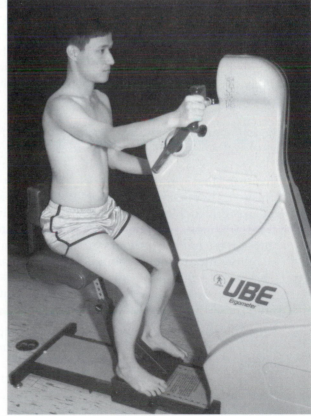

B

Figure 5–20. General capacity exercises: **(A)** Lower-body ergometry, bike; **(B)** Upper-body ergometry, arm bike.

Pulleys, free weights, and Theraband promote primarily concentric–eccentric contractions; both angle and direction can be altered to emphasize particular portions of the range. These forms of resistance are easily adapted to a home program. In performing a home exercise program the patient should understand how to increase or decrease the difficulty of each exercise, by altering either the amount of weight, the number of repetitions, the duration of the contraction, or the length of the lever arm.

Many isokinetic devices can resist concentric reversals, as well as eccentric contractions. The advantage of isokinetic exercise is an objective record of various parameters of muscle performance; the disadvantage is lack of adaptability and cost. Many patients may return to a weight program with other resistive equipment. The therapist should carefully review all movements to prevent excessive strain to particular structures.

► SUMMARY

The general strategy of the intervention model is to gradually increase the difficulty of each of the three units of the procedure. Many patients respond best if only one component is changed at a time. For example, when the activity is made more challenging by progressing from modified plantigrade to quadruped, the difficulty of the technique is either maintained or decreased.

The following intervention principles and factors are considered when sequencing **activities:**

► Postures that provide support during early phases of treatment, when mobility is the goal, are integrated with those that incorporate increasing amount of range and weight bearing through the joint to promote proximal dynamic stability and motions required for function. This sequencing of postures may include supine, sidelying, prone, sitting, modified plantigrade, quadruped, and standing.

► Kinesiological and biomechanical relationships of the shoulder complex, combined with an understanding of those motions that can exacerbate or alleviate the symptoms, provide the basis for determining the movements in treatment. This knowledge leads to a progression of movements in which shoulder flexion with ad-

duction usually precedes flexion, abduction, and external rotation.

► Movement combinations can be performed to provide assistance or to promote overflow from the uninvolved to the involved limb. Movement sequences usually begin with trunk and bilateral combinations, followed by unilateral activities. Resistance is gradually increased during all movement combinations as ability progresses.

The sequencing of **techniques** is determined by the type of tissue involvement and the treatment goals:

► Mobility: When ROM is limited by contractile tissue, techniques of hold relax and contract relax are indicated. Extensibility of noncontractile tissue can be increased by techniques including massage and joint mobilization.

► Stability of the scapula and shoulder in functional ranges and increases in proprioceptive feedback can be enhanced with the techniques of SHRC, AI, and RS.

► Concentric and eccentric dynamic control to promote normal scapulohumeral rhythm is achieved in the controlled mobility and static–dynamic stages with SRH, SR, and AR.

► The timing, sequencing, and strength of movement required for skilled movement and function are promoted by SR, AR, TE, and RC.

► Sensory inputs and adjunctive techniques such as heat, ice, or electrical stimulation are useful in the early phases of treatment to relieve pain, reduce swelling, and promote healing but are withdrawn as more advanced goals are emphasized.

The **parameters** of exercise are determined by the tissue's reactivity, the need for specific learning strategies, and the physiological stress appropriate for that individual. For example:

► The intensity of stretching techniques is determined by the extent of insult and the course of healing. The intensity of the contraction is determined by the response desired, below 40% of a maximum contraction for stability and endurance and above 40% to achieve increased anaerobic strength.[23] These intensity levels may vary if the person is deconditioned. A deconditioned person may reach anaerobic threshold sooner, an indication that the intensity level needs to be lowered. Manual, mechanical, free-weight, or elastic resistance can all be employed to achieve the intensity desired and the appropriate type of contraction.

▶ The duration of each procedure is determined by the ability of the circulatory system to replenish the tissues and the extent of sensory stimulation related to the relief of pain. The duration of each treatment session should be long enough to include a brief reassessment, a warm-up, the overlapping of various treatment procedures, a review of the home exercise program, and if needed, an endurance program. The warm-up, combined with the general and specific endurance program, can be conducted independently, leaving about 20 to 30 minutes for the direct, hands-on, session.

▶ The frequency, the number of repetitions of a movement or contraction, should allow for a summation of stimuli to enhance and reinforce learning and appropriately stress the tissues to allow the achievement of the desired responses. However, the procedure should not produce pain or lead to fatigue. The following guidelines may be helpful: when the patient is very reactive or painful, movements are performed slowly with few repetitions. As healing occurs, the tissues can be progressively stressed by increasing the speed of movement. In addition, because the treatment goals require learning of movements and improved movement endurance, the number of repetitions is increased, for example up to 10 to 20. When anaerobic "strength" is desired, the repetitions are few but the intensity is high. Those procedures that the patient can perform independently can be incorporated into the home program.

The total intervention plan should provide for a balance of procedures that directly focus on the involved tissues, emphasize reinforcement or overflow from surrounding tissues, and focus on aerobic endurance and anaerobic strengthening of the specific shoulder movements and of the body in general.

The general program for patients with shoulder dysfunction described in this chapter illustrates how the overlapping of procedures can occur to promote functional movement patterns, achieve the varied stages of movement control, and enhance movement capacity to achieve the treatment goals and functional outcomes.

▶ PATIENT CASE

Mr. D is a 55-year-old man who presents with pain in his right lateral shoulder noted during abduction movements. He is a painter and uses his shoulders daily in all planes of movement. He injured his arm when he fell off a ladder 1 month ago. Plane films are negative; MRI shows a slight tear of the right rotator cuff.

The patient states that he is limited in performing his painting activities and in other overhead activities.

▶ EVALUATION

Because the patient has involvement of his upper extremity, the functional capability that the evaluation will assess reflects his ability to "manipulate" the environment including occupational tasks and components of ADL (Fig. 5–21).

Environmental, Social Factors

Divorced with two children. Lives alone in an apartment.

No reported recreational activities or hobbies.

Psychological, Medical Factors

States he is depressed because of inability to work. He is not covered by workers' compensation and needs to return to work as soon as possible. He reports that the physician initially told him to rest his

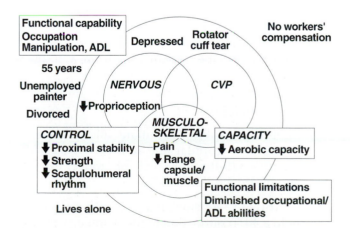

Figure 5–21. The patient findings included in the Evaluation Model.

arm and perform only pendulum exercises. His medical history is unremarkable.

Because of the history and medical report, the assumption is that the primary problem is in the musculoskeletal system. The assessment of the physical systems will begin with the ANS to determine if pain threshold or abnormal circulation could be related to an imbalance in the ANS and to measure vital physiological parameters; the musculoskeletal (MS) system is assessed in detail to determine the contribution of the various tissues to range limitations, to instability, and to pain; the area of movement control is measured to determine the quality of movement; movement capacity is assessed to ascertain the quantity of both general and specific segment movement.

The findings include:

Physical Systems

ANS:
Heart rate 75; blood pressure 120/90; dry blotchy skin; cold hands. Pain threshold appears low.

MS:

▶ No restrictions in neck movements; cervical movements do not produce pain in the shoulder.

▶ Thoracic spine: slight increase in kyphosis; no (areas of) tenderness in paraspinal muscles.

▶ R scapula: maintained in abduction and elevation. The R upper trapezius and levator scapulae are tight and tender to palpation. No pain or restriction in the acromio clavicular (A-C) and sterno clavicular (S-C) joints.

▶ Shoulder: Passive ROM (supine) flexion 120°, abduction 90°, external rotation 10°, internal rotation 70°. All motions limited by capsular and muscular tightness. Active external rotation and abduction reproduce the primary pain and are rated by the patient as a 6 on a 10-point scale.

Movement Control:

▶ MOBILITY—Able to initiate all movements. Strength of scapular and uninvolved shoulder muscles 3/5 through available range; external and internal rotation 3/5.

▶ STABILITY—In sidelying and sitting unable to hold a 40% contraction of the scapula adductors in their shortened ranges longer than 10 seconds before fatiguing. An isometric contraction

of the external rotators in shortened ranges is limited to 1 to 2 seconds because of pain. The scapular muscles and external rotators of the shoulder do not immediately respond when resistance is applied, suggesting that proprioception is decreased.

▶ SCAPULOHUMERAL RHYTHM is abnormal, with excessive scapula elevation at the initiation of shoulder flexion. Because of both pain and weakness, he is unable to lift arm beyond 90° in supine or sitting and complains of pain while lowering his arm.

Movement Capacity:

▶ He has been sedentary for the past month. He normally is not very active other than at work.

Functional Limitation

Unable to perform overhead limb movements required for occupation or for dressing and hygiene. He has difficulty reaching behind his back, putting on a coat, and combing his hair.

The **Physical Impairments** related to the functional limitation are:

▶ Decreased ROM, both passive and active,

▶ pain that seems to be of biomechanical origin,

▶ decreased dynamic stability of the scapula and rotator cuff,

▶ decreased general capacity for exercise and particular ability to perform repetitive upper-extremity movements.

Associated **environmental, medical factors** are:

▶ No prior shoulder injury,

▶ has performed repetitive shoulder movements as part of occupation for 20 years,

▶ out of work and motivated to return to work,

▶ lives alone, without family support,

▶ self-report of depression,

▶ healing tear of rotator cuff,

▶ no other associated medical problems.

Clinical Impression:

The association of the impairments to the functional limitation:

▶ Primary rotator cuff involvement leading to pain from abnormal tissue integrity and "impingement pain" from the abnormal biomechanical forces,

▶ Decreased ROM, weakness, and abnormal scapulohumeral rhythm related to both the tear and the subsequent disuse.

The functional outcome is determined by assessing the extent to which the impairments that contribute to the functional limitation can be changed or if the limitation can be reversed by modifying the environmental challenges.

Functional Outcome

Patient will be able to return to occupation and be independent in all ADLs. He may need to adapt some painting implements to reduce strain on his shoulder.

This outcome anticipates that changes will be made in the physical impairments, although minimal environmental modifications may be needed. This determination is made because the partial tear will heal and his movement control and capacity will improve. At his age, the healing will not occur as quickly as with a younger person but he should have sufficient circulation in the tissues to promote healing and withstand the repetitive movements that occur with his job. His sedentary behavior should respond to a conditioning program, and he is motivated to return to work.

Anticipated treatment frequency is 2 times tapering to 1 per week for a duration of 10 to 12 weeks.

Determination of frequency is made by assessing his ability to follow directions and comply with a home program. The 10 to 12 weeks' duration of treatment takes into consideration the time since injury, the anticipated healing time, and the time needed to develop control and capacity and to reverse the effects of the trauma and disuse.

The impairments found during the evaluation are transposed into the classifications within the intervention model, particularly the stages of control.

Mobility	Stability	Controlled Mobility	Skill
Decreased ROM of scapula into adduction, and shoulder into flexion, abduction external rotation	Decreased holding at scapula and shoulder	Poor scapulo-humeral rhythm	Abnormal timing and sequencing concentric eccentric movement

The **treatment goals** delineate the movement and its quality and the quantity to be achieved. Both quality and quantity of movement can be categorized by the stages of control and parameters of movement including ROM, the ability to sustain isometric contractions, the ability to maintain and then move within progressively more difficult postures, and to move the limb during functional tasks.

The sum of all the treatment goals should achieve the functional outcome.

The following are examples of statements that may be included in the narrative portion of the chart.

▶ INITIAL TREATMENTS (WEEKS ONE TO FOUR)

Documentation in S.O.A.P. (Subjective, Objective, Assessment, Plan) format:

S. "My shoulder feels stiff and it hurts when I put on my coat or try to reach overhead but after the last visit I had less discomfort, and the home program is working OK."

O. Range and strength measures as above.

Treatment to Increase ROM (Fig. 5–22):

▶ 5 minutes ultrasound with tight muscles maintained in an elongated position.

▶ Massage applied around shoulder, to pectoralis major and minor, and to teres major.

▶ Hold relax to the agonist performed with the limb moving into flexion adduction, then into flexion abduction.

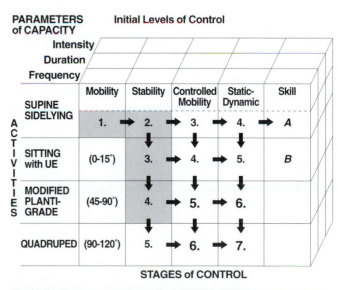

Figure 5–22. The procedures emphasized at the beginning phase of rehabilitation.

▶ Joint distraction, glides and oscillations, grade III, performed to increase extensibility of capsule.

To Increase Proximal Stability:

▶ Isometric contractions of the scapula adductors in shortened range, and the rotator cuff in neutral position (to avoid pain). Contractions performed with increasing duration, now holding up to 10 seconds while non-weight–bearing in supine and sidelying and weight bearing in sitting.

▶ Alternating isometrics to the scapula and rotator cuff with the shoulder non-weight–bearing in increasing ranges of flexion and adduction and with weight bearing in sitting and modified plantigrade.

▶ Pulleys for scapula adductors, emphasizing holding in shortened ranges performed in sitting and standing.

To Improve Movement Capacity:

▶ Stationary bike and treadmill each for 10 minutes.

Home Program Consists of:

▶ Modifying pendulum exercises to include active movement.

▶ Isometrics of scapula adductors while supine and sitting using body weight and Theraband resistance.

▶ Isometrics with wand, resistance applied by uninvolved side, for shoulder rotators with shoulder up to 45° of flexion and adduction in supine or sitting.

▶ Small range rotational movements with the shoulder at 0° of flexion resisted with Theraband.

▶ Self-mobilization techniques in sitting with elbow supported on table.

▶ Ice applied after exercises to prevent swelling.

▶ Walking program for 30 to 45 minutes 3 times per week encouraged for general capacity.

▶ Patient education includes the importance of avoiding pain-producing movements. Instructed to put his right arm into shirt and coat first to avoid painful abduction and to restrict arm movements to the front of his body.

A. The goals include:

▶ Increasing ROM by increasing the length of the capsule and soft tissue. Should achieve 140°

flexion, abduction 120°, external rotation 30° by end of third week;

▶ Improving proximal dynamic stability as demonstrated by maintenance of scapula position in modified plantigrade and during the first 45° of shoulder elevation;

▶ Increasing time and intensity on the stationary bike to 20 minutes and increasing speed and distance of home walking program;

▶ Increasing the repetitions of movement and the duration of the isometric contractions.

P. Continue with program to increase range and muscular stability. Progress dynamic control in modified plantigrade and quadruped as tolerated. Initiate free, open-chain, movements when healing and proximal control allows to avoid reinforcement of abnormal scapulohumeral movements. Continue to encourage performance of home program and to increase outside exercise activities.

▶ **SECOND PHASE (WEEKS 4 TO 8) (FIG. 5-23)**

S. Patient states he is able to comb his hair with less pain but still cannot reach overhead or behind back. "I walk outside more, up to 2 miles now. I can't go back to work until I can perform all arm movements."

O. Passive range measured in supine: 145° flexion, 120° abduction, 45° external rotation, extension 35°, can reach to back pocket.

MMT: (within available range) flexion 4/5, abduction, external and internal rotation 4-/5.

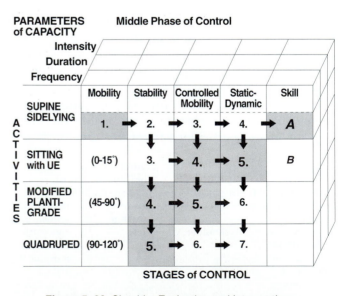

Figure 5–23. Shoulder Evaluation and Intervention.

Pain with passive and active external rotation less than previously reported: 4/10.

Treatment to Increase ROM:

▶ Hold relax to pectoralis minor to achieve full scapula motion and proper postural alignment.

▶ Oscillations and distractions grade 3–4 to increase shoulder capsule length.

▶ Hold relax and contract relax to increase range into shoulder flexion, abduction and external rotation, and extension and internal rotation performed in supine and sitting.

To Increase Stability:

▶ In supine and sitting AI and RS to rotation during shoulder flexion and abduction to increase isometric control of the scapula muscles and rotator cuff in increasing ranges of shoulder flexion. In supine, he is able to contract through a 130° pain-free arc.

▶ AI and RS in modified plantigrade and quadruped.

To Improve Dynamic Stability, Controlled Scapulohumeral Rhythm:

▶ Bilateral D1 thrust and reversal with manual and mechanical (pulleys and Theraband) resistance to increase strength of serratus and scapula adductors and strength of shoulder muscles.

▶ Modified plantigrade weight shifting performed through increasing range with increased weight bearing over involved shoulder. When other limb is raised, the weight-bearing scapula can hold for up to 10 seconds before scapular and shoulder muscles begin to "flicker."

To Increase Movement Capacity:

▶ Upper body ergometry (UBE) with both forward and backward resistance at fast speeds for 10 minutes.

Home Program Includes:

▶ Isometrics of rotator cuff in increasing ranges of shoulder flexion, abduction, and external rotation with Theraband.

▶ Weight shifting in modified plantigrade.

▶ Resisted shoulder extension with scapula adduction, shoulder flexion with scapula abduction, and both internal and external rotation with Theraband. Movements are performed through increasing ranges to improve concentric–eccentric control. Shoulder movements are

performed with elbow flexion progressing to elbow extension.

▶ The walking program is increasing and he is now swimming with modification in both the breast- and backstroke. The painful movements of flexion and abduction above 130° are avoided.

A. Program is progressing as anticipated: tissue extensibility has increased. Range in flexion has progressed from 120° to 145°; proximal dynamic stability is improving with isometric and isotonic resistance in weight-bearing postures progressed from modified plantigrade to quadruped; strength of scapula and shoulder improving with progressively increasing resistance to bilateral and unilateral limb movements with extended elbow.

P. Patient encouraged to adapt equipment by extending brush handles in preparation for return to work. Home program continues to emphasize development of movement control and capacity. Goals now emphasize proximal dynamic stability in the weight-bearing postures of modified plantigrade and quadruped and strengthening scapula and shoulder muscles through range.

▶ END PHASES OF REHABILITATION (WEEKS 9 TO 12) (FIG. 5–24)

S. "I can reach overhead better, but my arm gets tired at the end of the day and I still have pain reaching behind my back. I'm up to 3 miles walking and ride the stationary bike for 30 minutes."

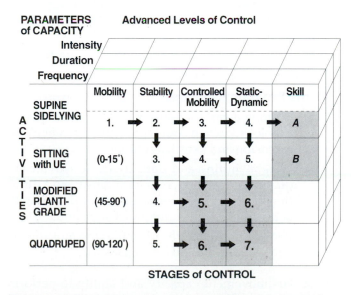

Figure 5–24. Procedures emphasized at the advanced phases of rehabilitation.

O. Range: flexion 170°, abduction to 160°, external rotation 70°, reaches behind back with thumb at level of T$_{10}$, two inches below reach of other arm. Strength 4+/5 all shoulder and scapular muscles. Has less endurance on involved side as measured by onset of pain and decreased scapulohumeral rhythm after 5 repetitions of shoulder flexion with 5-lb weight.

Treatment Program for ROM:

- ▶ Contract relax into D2 flexion and soft-tissue stretching of anterior chest muscles, performed in sitting to allow full scapular movement.

- ▶ Joint mobilization with emphasis on grade IV oscillations to increase ranges of shoulder extension and internal rotation.

To Improve Dynamic Stability (Fig. 5–22):

- ▶ To improve rotator cuff control, AI and RS are performed in sitting, with the arm near full range of shoulder flexion and abduction.

- ▶ Weight shifting in modified plantigrade and quadruped with increasing amounts of weight bearing on involved limb and with other limb moving against resistance of weights or Theraband.

- ▶ AI and RS with shoulders at 140° to 160° of flexion performed at the stall bars.

- ▶ Bilateral and unilateral shoulder flexion with abduction and external rotation in supine and sitting to strengthen trapezius, middle deltoid, and rotator cuff. Resistance applied manually, with pulleys and Theraband to enhance both concentric and eccentric control.

- ▶ In prone, manual resistance applied to scapula adduction and shoulder hyperextension to promote concentric–eccentric control.

- ▶ UBE, at slower speeds for longer durations to increase endurance.

Home Program Includes:

- ▶ Turning away from arm which is supported on a table or kitchen counter to maintain range into extension and external rotation.

- ▶ Weight shifting and static dynamic activities in quadruped with increasing intensity and duration of resistance; resisted shoulder flexion with abduction with weights and Theraband.

- ▶ Performing all overhead swimming movements and walking and bike exercises.

A. His movement capacity and ability to perform repetitive movements have improved; his control of shoulder movements is now sufficient for his daily activities. He is compliant with his independent home program. He is encouraged to continue his control and capacity program; proper use of health club equipment has been discussed. He is able to perform all ADL- and work-related movements.

P. Discharge from physical therapy.

▶ REVIEW QUESTIONS

1. Why might patients have less difficulty moving into flexion and adduction in comparison to flexion and abduction? Which patients may demonstrate pain with flexion and adduction?

2. What is the progression of extremity combinations that promotes progression from the least to the most difficult movements? What are the advantages of each?

3. Why is progressing through a sequence of weight-bearing, closed-chain procedures important?

4. What are the stabilizing muscles of the scapula? How would you detect deficits in function? Which procedures could be used to remedy these deficits?

5. What sequence of procedures could be used to promote control and endurance of the rotator cuff muscles?

REFERENCES

1. Rowe CR: The Shoulder. New York, NY: Churchill Livingstone, 1988.

2. Neumann DA. Arthrokinesiologic considerations in the aged adult. In: Guccione AP, ed. *Geriatric Physical Therapy.* St. Louis, Mo: CV Mosby Co; 1993.

3. Jobe FW, Perry J, Pink M. Electromyographic shoulder activity in men and women professional golfers. *Am J Sports Med.* 1989;17:782–787.

4. Meister K, Andrews JR. Classification and treatment of rotator cuff in the overhand athlete. *J Orthop Sports Phys Ther.* 1993;18:413–421.

5. Rowe CR, Pierce DS, Clark JG: Voluntary dislocation of the shoulder. A preliminary report on a clinical electromyographic and psychiatric study of twenty-six patients. *J Bone Joint Surg [Am].* 1973; 55:455–460.

6. Caillet R: *Shoulder Pain,* 2nd ed. Philadelphia, Pa: FA Davis, 1981.

7. Elvey RL. Treatment of arm pain with abnormal brachial plexus tension. *Aust J Physiother.* 1986;32:225–230.

8. Wright H: Evaluation and management of thoracic outlet syndrome. In: Donatelli R, ed: Clinics in Physical Therapy—Physical Therapy of the Shoulder, 2nd ed. New York, NY: Churchill Livingstone, 1991.

9. Smith RL, Brunolli J: Shoulder kinesthesia after anterior glenohumeral joint dislocation. *Phys Ther.* 1989;69: 106–112.

10. Warner JP, Micheli LJ, Arslandian LE, et al. Patterns of flexibility, laxity and strength in normal shoulders with instability and impingement. *Am J Sports Med.* 1990; 18:366–375.

11. Culham E. The relationship of age and thoracic posture to the resting position and mobility of the shoulder complex. Kingston, Ont, Canada: Queen's University; 1992. PhD Thesis.

12. Paine RM, Voight M. The role of the scapula. *J Orthop Sports Phys Ther.* 1993;18:386–391.

13. Inman VT, Saunders JB, Abbott LC. Observations on the function of the shoulder joint. *J Bone Joint Surg.* 1944;26:1.

14. Maitland GD. *Peripheral Manipulation,* 3rd ed. Boston, Mass: Butterworth-Heinemann Ltd; 1991.

15. Peat M: Functional anatomy of the shoulder complex. *Phys Ther.* 1986;66:1855–1865.

16. Kamkar A, Irrgang JJ, Whitney SL. Nonoperative management of secondary shoulder impingement syndrome. *J Orthop Sports Phys Ther.* 1993;17:212–224.

17. Matzen FA, Thomas SC, Rockwood CA. Anterior Glenohumeral Instability. In: Rockwood CA, Matzen FA, eds. *The Shoulder.* Philadelphia, Pa: WB Saunders Co; 1990.

18. Kaada B. Treatment of peritendinitis calcarea of the shoulder by transcutaneous nerve stimulation. *Acupunct Electrother Res.* 1984; 9:115–125.

19. Portney LG, Sullivan PE. EMG Analysis of Ipsilateral and Contralateral Shoulder and Elbow Muscles During the Performance of PNF Patterns. Presented at the Annual Conference of the Society for Behavioral Kinesiology, Boston, Mass; 1980.

20. Sullivan PE, Portney LG. EMG activity of shoulder muscles during unilateral upper extremity PNF patterns. *Phys Ther.* 1980;60:283–288.

21. Mosely BJ, Jobe FW, Pink M, et al. EMG analysis of the scapular muscles during a shoulder rehabilitation program. *Am J Sports Med.* 1992;20:128–134.

22. Townsend H, Jobe FW, Pink M, et al. EMG analysis of the glenohumeral muscles during a baseball rehabilitation program. *Am J Sports Med.* 1991;19:264–272.

23. Astrand PO, Rodahl K. *Textbook of Work Physiology; Physiological Bases of Exercise.* New York, NY; McGraw-Hill; 1986.

EXAMPLE OF FLOW SHEET DOCUMENTATION _____

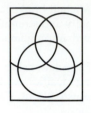

FUNCTIONAL LIMITATION

Decreased ability to perform ADL, particularly putting on coat, combing hair, and reaching overhead to perform occupational tasks.

Impairment	date	date	date	Tx. Goal
Decreased ROM of muscles and capsule into flexion, abduction, ext. and int. rotation and extension	O T			ROM WFL
Decreased scapula and GH stability	O T			Equal scapula position in quad. No lat. GH pain.
Decreased dynamic control	O T			Normal scap-hum rhythm
Decreased strength and endurance scap. and GH muscles	O T			↓Fatigue lift arm 10x against 10 lbs. 5/5 MMT

O = Objective measure, eg., ROM to 140° flexion; scapula 2 in. more lateral than other limb in quadruped, able to lift arm 5 times against 5 lb. resistance.

T = The treatment procedures, eg., joint mob. and HR to increase ROM, heat.

FUNCTIONAL OUTCOME:

Will be able to perform all occupational movements and activities of daily living.

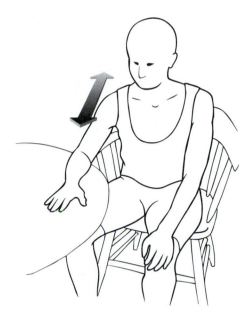

**Rock shoulder forward
and back over elbow.**

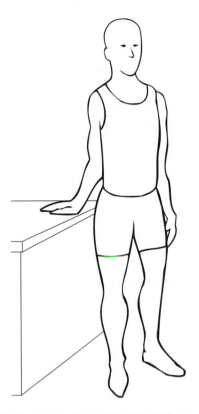

**Twist away from hand until you
feel some tightness.**

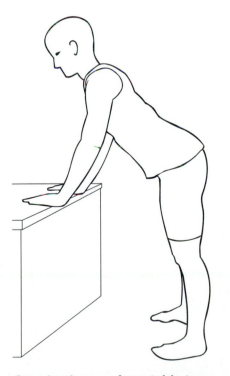

Step back away from table top.

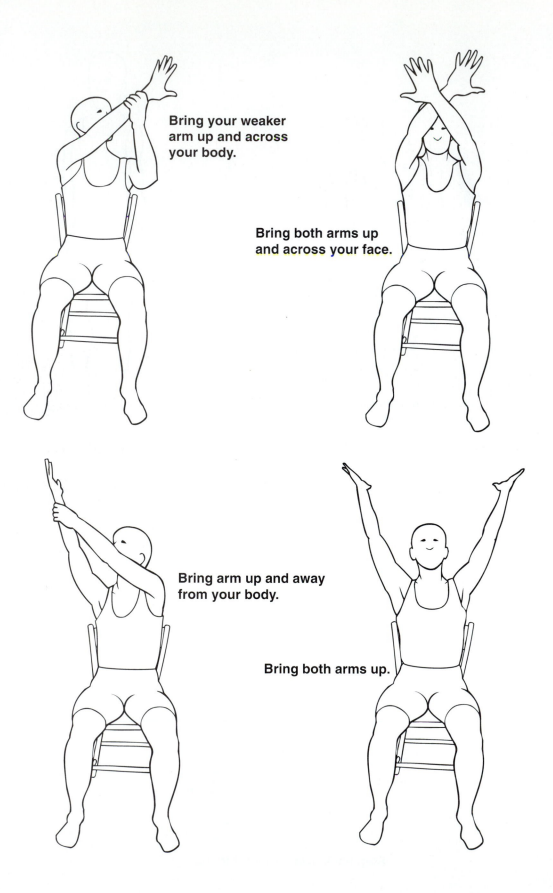

Bring your weaker arm up and across your body.

Bring both arms up and across your face.

Bring arm up and away from your body.

Bring both arms up.

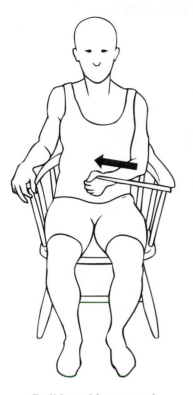

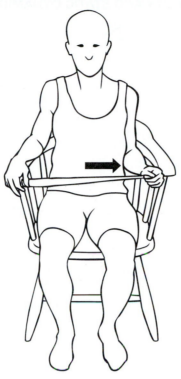

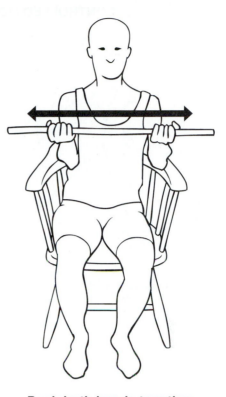

**Pull hand in toward
your stomach.**

**Push arm out away
from your body.**

**Push both hands together,
pull both hands apart.**

**Pinch shoulder blades
together. Hold position
for 3 breaths.**

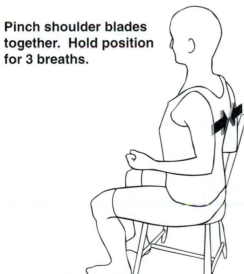

**Pinch shoulder blades
together. Pull elbows back.
Release slowly.**

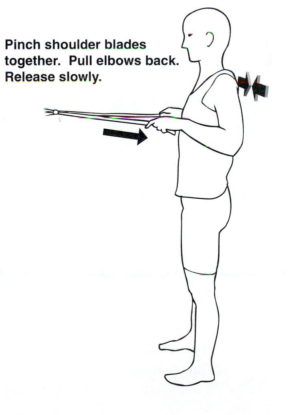

CONTROLLED MOBILITY AND STATIC DYNAMIC EXERCISES

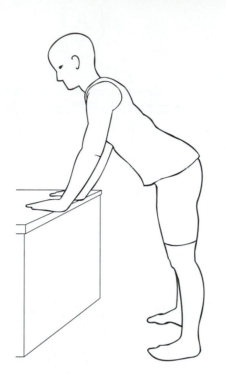

Stand with hands on counter or on a table. Rock forward over your hands then back.

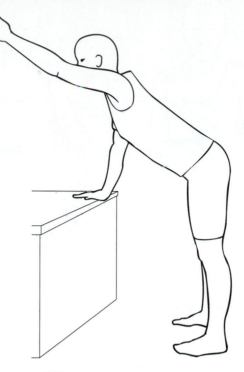

Lift your stronger arm up.

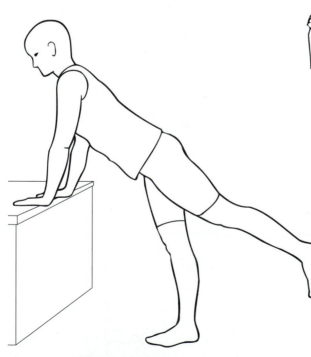

Lift one foot up.

Lift up against the band with your stronger arm, holding the band down with your weaker arm.

WEIGHT BEARING ON HANDS AND KNEES

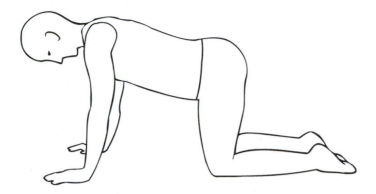

Rock forward and backward.

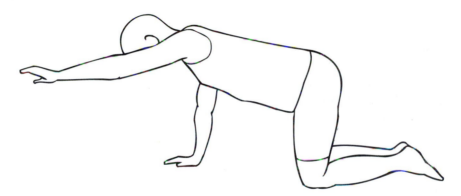

Lift your stronger arm up. Rock forward and backward over your weaker arm.

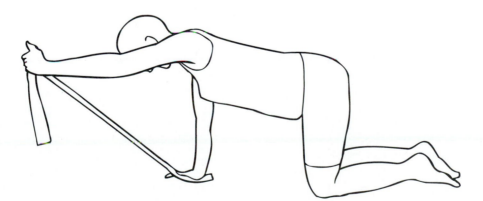

Lift your stronger arm up, hold the band down with your weaker arm.

CHAPTER 6

Knee

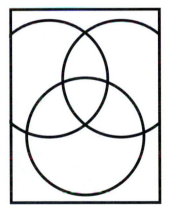

Knee dysfunction can result from various etiologies affecting a wide age range of patients (Fig. 6–1). Athletic injuries occur primarily in younger patients, whereas arthritic conditions are common in the older age group. The amount of functional limitation and the type of tissue involvement will determine the appropriateness of physical therapy and other disciplines.

Common diagnoses for which the patient may be referred to physical therapy include: ligamentous and capsular sprain, disruption of the meniscus, patellofemoral dysfunction, tendinitis, or arthritic conditions. In addition, referrals may follow surgical repair of ligamentous or capsular tears or avulsions, meniscectomy, partial or complete patellectomy, "shaving" the undersurface of the patella, arthrotomy, partial or complete joint replacement, or relocation of the quadriceps or other tendons. Knee function can be affected not only by these conditions but by any problem that results in prolonged immobilization of the lower extremity.

Independent ambulation on all surfaces is the functional outcome desired with most knee conditions. Many persons may be limited in weight bearing, have difficulty walking on uneven surfaces, climbing and descending stairs, moving between sitting and standing, and increasing the speed of ambulation. These limitations may be due to various impairments, many of which can be improved with physical therapy, such as decreased mobility, decreased stability, malalignment of the articulations of the knee, and weakness or diminished control of quadriceps and hamstrings.

EVALUATION

The specific evaluative measures used by the therapist will depend on the patient's condition at the time of referral. During the evaluation, medical conditions, such as bone tumors, that can have adverse health consequences need to be ruled out.[1] Those impairments for which physical therapy is appropriate, most commonly those of biomechanical origin, need to be assessed to determine the impairments that contribute to the limitation and can be remedied by physical therapy.

Patient Report of Problem and Functional Limitations

The description of the problem is obtained from the patient. The medical record or referral may have additional information, particularly concerning surgical repair. The disability may have been caused by a traumatic incident or may have evolved gradually. Recent changes in activity level or type of shoes worn are noted. The extent to which activities of daily living (ADL) are limited is evaluated both by questioning and observation.

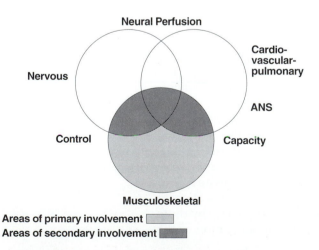

Areas of primary involvement ▢
Areas of secondary involvement ▮

Figure 6-1. Areas of primary and secondary involvement.

The patient is questioned as to the symptoms of the disability to begin to determine which tissues are involved and their reactivity. The description of pain or discomfort should include the type, frequency, and duration, and the activities or movements that aggravate or relieve the pain. The presence of knee discomfort with no other positive findings in that area indicates that a careful evaluation of hip function be included and a referral be made to an orthopedic surgeon.[2]

Environmental, Social, and Medical Factors

Occupational, social, and recreational activities, particularly repetitive, stressful movements such as climbing stairs, squatting, jogging, and dancing, are assessed. Medical conditions such as arthritis, diabetes, and obesity need to be noted. The results of special diagnostic tests and surgical history should be obtained.

Physical Systems

Musculoskeletal System

There needs to be an assessment of proximal and distal segments as well as the performance of an indepth examination of the involved knee. The findings are compared with those for the corresponding segments on the other limb.

Tissue Palpation. The structures of the knee are systematically palpated to determine tissue density, alignment, and points of increased tenderness and elevated temperature.

Range of Motion. Passive and active hip, knee, and ankle ranges are compared with these for the uninvolved limb. Malalignment, laxity, or tightness at the hip and ankle may transmit abnormal biomechanical forces through the knee and result in tissue stress, particularly during weight bearing.[3]

Assessment of knee motion includes osteokinematic movements of knee flexion and extension and arthrokinematic movements of the patella in cephalo–caudal and medial–lateral directions, anterior–posterior and rotational gliding of the tibia on the femur, and gliding of the fibula on the tibia.[4] Findings may include tightness, stiffness, or laxity in contractile and noncontractile structures. The direction of laxity may direct the assessment of specific ligamentous structures. Care must be taken that the amount of force is not excessive to avoid further damage to tissues.

Alignment. The angular alignment of the patellofemoral and femorotibial joints is assessed.[5,6] These values are considered in conjunction with those of the hip, ankle, and foot in non–weight-bearing and particularly weight-bearing postures. Abnormal alignment may increase tissue stress over time and, with repetitive strain, result in clinically significant symptoms. For example, tightness in the lateral muscular and fascial structures or weak medial musculature may result in abnormal patellar tracking during knee motion. The unequal patellar pressure against the femoral condyles may aggravate symptoms during resisted movement through range. Pain may be evident when lifting or raising from the flexed position or when going up or down stairs. Involvements of contractile tissues and noncontractile tissues and medial structures and lateral structures are differentiated to determine the appropriate treatment plan. If, for example, lateral patellar tracking occurs during passive knee flexion, the flexibility and length of the lateral capsule and iliotibial band are implicated. If, however, lateral tracking occurs primarily during active extension, vastus medialis control may be more involved. Other alignment abnormalities that can affect the knee include unequal hip rotations and excessive pronation or hindfoot valgus, for which stretching the hip or strengthening the medial ankle structures and posting wedges or inserts in the shoe may be indicated. Weight-bearing activities are assessed with frequently worn shoes on and off to determine functional alignment.

Girth Measurements. The circumference of the leg can be measured at the knee and at various proximal and distal points to assess the presence of edema, swelling, and atrophy.

Movement Control

Strength. The strength of the knee musculature can be assessed in many ways.[7,8] Of functional concern is the ability to perform fast reversals of controlled concentric and eccentric contractions of the quadriceps and hamstrings, which normally occur during weight-bearing activities. The assessment of the pre-

requisite muscle functions can be guided by the stages of control.

Mobility–ROM. Range of motion (ROM) has been assessed with the measurement of musculoskeletal structures. The therapist needs to be aware of ROM requirements for anticipated functional activities.[9,10]

Mobility–Initiation. Immediately following surgery, patients may have difficulty voluntarily activating the quadriceps because of reflexive inhibition from pain and joint edema. When the pain subsides, most patients are capable of activating the quadriceps to some extent but usually have difficulty with the oblique portion of the vastus medialis (VMO).[5] VMO activity is assessed by palpating the patella's superior medial border and observing patella tracking during an active contraction or by use of electromyographic (EMG) biofeedback.

Stability–Holding. The patient should be able to sustain a "quad set" for at least 10 seconds without fatigue,[11] which can be noted as "flickering" of the muscle. The inability to contract in the shortened range and the active lag commonly found during leg raising may be due to adaptive lengthening, pain, or decreased ability to activate a sufficient number of motor units to sustain the contraction. Sufficient stretch sensitivity of muscle spindles is a prerequisite to appropriate muscle responses.[12]

Stability–Maintenance of Weight Bearing. The ability to maintain the knee in a neutral position during weight-bearing activities requires isometric contraction of both the quadriceps and hamstrings. The prerequisites for postural stability are the previous stages of control: sufficient ROM to assume a position and the ability to sustain an isometric contraction while non–weight-bearing. If quadriceps or hamstring control is lacking or position sense diminished, many patients will hyperextend the knee and stabilize with capsular and ligamentous structures, causing increased stress on these tissues.[13–15] Postural stability is commonly assessed in standing with gradual increases in the amount of weight bearing on the limb as tolerated. Patients may be able to control the knee position, for example, with 50% weight bearing for short durations but may demonstrate difficulty noted as hyperextension or buckling with 75% or 100% weight bearing for 10 seconds.

Controlled Mobility. The ability of the quadriceps and hamstrings to contract concentrically and eccentrically through range in weight-bearing positions indicates the presence of controlled mobility. Movements such as short-arc squats, ascending and descending stairs, and moving between sitting and standing are performed repeatedly during the assessment while knee alignment is observed. If movements can be performed with control and without pain, the activities are repeated with increased speed. Increased "flickering" in the quadriceps or reduced smoothness of the movement denotes fatigue or weakness. Hamstring eccentric control near full knee extension is essential to protect the ligamentous and capsular structures from overstretching.

Static–Dynamic. Unilateral weight bearing increases the body-weight resistance through the supporting limb. Unilateral standing is assessed statically, then dynamically by having the patient shift weight onto the affected limb, control a squat, or balance on a balance board. Control can be further challenged by weight bearing on the ball or heel of the foot, which decreases the base of support (BoS).

Skill. A **gait evaluation** is incorporated within the skill stage. The control of the timing and sequencing of movement is assessed during the performance of functional activities such as walking or jogging. If appropriate, the "cutting" or lunging movements that occur during sports activities should be observed. Previously assessed problems such as lack of ROM, pain, or reduced movement control may be manifested as unequal weight bearing and stride length, and altered cadence. Bilateral equality ascending and, particularly, descending stairs is assessed.

Mechanical devices can be used to measure torque, work, and power.[8] An isokinetic assessment will provide various information, including the amount of peak torque and the range in which it occurs, the smoothness of the contraction, and the time required to reverse antagonists. During the assessment, the speed of movement must be commensurate with the amount of tissue healing and the patient's general exercise capacity. For example, slow speeds, which increase the intensity of effort, may be indicated only if the tissues are well healed and the cardiovascular pulmonary (CVP) system can cope with that intensity of effort. Weights can be used to assess the ability to resist one maximum effort or repetitions of various intensities. Assessing repetitive activity at less than maximum effort will measure the aerobic power needed for most functional activities.

Sensation. Particularly important for function is the sensory input from the joint and, particularly, muscle receptors that monitor the knee position and reflexively activate the surrounding quadriceps and hamstrings.[13–15] The assessment of passive and active position sense is performed to detect proprioceptive loss.

Movement Capacity

The capacity to perform functional activities requires muscle endurance and general aerobic ability. Muscle endurance is measured by the ability to sustain a "quad set" for at least 30 seconds and to perform some of the previously assessed control measures repeatedly and with longer duration.[16,17] For example, the patient can perform 10 short-arc squats unilaterally before being limited by muscle fatigue or pain; the patient can move between sitting and standing with equal weight bearing five times. Endurance also may be measured on isokinetic devices by determining the number of repetitions or the length of time before peak torque is reduced by half.[18] General body endurance can be measured on an upper-body ergometer when lower-extremity impairments are present.

Functional Activities

Assessment of ADL may reveal limitations in dressing—for example, in donning socks or shoes. The patient may also demonstrate difficulty with sitting, standing, or more strenuous activities. Functional limitations are commonly the result of multiple impairments including deficits in both movement control and capacity (Fig. 6–2). To determine the achievable functional outcomes, the therapist must have certain knowledge to assess the extent to which the physical impairments can be improved. For example, how much range can be expected after a total knee replacement? How much muscle stability

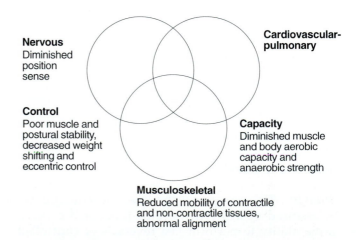

Figure 6–2. Commonly found impairments categorized according to physical systems.

TABLE 6–1. PHYSICAL IMPAIRMENTS CLASSIFIED ACCORDING TO STAGES OF MOVEMENT CONTROL WITHIN THE INTERVENTION MODEL

Mobility	Stability	Controlled Mobility	Skill
Decreased ROM resulting from reduced flexibility in the quadriceps, hamstrings, capsule, ligaments	Decreased or unbalanced muscle stability of quadriceps in shortened range and hamstrings in lengthened range Poor postural stability in standing	Impaired ability to control increased weight bearing Poor eccentric control in both quadriceps and hamstrings	Decreased speed of movement

ROM, range of motion.

can be achieved after a partial tear of the anterior cruciate ligament (ACL)? When procedures directed toward changing the physical impairments cannot provide satisfactory outcomes, other means must be considered, such as compensatory mechanisms and modification of the environment. To continue with the above two examples, if knee range cannot be increased, function can be improved by a raised toilet seat; stability and function of an unstable knee may be improved by an orthotic device; stair climbing technique can be altered to minimize stress and knee buckling.

The impairments found during the evaluation are transposed into the classifications of the intervention model so the treatment plan can be developed (Table 6–1).

INTERVENTION PLAN

Special Considerations. The quadriceps, like most muscles, are composed of two main categories of extrafusal muscle fibers: type I and type II. The type I, slow-twitch fibers have a low threshold of stimulation, do not easily fatigue, and are recruited during postural and aerobic activities.[17] After prolonged immobilization, these fibers tend to atrophy, reducing the ability to sustain an isometric contraction in the shortened range.[19] Clinically this deficit may be reported as quadriceps fatigue and an inability to control knee position. Increases in pain with the repeated performance of functional activities may be noted. Throughout the entire rehabilitative process the improvement of quadriceps control and the capacity to sustain movement is essential. To improve **control** of this "postural" muscle during initial stages of the rehabilitative process, low-intensity isometric contractions in shortened ranges are performed to increase the stretch sensitivity of muscle spindles. This ability is required before increasing inhibitory influences, which can be produced by the application of prolonged stretch and weight bearing. To minimize inhibitory effects, full unprotected weight bearing

should not be performed until the quadriceps muscle can sustain isometric contractions in shortened ranges. The **capacity** to sustain the contraction requires sufficient circulatory supply, and the ability to extract and utilize oxygen and nutrients which is developed with low-intensity, long-duration contractions.[17]

The intervention procedures are divided into three phases: initial, middle, and advanced. The goals presented at the beginning of each level indicate the focus of each treatment progression (Fig. 6–3).

Initial Phase

The goals of the initial phase, which may include postoperative care, are (Table 6–2):

▶ To facilitate quadriceps control so that a straight leg raise (SLR) can be performed to move the limb safely in and out of bed.

▶ To increase ROM.

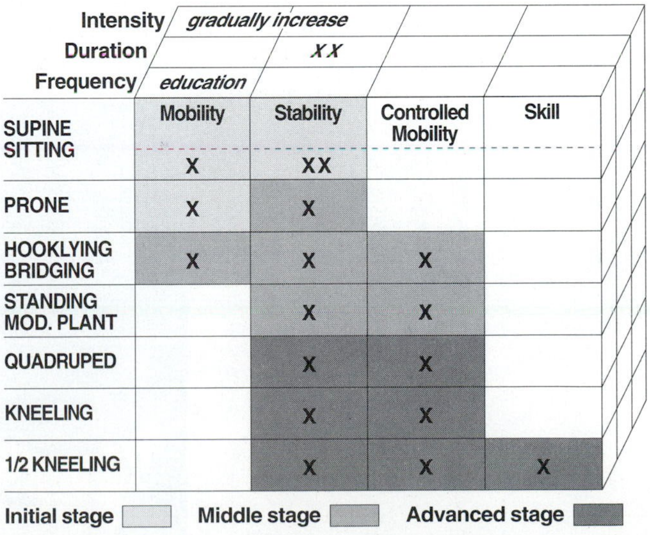

Figure 6–3. Intervention model including all treatment procedures.

TABLE 6–2. TREATMENT GOALS THAT CAN BE ACHIEVED WITHIN THE DIFFERENT STAGES OF CONTROL

Mobility		Stability	Skill
▶ ROM	▶ INITIATION	▶ MUSCLE	Ambulation with assistive device
Reduce pain, reduce edema, increase tissue extensibility	Facilitate: isometric quads, VMO in shortened range, isotonic hamstrings in lengthened range	Sustain: quad set for 10 seconds in shortened range for 5–10 repetitions, hamstring contraction in lengthened range	

ROM, range of motion; VMO, vastus medialis oblique.

▶ To strengthen the trunk, upper extremities, and uninvolved lower extremity as needed.

▶ To promote ambulation with appropriate weight bearing and use of assistive devices.

Acute

Mobility–ROM. This may be limited by pain and swelling during initial treatments (Table 6–3). Interventions may include the techniques of prolonged ice, neutral warmth, transcutaneous nerve stimulation (TNS), or other electrical modalities to block the pain cycle. Ice, compression, and elevation may help reduce or limit swelling in or around the joint. Because an increase in pain is usually indicative of tissue stress, treatment procedures are performed within the patient's pain tolerance. To reduce further tissue trauma that can occur if the pain threshold has been raised by modalities or pharmacological agents, the therapist must proceed with caution during ROM and strengthening procedures.

Mobility–Initiation of Active Movement. Depending on the injury or type of surgery, the initial goals may

TABLE 6–3. ASSOCIATION AMONG PHYSICAL IMPAIRMENTS, INVOLVED TISSUES, AND TREATMENT OPTIONS

Impairment	Tissue	Treatment
Edema Swelling		Compression, ice, elevation, e-stim, low-intensity mobilization and isometric contractions
Pain	Joint, soft tissue	Heat or ice, improve alignment or flexibility, e-stim
Decreased extensibility		Heat, massage, hold relax, low intensity joint mobilization

be to initiate quadriceps contractions prior to teaching ambulation with an assistive device. The quadriceps ability must be sufficient to allow the patient to maneuver the leg in and out of bed. Posttraumatic or postsurgical pain and joint effusion may cause reflex inhibition of the quadriceps in addition to reducing ROM.[20,21] An **indirect approach** promoting overflow from intact, uninvolved areas may be the only way to initiate quadriceps contractions at this stage. This may be accomplished by resistance applied to: trunk patterns (Fig. 6–4), an extensor pattern of the un-

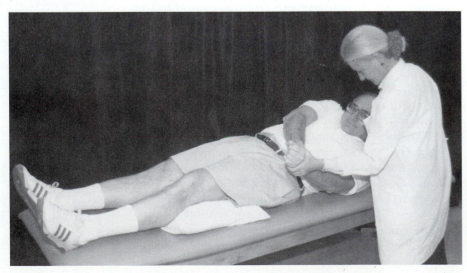

Figure 6–4. A: Supine; upper trunk pattern. T: TE.

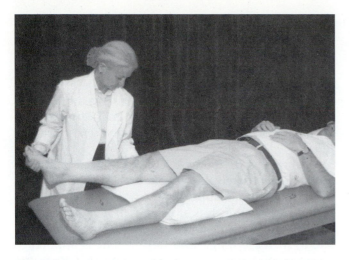

Figure 6–5. S: Supine; extensor pattern contralateral limb. T: TE.

involved lower extremity (Fig. 6–5), or bilateral dorsi or plantarflexion.[22,23] A secondary goal of these procedures is to strengthen the trunk and other extremities for ambulation.

A **direct approach** can be initiated once the patient has experienced the sensation of the quadriceps contraction and can voluntarily activate the quadriceps. Activation of knee extensors may be assisted by biofeedback, which will augment the sensation of muscle contraction. Quadriceps setting exercises and active terminal extension will promote initial phases of stability and knee control to begin assisted ambulation. Patients who have undergone surgical repair of ligamentous and capsular structures may require prolonged immobilization. However, when not contraindicated, isometric holding of the quadriceps can still be promoted and is an important goal of initial treatment sessions.

As healing progresses, treatment may be directed at further improving quadriceps control and ROM. In some cases ROM may be the most critical factor; in others, quadriceps control may be the primary goal while increases in ROM may need to be delayed until adequate healing occurs to cope with the stress of active or passive movement.

Subacute

Goal: To Increase Passive ROM

Procedure:

A: Sitting, supine, prone; unilateral knee extension and flexion, D1, D2

T: Hold relax (HR), contract relax (CR), joint mobilization, massage, heat, compression, ice

P: Low intensity, duration, and frequency according to tissue response

Normal mobility requires extensibility of both the noncontractile and contractile tissues. To achieve full passive osteokinematic movement into knee extension, hamstring length must be optimal, the tibia must rotate externally and glide anteriorly as well as roll on the femur and the patella must glide in a superior direction. For passive flexion, the quadriceps must be extensible, the patella must move in an inferior direction, and the tibia must rotate internally, glide, and roll posteriorly on the femur.[4]

To increase range, intervention needs to be directed at increasing the extensibility of the limiting contractile and noncontractile tissues. After the initial healing has occurred, heat applied at the depth of the involved tissue may be indicated before the application of procedures to elongate that tissue. However, heat may be contraindicated if an increase in swelling results. Techniques that reduce swelling may need to be continued as part of the program. To reduce adhesions between the skin and the underlying tissue, massage can be applied, but with caution to avoid separation of the healing tissue. To promote full mobility of the noncontractile fascial and joint tissues, massage, traction, joint mobilization, and rotational motions can be progressively applied. To promote full range in the contractile tissues, the techniques of HR, rhythmic stabilization (RS), and CR are indicated (see Chapter 3).

To gain range into **knee extension,** the extensibility of the hamstrings may need to be increased. The technique of choice is HR with the isometric contraction applied to the agonistic quadriceps (Fig. 6–6). Applied in this manner, HR can produce gains in hamstring length as well as promote an anterior glide of the tibia on the femur. Quadriceps control in the shortened range is also achieved with this technique, which is consistent with treatment goals. An alternative method for increasing the extensibility of the hamstrings is the direct application of HR to the hamstrings. This technique may be as effective in gaining range but does not promote the goal of improving isometric quadriceps contractions. Only when pain has subsided should CR, which emphasizes the rotatory component of the joint, be performed. With CR, a high-intensity isometric flexion and isotonic rotational force of hamstrings is produced. If CR is applied too early in the rehabilitation process, the rapid development of muscle tension and the rotatory movement may aggravate the patient's pain, resulting in unwanted splinting around the joint.

To increase range into **knee flexion,** extensibility of the quadriceps initially can be promoted by the

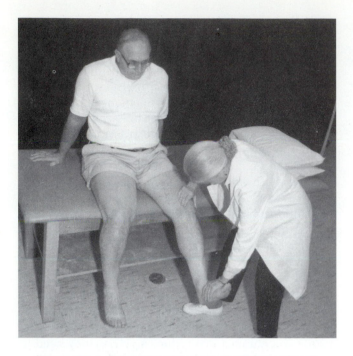

Figure 6–6. A: Sitting; knee extension. T: HR to quadriceps.

technique of HR applied to the agonistic hamstrings (Fig. 6–7).[24] During the hamstring contraction, the tibia glides posteriorly on the femur, enhancing the knee flexion motion. To gain range into knee flexion, we recommend that HR to the tight quadriceps **not** be performed for the following reasons: As range into knee flexion is gained, the quadriceps are placed in more lengthened ranges. This prolonged stretch cou-

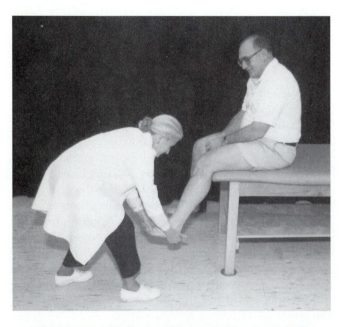

Figure 6–7. A: Sitting; knee flexion. T: HR to hamstrings.

pled with the addition of an isometric contraction may overly inhibit a weakened quadriceps. In addition, the quadriceps contraction with the knee in flexion may increase the compression of the patella on the femoral condyles. Although increased extensibility of the quadriceps is desired, excessive inhibition is not consistent with the treatment goal of increasing isometric control of the quadriceps in their shortened range.

To review, to increase knee ROM that is limited by decreased extensibility of muscle, HR to the agonist, or the muscle opposing the tight-muscle groups, is the treatment of choice. To gain movement into extension, HR to the agonistic quadriceps is appropriate; to increase range into flexion, HR is applied to the agonistic hamstrings. The technique of CR may be applied directly to the hamstrings to gain extensibility into extension when pain has decreased.

The mobility techniques are most frequently applied to a unilateral lower extremity pattern either in supine, sitting, or prone. The unilateral pattern allows the therapist to have more effective control of joint movement, since both manual contacts are placed on the involved limb. However, if voluntary contraction is limited, use of trunk or bilateral patterns can promote overflow to the involved limb to enhance muscular contractions and indirectly increase ROM. During the early stages of treatment following most ligamentous repairs, when rotational motions of the knee are contraindicated, flexion and extension are limited to straight plane movements. When internal or external rotation of the tibia on the femur can be emphasized, diagonal patterns can be incorporated into the program.

The **intensity** of resistance is usually limited to the minimal-to-moderate range as tissue healing occurs to avoid pain and minimize swelling. Producing pain can be counterproductive because it increases the tendency to abnormally guard or splint, reducing the muscle's extensibility and joint ROM.

In summary, the treatment goals that can be promoted during the initial stages of intervention include: 1) increased knee mobility–ROM by reducing pain, swelling, and increasing tissue extensibility; 2) initiation of active quadriceps contraction through indirect activation of the quadriceps if voluntary control is lacking; 3) initiation of stability by focusing on isometric contractions of the quadriceps in shortened ranges; 4) improved function of the trunk and uninvolved extremities. The treatment described in this section is appropriate for patients with postsurgical, posttraumatic, and degenerative conditions. Ambulation is performed only with assistive devices to limit the amount of weight bearing. Closed-chain activities should be minimized and carefully monitored during initial procedures. As quadriceps control is gained, weight-bearing activities can be emphasized.

Middle Phase

For many nonsurgical patients treatment may begin at this phase. Impairments and typical findings may include:

▶ Mobility–passive ROM: 210° to 90° limited by contractile and noncontractile tissue;

▶ Mobility–active ROM: quadriceps strength 3/5 although may lack active terminal extension; hamstrings 3/5 but with poor control in lengthened ranges;

▶ Stability of the muscle: quadriceps cannot sustain a quad set for longer than 10 seconds or against more than minimal weight;

▶ Stability in weight-bearing postures: quadriceps and hamstring contractions difficult to maintain with more than 50% body weight.

The treatment goals of the middle stage are:

▶ To further increase ROM.

▶ To increase quadriceps and hamstring isometric control in shortened and lengthened ranges respectively; improve isometric and isotonic control of both the quadriceps and hamstrings throughout range with emphasis in weight bearing.

▶ To increase power, strength, and endurance of the quadriceps and hamstrings.

The functional outcomes that may be achieved include:

▶ Ambulation without an assistive device on most surfaces.

▶ Stair climbing with use of the bannister.

▶ Independence in donning shoes and socks.

The ROM procedures described in the initial phase may need to continue, but if pain is diminished treatment may be more aggressive at this phase.

Treatment, although modified for the needs of each patient, also focuses on further increasing isometric control of the quadriceps and introducing weight-bearing postures in which stretch and the intensity and duration of the contractions can be increased.

Procedure:

A: Supine or long sitting, knee extension, and short-arc movements

T: Shortened held resisted contractions (SHRC), alternating isometrics (AI), rhythmic stabilization (RS), agonistic reversals (AR)

Isometric quadriceps contractions in the shortened range can be promoted with bilateral or unilateral movements. Combinations are chosen to enhance overflow from stronger segments. Isometric control is promoted with the sequence of stability techniques, SHRC, AI, and RS. AI and RS also promote hamstring control in lengthened ranges. *Holding a low-intensity isometric contraction in the shortened range for approximately 10 seconds will improve muscle spindle stretch sensitivity and reduce the active lag; holding up to 1 minute will improve the muscle's endurance.* As treatment progresses and more difficult procedures are attempted, sustained quad sets may need to be reemphasized to ensure muscle stability. If activity in the vastus medialis is specifically desired, as it may be for patients with patellofemoral dysfunction, diagonal resistance can be incorporated into the patterns to attempt to enhance muscle responses. In addition to exercise, taping may help to correct patellar alignment during ambulation.[5] With these patients, a treatment goal is to promote pain-free knee extension and flexion, which requires a neutral position of the patella. This is developed by balancing the medial and lateral structures during passive and active movements. Short-arc movements are emphasized before the range is gradually increased.

Home Program

The reader is referred to the visuals for the home exercises at the end of the chapter (pp. 154–158). At home the patient is instructed to put a pillow or bolster under the knee and extend the hip and knee (Fig. 6–8). An elastic band can be looped around the foot to resist short-arc quadriceps contractions, or the patient can extend the hip and knee against a band positioned at the foot, with another band providing resistance at the knee (Fig. 6–9).

When resisted movement through range is indicated, bilateral patterns in sitting and prone can be performed. When muscle strength is less than 3/5, the application of bilateral patterns in combination with gravity-assisted movement are the best options to maximize muscle contractions. Manual resistance can be applied throughout range varying the intensity as needed. Resistance is important for the facilitation of alpha-gamma coactivation, proprioceptive feedback and enhancement of a muscle's response. If

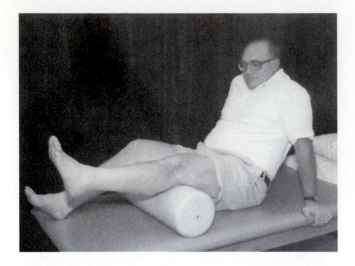

Figure 6–8. A: Long sitting; unilateral knee extension, support under knee. T: SHRC.

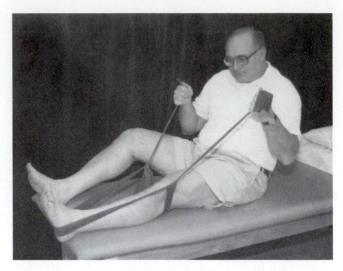

Figure 6–9. A: Long sitting; knee extension, short-arc quad. T: SHRC → AR with elastic resistance.

the movement is resisted by gravity, manual assistance may be required. Excessive resistance, particularly to weakened postural muscles, can reduce the muscle's ability to overcome the resistance and result in inhibition through stimulation of peripheral receptors such as the Golgi tendon organs (GTOs), Renshaw cells, and possibly spindle secondary endings.[21] If the muscle grade is 3/5, gravity-assisted, manually resisted activities may be appropriate when repetitive exercise is performed. When the muscle grade is 4/5 or above, gravity plus manual or mechanical forces are indicated.

Procedure:

A: Prone; bilateral symmetrical knee flexion and extension

T: Slow reversal hold (SRH), repeated contractions (RC), timing for emphasis (TE), agonistic reversals (AR)

In prone, gravity assists knee extension and resists knee flexion. As the knee flexes toward the shortened range, the hamstrings may become actively insufficient and the quadriceps, particularly the rectus femoris, can become passively insufficient. The hamstrings can be resisted against gravity through the full range of knee flexion with strengthening techniques of SRH, RC, or TE. Eccentric control of the hamstrings can be promoted with the technique of agonist reversals through increments of range with emphasis on lengthened ranges (Fig. 6–10). In comparison to movements performed in sitting, the hip is maintained in extension. Thus, when

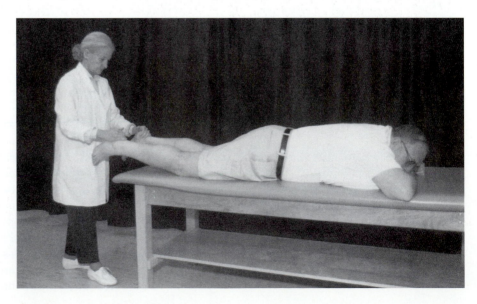

Figure 6–10. A: Prone; bilateral symmetrical knee flexion. T: AR emphasizing lengthened range.

quadriceps contraction is resisted, active insufficiency of the rectus femoris does not occur, allowing this portion of the muscle to assist with knee extension.

Procedure:

A: Sitting; bilateral symmetrical or reciprocal knee extension and flexion
T: SRH, slow reversal (SR), TE, AR

In sitting, active insufficiency of the rectus femoris may occur during knee extension; full knee extension may be limited by passive insufficiency of the hamstrings. Bilateral symmetrical (Fig. 6–11) or reciprocal (Fig. 6–12) combinations can be easily performed in this posture to promote overflow from the contralateral limb. For example, quadriceps on the stronger limb can be used to facilitate quadriceps on the weaker limb, a bilateral symmetrical combination, or hamstrings on the stronger limb can reinforce the quadriceps contraction, a reciprocal combination. Choice of a symmetrical or reciprocal pattern depends on which combination provides the best response. The techniques of RC and TE first emphasize strengthening of the quadriceps in the shortened ranges of knee extension. Resistance is then applied through increments of range until resistance through full range of knee extension can be accomplished. Bilateral and reciprocal combinations and strengthening techniques of RC, TE, and AR can be applied to improve hamstring as well as quadriceps control, but with emphasis on more lengthened ranges for the hamstrings.

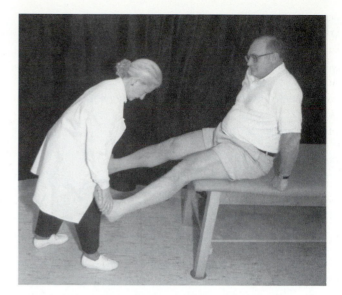

Figure 6–11. A: Sitting; bilateral symmetrical knee extension. T: TE.

Procedure:

A: Sitting; unilateral patterns
T: AR, SRH, SR
P: Increasing speed

Unilateral movements in sitting are used to emphasize more specific control of the quadriceps and hamstrings. For example, emphasis can be placed on concentric–eccentric quadriceps control near the shortened range of knee extension with the technique of AR. During this movement, external rotation of the tibia in relation to the femur and diagonal resistance

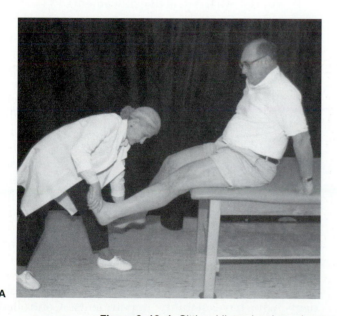

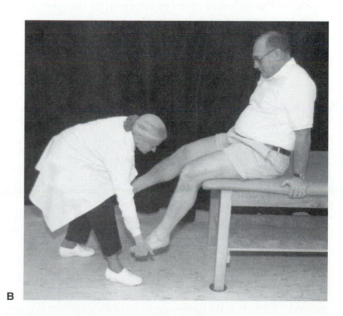

A   **B**

Figure 6–12. A: Sitting; bilateral reciprocal patterns. T: TE on **(A)** knee extension; **(B)** knee flexion.

can be emphasized with manual contacts to enhance VMO activity.

For those patients experiencing difficulty with quick activation of the antagonistic muscle, reversal movements are indicated. The speed of the reversal can be increased and resistance decreased to emphasize phasic control and automatic responses throughout the range.

Procedure:

A: Modified plantigrade or standing; bilateral progressing to unilateral weight bearing, knee straight progressing to short-arc squats

T: AI, RS → SRH → AR

An increase in proprioceptive sensitivity of the quadriceps and hamstrings is a goal during all procedures. This sensory motor connection is promoted initially, along with further enhancement of muscle spindle stretch sensitivity during the application of low-intensity, long-duration contractions. Non–weight-bearing activities may be less difficult for the patient to perform in early stages than the more challenging closed-chain postures where body weight must be controlled. In weight-bearing postures, knee position must be carefully monitored for hyperextension or oscillation. These abnormalities suggest that the posture may be too difficult and that less-challenging activities are indicated.

When it becomes evident that the patient can tolerate the resistance of weight-bearing, isometric control of the quadriceps and hamstrings can be promoted in the shortened range of knee extension in **modified plantigrade** or **standing.** In these postures, isometric resistance can be applied to the pelvis or knee to improve stability with the techniques of AI and RS and controlled movement with AR. In addition to manual resistance, pulleys, a sport cord, or elastic bands can be used to resist quadriceps and hamstring contractions (Figs. 6–13, 6–14). The intensity of the body-weight resistance can be increased by weight shifting over the involved limb, then lifting the uninvolved limb: controlled mobility to static–dynamic control. Isometric resistance in the shortened range is followed by short-range eccentric–concentric contractions. The goals of these procedures are to develop the quadriceps ability to eccentrically control body weight and hamstring ability to eccentrically control the rate of knee extension. The challenge is increased further by having the patient repeat these activities on a balance board (Fig. 6-15). To increase the reliance on proprioception for balance control, the patient can perform the above sequence with eyes closed. Additional challenge to proprioception is pro-

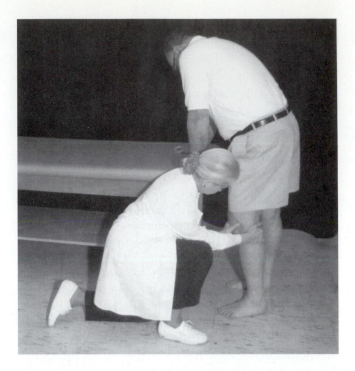

Figure 6–13. A: Modified plantigrade. T: AI to stabilize knee.

vided when the patient stands on foam. Automatic control is promoted by throwing and catching a ball while on the balance board. Quick movements can be promoted under controlled conditions by bouncing, jumping, then running on a small trampoline.

Procedure:

A: Bridging; pelvic motions, varying knee range, unilateral weight bearing

T: AI, RS, SRH, AR, active movement

Bridging incorporates stretch to the quadriceps and weight bearing through the knee joint. The amount of stretch is varied by the position of the knee and the weight bearing is increased by lateral shifting and lifting of the *uninvolved* leg. The activity, the techniques, and parameters can be varied to change the stress. To illustrate, the activity can be varied by changing the BoS from a solid surface to a moveable support such as a ball. For further challenge the patient can be positioned on elbows or hands. When the lever arm is lengthened by extending the knee, increased hamstring control is required.[25] In this posture, stability is first promoted by the techniques of AI and RS, with resistance applied at the pelvis, progressing to the knee, and then the ankle (Fig. 6–16). Muscular stability can be promoted with the knee in varying ranges of flexion, an important factor for patients who have stability impairments. Controlled

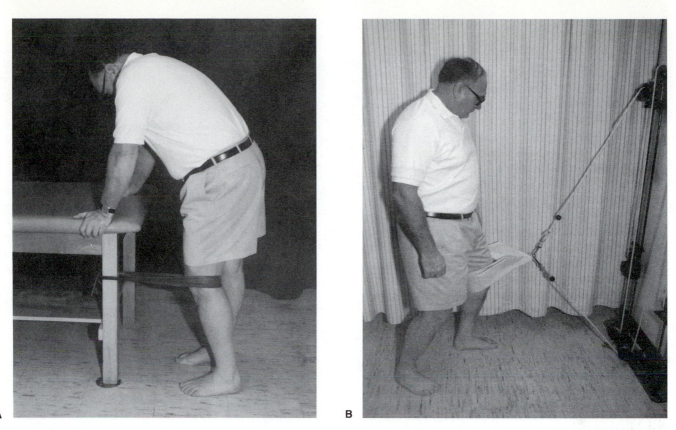

Figure 6–14. A: Modified plantigrade; short-arc squats. T: AR with **(A)** elastic resistance; **(B)** pulley resistance.

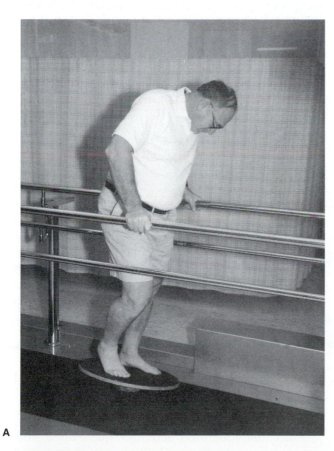

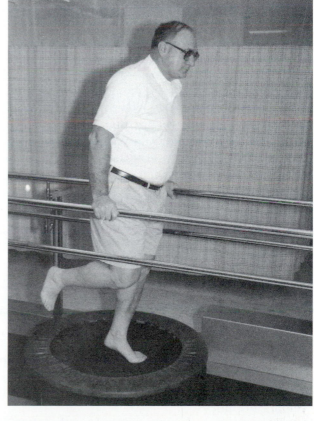

Figure 6–15. (A) A: Standing, on a balance board. T: Active movement. **(B)** A: Standing, jumping on trampoline. T: Active movement.

mobility or weight shifting is promoted further with SRH to pelvic rotation and lateral shifting. AR will promote concentric–eccentric control of the hip extensors and hamstrings as the hips are slowly lowered to the supporting surface. This hamstring control is critical for those with translatory ligamentous instability. Isometric resistance can be applied in a symmetrical or reciprocal fashion with the knee in various ranges to further enhance knee stability. Excessive resistance applied in the shortened range of knee flexion often results in cramping of the hamstrings and should be avoided.

More difficult procedures can include quick alternating weight bearing on the lower extremities, running in place, then laterally with the knee position varying from flexion to near full extension. These procedures will simulate the fast bursts of muscular activity that are needed for running. These advanced procedures are appropriate for patients returning to strenuous activities and may not be suitable for the older or sedentary population.

Advanced Phase

At this phase the isometric and isotonic strength of the quadriceps and hamstrings have improved, although some difficulty with active terminal extension may still remain. Complete ROM into flexion may be lacking. Pain is usually diminished and not a factor.

Return to full function should be achieved at this stage. The treatment goals of the advanced stage are:

▶ To further improve eccentric control of the quadriceps and hamstrings in progressively more difficult weight-bearing postures.

▶ To promote advanced movements with the normal timing, sequencing, and speed of responses.

▶ To restore normal quadriceps:hamstring ratio.

▶ To increase muscle endurance.

Functional outcomes may include:

▶ Ambulation on all surfaces.

▶ Step-over-step ascent and descent of stairs.

▶ Running in all directions.

Strength and endurance of the quadriceps and hamstrings can be promoted with resistance supplied by mechanical devices such as isokinetic equipment, weights, or pulleys.

The mat procedures suggested for this stage incorporate knee flexion and weight bearing into most of the activities. Therefore these procedures probably would not be indicated for those complaining of patellofemoral pain or for whom range into knee flexion beyond 90° is not possible.

The progression of activities at this stage is designed to further improve quadriceps control by gradually increasing and combining: (1) the amount of weight bearing on the involved limb, (2) the prolonged stretch on the quadriceps, and (3) the amount of body weight borne directly on the quadriceps tendon. All three factors tend to increase inhibitory influences to the quadriceps.[26] When the postures and the movements performed in those postures are altered, the effects of inhibitory influences can be gradually increased. This progression is important for those patients still experiencing difficulty controlling the lowering of body weight, as occurs during stair descent or stepping down off a high curb.

The postures discussed in this section are sequenced according to the progressive difficulty of demands placed upon the quadriceps. At this point in the treatment program, standing and modified plantigrade have already been incorporated to improve quadriceps–hamstring activity near the shortened range of knee extension. An increase in body-weight resistance has been achieved by lateral weight shifting and unilateral weight bearing. In the advanced stage of treatment, weight bearing on a partially flexed knee is added. When the body-weight resistance is increased, the challenge to maintain the knee position increases as the quadriceps are placed on stretch.

Procedure:
   A: Half-kneeling, involved limb anterior
   T: AI, RS, SRH, AR

Half-kneeling, with the involved leg placed anteriorly, results in 90° of knee flexion (Fig. 6–17). As with bridging, weight bearing on the quadriceps tendon is not a factor. As the patient rocks forward over the involved limb, the amount of knee flexion and the amount of weight bearing on that limb increases. Weight shifting can be promoted with the controlled mobility technique of SR.

Procedure:
   A: Quadruped, kneeling, half-kneeling involved limb posterior
   T: AI, RS, SRH, AR

The following three activities, quadruped, kneeling, and half-kneeling with the involved limb posterior, require weight bearing on the involved knee. A

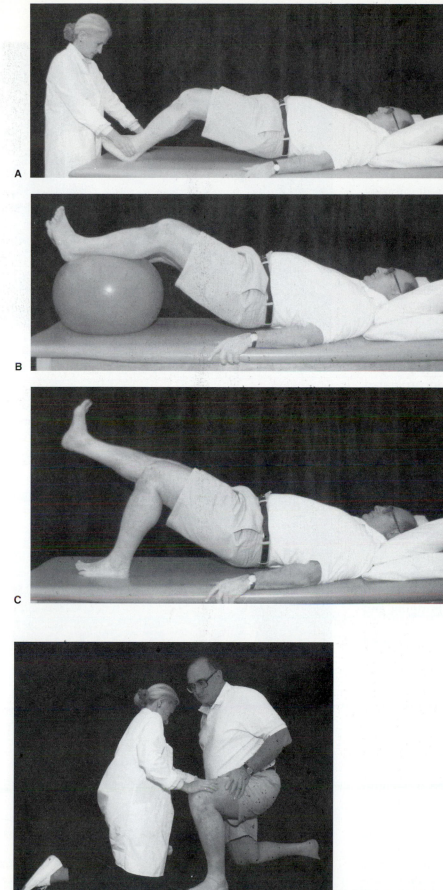

Figure 6–16. (A) A: Bridging, knees in 30° of flexion. T: RS, manual contacts on ankles. **(B)** A: bridging, weight bearing on ball. T: active movement. **(C)** A: bridging, unilateral weight bearing. T: active movement.

A

B

C

Figure 6–17. A: Half-kneeling, involved limb anterior, T: AI → SR → AR.

pillow or piece of foam placed under the knee may alleviate any discomfort caused by the pressure.

In **quadruped,** the knee is flexed to 90° and can be further flexed by rocking in a posterior direction; weight bearing occurs on the quadriceps tendon, and body-weight resistance can be accentuated by weight shifting onto the affected knee and lifting the unaffected limb. AI and RS can be applied to the pelvis for enhancement of muscular stability around the knee. SRH superimposed on rocking motions will improve both isotonic control as well as functional range of motion. Static–dynamic activities will increase the stability demands of the involved limb when it is weight bearing; dynamic control of the involved limb is promoted when resisted isotonic movements are performed. Resistance can be applied to the dynamic limb either manually or mechanically with pulleys or weighted cuffs. If the inhibitory influences produced by these procedures appear to reduce quadriceps control, a return to resisted terminal extension exercises in supine may be indicated. For many patients, terminal extension exercises must be incorporated into all stages of rehabilitation.

Kneeling is more strenuous than quadruped because of the increased weight borne on the quadriceps tendon. As in the other postures, stability is enhanced first with AI and RS; controlled mobility with SRH is used to promote concentric control of antagonists; concentric–eccentric quadriceps activity is promoted with AR through increments of range until the heelsitting position is attained. If full range is lacking, mobility techniques can be applied in non–weight-bearing postures to elongate particular tissues. The amount of quadriceps activity that occurs during these kneeling procedures seems to be greater than in the previous procedures performed in bridging and quadruped.

Half-kneeling with the involved limb placed posteriorly is a progression from kneeling. More weight bearing occurs on the supporting limb than in the previous postures, making rocking in half-kneeling quite difficult for some patients (Fig. 6–18).

For those who are returning to strenuous athletic events, additional procedures to improve the speed of quadriceps activity are necessary. Although fast bursts of activity can be promoted by some mechanical devices,[18] timing exercises performed in weight-bearing postures are important to stimulate the control needed for most athletic endeavors and to emphasize a specificity of training. Fast alternating weight bearing, such as described in bridging, can be performed in standing or the patient can practice jumping up and down a small curb (Fig. 6–19) or running on a mini trampoline. Parallel bars may be used initially for support while balancing on a board.

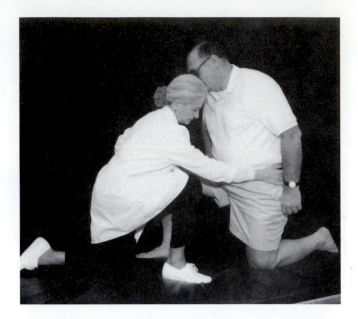

Figure 6–18. A: Half-kneeling, involved limb posterior. T: AI → SR → AR.

These procedures are strenuous and require normal quadriceps strength, completely free range, good eccentric control, and the ability to produce fast bursts of quadriceps activity. Sideward, backward,

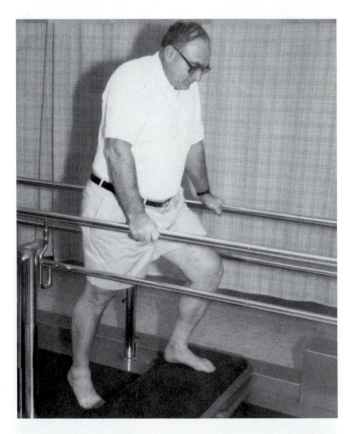

Figure 6–19. A: Standing, jumping up a curb. T: Active movement.

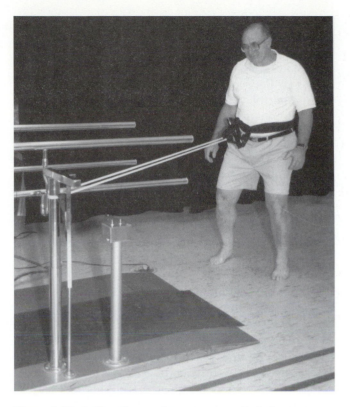

Figure 6–20. A: Standing, cutting movements. T: Active movement or against sports cord.

rotational, and cutting movements may be added to further simulate the control needed for the specific athletic event. These movements can be practiced actively, against resistance of a sports cord (Fig. 6–20) or combined with endurance training on a treadmill. The high degree of control needed to perform these last exercises make them the culmination of most physical therapy treatments, and they should be attempted only toward the end of rehabilitation.

▶ *SUMMARY*

To summarize, the sequence of procedures for the rehabilitation of a patient with knee disability has been:

1. To increase ROM using techniques to increase tissue extensibility.
2. To increase quadriceps control by first emphasizing holding in the shortened range, then progressing to resistance of concentric–eccentric contractions through range with emphasis on weight bearing.
3. To increase the stress on the quadriceps by progressing the influences of weight bearing and prolonged stretch.
4. To improve hamstring control to stabilize the knee posteriorly and to provide controlled deceleration.
5. To improve stability, controlled mobility, and skill levels of control.

CLINICAL PERSPECTIVE _____

Common Physical Impairments Associated with Knee Dysfunction

1. Problem: Active lag of quadriceps during leg raising.

Analysis:
a. The muscles are inhibited by swelling and pain in the knee.
b. The muscle may be adaptively lengthened following prolonged positioning in flexion.
c. Alpha-gamma coactivation may be deficient.

Solution:
a. To reduce the swelling: compression, ice, elevation, and electrical modalities
b,c. To enhance muscle shortening and alpha-gamma coactivation, a SHRC is performed in progressively more shortened ranges. Because the patient may have difficulty voluntarily isolating the quadriceps contraction, the response is enhanced with overflow by performing the exercise bilaterally and including hip extension. This can be accomplished by encouraging the patient to push the knees down into a firm pillow placed under the knees rather than to tighten the knee cap and lift the leg up. To enhance gamma activation and shortening of the intrafusal fibers, the contraction is maintained for 10 seconds. This should be performed frequently throughout the day, for example 10 repetitions, three or more times per day. When the "quad set" can be maintained, the duration of the contraction is increased to improve the muscles aerobic endurance. The intensity of the contraction under both time conditions should not exceed 40% to 50% of a maximum effort to promote gamma firing and to ensure that the contraction is primarily performed by type I motor units. As the efficiency of motor unit activation occurs and aerobic ability improves, resistance can be increased by the use of elastic bands or cuff weights. Progressive increase in the body-weight resistance follows with a simultaneous increase in approximation force to facilitate the response. Isometric and short-arc quadriceps contractions are resisted further by progressive elastic resistance in the standing or modified plantigrade position. Biofeedback may augment the patient's response.

Activation in the shortened range can also be resisted during bilateral symmetrical or reciprocal knee extension movements in sitting. The technique of TE can enhance overflow from ipsilateral dorsiflexors and from the stronger contralateral limb.

2. Problem: Poor eccentric control of the quadriceps noted during stair descent.

Analysis:
a. The quadriceps may be tight, resulting in increased patellar compression into the femoral condyles, as the quadriceps are lengthened during eccentric contractions.
b. Abnormal patellar tracking can result from an imbalance of passive extensibility of the quadriceps and iliotibial band or tensor fascia lata, or an imbalance of strength of medial and lateral portions of the quadriceps. Both can increase asymmetric pressure on the femoral condyles and result in pain.
c. The combined inhibitory influences of body weight plus stretch may reduce quadriceps strength.

Solution:
a. Increase the overall length of the quadriceps with HR in non–weight-bearing postures such as in supine, sitting, or prone to reduce patellar compression.
b. Determine if the abnormal tracking results from passive as opposed to active elements. Increase extensibility of range-limiting tissues; if decreased medial control exists, facilitate vastus medialis during SHRC as in problem **1.**
c. The stretch sensitivity of the muscle spindle needs to be increased so the quadriceps can respond to the added demands of body-weight resistance in more lengthened ranges (see problem **1**). Resistance in shortened ranges is increased by gradually progressing from bilateral to unilateral weight bearing, either independently or in combination with external resistance. To gradually increase stretch, short-arc eccentric contractions in non–weight-bearing postures precede short-arc squats in upright postures. This last procedure is the most difficult because it combines body-weight resistance with stretch.

3. Problem: Hyperextended knee during standing and ambulation.

Analysis:
a. Poor quadriceps control.
b. Decreased range of ankle dorsiflexion.
c. Decreased position sense.
d. Poor hamstring control.

Solution:
a. To improve quadriceps control see problems **1** and **2 c.**

b. To increase range of ankle dorsiflexion combine heat to increase tissue extensibility with joint mobilization, HR, and prolonged passive stretch in modified plantigrade or in non–weight-bearing postures.
c. and **d.** Poor position sense and diminished hamstring control usually occur together. Position sense may be enhanced by increasing the muscle spindle feedback. To promote this control low-intensity isometric contractions are elicited in various portions of the range. Alternating isometrics are performed in non–weight-bearing and weight-bearing positions with the addition of other verbal and visual stimuli to promote low-intensity, long-duration quadriceps and hamstring contractions. To specifically enhance hamstring control, short-arc concentric–eccentric contractions can be performed against resistance in prone, modified plantigrade, standing, and bridging with the knees progressively in more extension. To challenge and further develop position sense, procedures can be performed on the balance board and then on the mini trampoline. Progressions include decreasing the size of the BoS, performing automatic movement such as throwing and catching a ball, and a gradual reduction in visual input (see Chapter 2, Postural Control).

▶ *REVIEW QUESTIONS*

1. What is the exercise technique of choice to increase range into knee flexion? Provide neurophysiological and biomechanical reasons.

2. Describe a progressive program to increase muscular stability around the knee.

3. Why can going down stairs be so difficult? Describe a program to improve this control.

4. What are the different control and capacity requirements for a long distance runner in contrast to a lineman on a football team? Describe a program to meet those requirements.

REFERENCES

1. Mankin HJ, Springfield DS, Gebhardt MC: Current status of allografting for bone tumors. *Orthopedics.* 1992; 15:1147–1154.
2. Hoppenfeld S. *Physical Examination of the Spine and Extremities.* Norwalk, Conn: Appleton-Century-Crofts; 1976.
3. Tiberio D: Effect of excessive subtalar pronation on patellofemoral mechanics: a theoretical model. *J Orthop Sports Phys Ther.* 1987;9:160–165.

4. Kaltenborn FM, Evjenth O. *Manual Mobilization of the Extremity Joints: Basic Examination and Treatment Techniques.* Oslo, Norway: Olaf Norlis Borhandel; 1989.

5. McConnell JC. The management of chondromolacia patellae: a long-term solution. *Aust J Physiol Ther.* 1986;32:215–223.

6. Chesworth BM, Culham EG, Tata GE, et al. Validation in outcome measures in patients with patello femoral syndrome. *J Orthop Sports Phys Ther.* 1989;10:302–308.

7. Kendall FP, McCreary EK, Provance PG. *Muscles: Testing and Function.* 4th ed. Baltimore, Md: Williams & Wilkins; 1993.

8. Rothstein JM, Lamb RL, Mayhew TP. Clinical uses of isokinetic measurements. *Phys Ther.* 1987;67:1840–1844.

9. Jevsevar DS, Riley PD, Hodge WA, et al. Knee kinematics and kinetics during locomotor activities of daily living in subjects with knee arthroplasty and in healthy control subjects. *Phys Ther.* 1993;73:229–242.

10. Rodosky MW, Andriacchi TP, Anderson GBJ. The influence of chair heights on lower limb mechanics during rising. *J Orthop Res.* 1989;7:266–271.

11. Macefield G, Hagbarth KE, Gorman R, et al. Decline in spindle support during sustained voluntary contractions. *J Physiol.* 1988;440:497–572.

12. Edin BB, Vallbo AB. Stretch sensitization of human muscle spindles. *J Physiol.* 1988;400:101–111.

13. Johansson H, Sjolander P, Sojka P. A sensory role for the cruciate ligaments. *Clin Orthop.* 1990;288:161–178.

14. Barrack RL, Skinner HB, Cook SD, et al. Effect of articular disease and total knee arthroplasty on knee-joint–position sense. *J Neurophysiol.* 1983;50:684–687.

15. Barrack RL, Skinner HB, Buckly SL. Proprioception in the anterior cruciate deficient knee. *Am J Sports Med.* 1989;17:1–6.

16. Smith JL, Hutton RS, Eldred E. Postcontraction changes in sensitivity of muscle afferents to static and dynamic stretch. *Brain Res.* 1974;78:193–202.

17. Astrand PO, Rodahl K. *Textbook of Work Physiology.* New York, NY: McGraw-Hill Book Co; 1986.

18. Davies GJ. *A Compendium of Isokinetics in Clinical Usage and Rehabilitation Techniques.* 2nd ed. La Crosse, Wis: S and S Publishing, Inc; 1984.

19. Edstrom L. Selective atrophy of red muscle fibers in the quadriceps in long-standing knee joint dysfunction injuries to the anterior cruciate ligaments. *J Neurol Sci.* 1970;11:551–558.

20. Wyke B. *Articular Neurology.* Presented at the National Conference of the American Physical Therapy Association; June 1979; Atlanta, Ga.

21. Crutchfield CA, Barnes MR. *The Neurophysiologic Basis of Patient Treatment.* Atlanta, Ga: Stokesville Publishing Co; 1984; 3.

22. Michaels J. *Exercise Overflow: An EMG Investigation.* Boston, Ma: Boston University Sargent College of Allied Health Professions; 1978. Thesis.

23. Markos PD. Ipsilateral and contralateral effects of proprioceptive neuromuscular facilitation techniques on hip motion and EMG activity. *Phys Ther.* 1979;59:1366–1373.

24. Iles JF, Robert RC. Inhibition of monosynaptic reflexes in the human lower limb. *J Physiol.* 1987;385:69–87.

25. Troy L. *EMG Study of Quadriceps and Hamstrings During Bridging.* Boston, Mass: Boston University, Sargent College of Allied Health Professions; 1981. Thesis.

26. Sullivan PE, Markos PE, Minor MAD. *Integrated Approach to Therapeutic Exercise: Theory and Clinical Application.* Reston, VA: Reston Publishing Co; 1982.

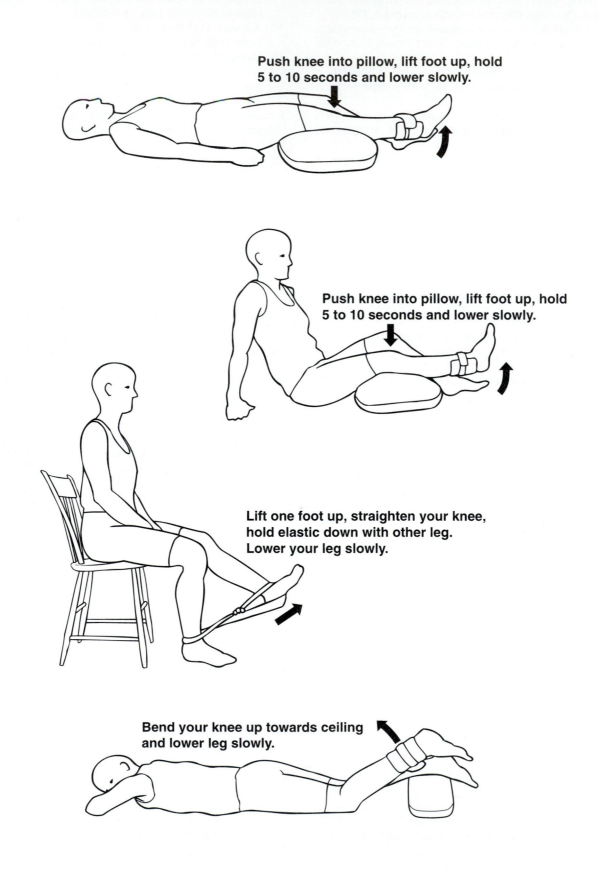

Push knee into pillow, lift foot up, hold 5 to 10 seconds and lower slowly.

Push knee into pillow, lift foot up, hold 5 to 10 seconds and lower slowly.

Lift one foot up, straighten your knee, hold elastic down with other leg. Lower your leg slowly.

Bend your knee up towards ceiling and lower leg slowly.

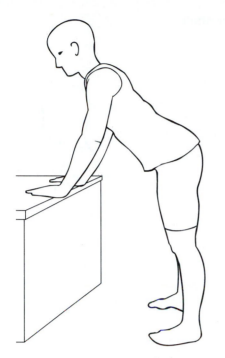

Stand and weight shift over your weaker leg.

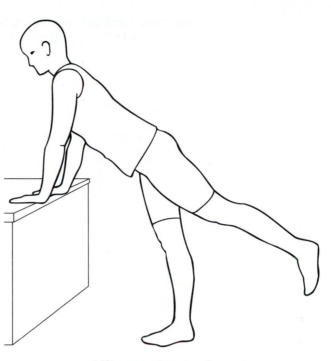

Lift your stronger leg.

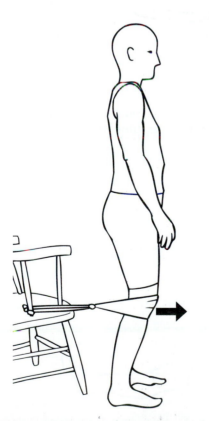

Bend your knee and let it slowly return to a straight position. Do *not* let your knee snap back.

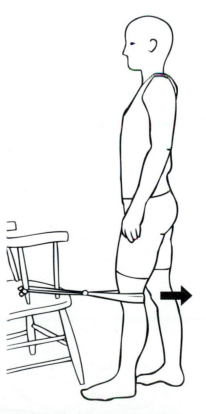

Pull your knee back against the elastic then let it slowly bend. Shift more weight onto your leg.

You may need to hold onto a table or chair while balancing on one foot.

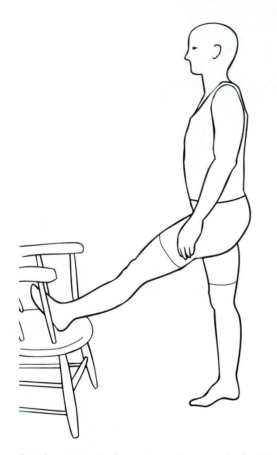

Put foot on chair to stretch muscle behind your thigh (hamstrings).

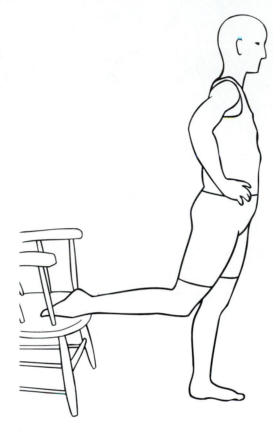

Put foot behind you on chair and try to bend your knee more.

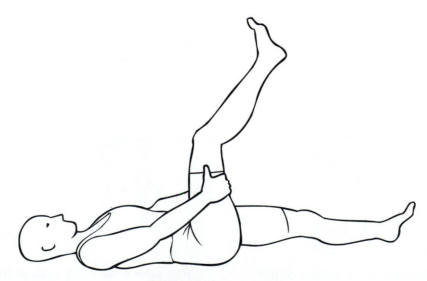

Straighten your knee.

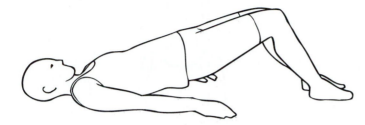

Lift your hips. Move your feet further out and repeat.

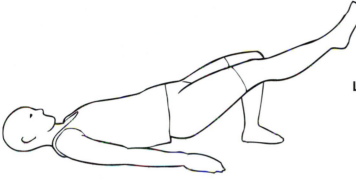

Lift your stronger leg up.

Move your foot further out and lift your stronger leg up.

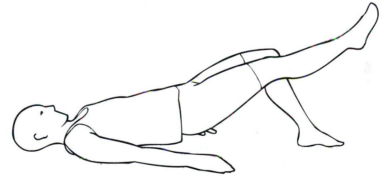

March in place moving your feet further out.

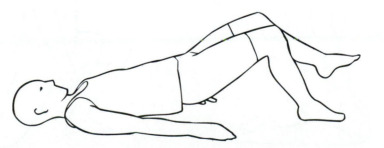

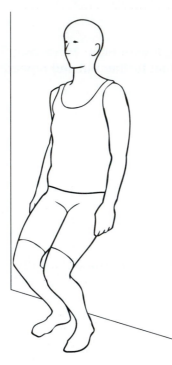

Slide down the wall putting more weight on your weaker leg.

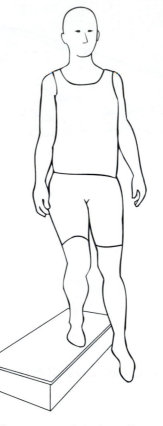

Step up and down off a step with your weaker leg supporting your body weight.

Move from kneeling toward sitting on your heels.

You may need to put a pillow under your knees.

With your weaker leg bent forward, rock forward to bend it more. With your weaker leg back, sit back toward your heel.

CHAPTER 7

Low Back

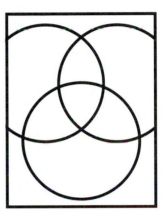

EVALUATION
PHYSICAL SYSTEMS
EVALUATION SUMMARY
INTERVENTION
PROCEDURES TO BALANCE THE AUTONOMIC NERVOUS SYSTEM
PROCEDURES TO IMPROVE CONTROL AND CAPACITY
SUMMARY
REVIEW QUESTIONS

Low back pain (LBP) is a common complaint that affects a wide variety of people regardless of age, occupation, or level of physical conditioning. However, rehabilitative and medical practice does not achieve rehabilitation of this group with consistent success.[1-7] Objective evaluative findings are not always correlated with the subjective reports or the intensity of the symptoms. In addition, with some patients, despite improved physical signs, the reports of pain persist.

The severity of disability can range from an acute, disabling problem to chronic discomfort. Involvement of muscles, joints, ligaments, disc, or capsule may lead to muscle spasm, tightness, weakness, and a pain-spasm cycle that results in disuse and reduced function. These physical deficits interact with many environmental, medical, and psychological factors.[8,9] Because of the many variables contributing to low back dysfunction, therapeutic, medical, or surgical interventions have not demonstrated a consistently high success rate.

The plan of care presented in this chapter recognizes the many variables that can influence the patient with LBP and the need to carefully apply and modify care according to the needs of the individual patient. The plan is sequenced according to the evaluative and intervention models described by the framework of clinical practice. During the evaluation, the many systems that could affect physical functioning are explored (Fig. 7–1). The environmental constraints and physical impairments that limit function are transposed into the intervention model, which, by integrating many perspectives, provides a comprehensive

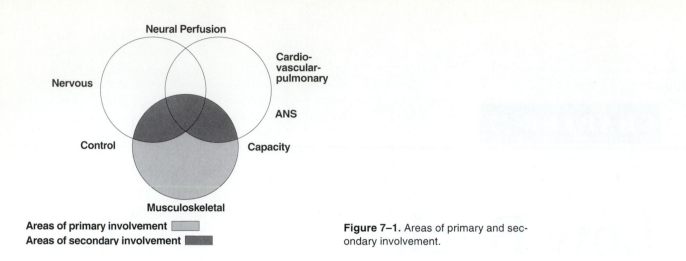

Figure 7–1. Areas of primary and secondary involvement.

treatment plan designed to alleviate the physical impairments and modify environmental strains associated with the dysfunction. The therapist must develop sufficient skill and sensitivity to understand the complexity of behaviors, in addition to the physical impairments, that are associated with LBP.

EVALUATION

A careful evaluation is performed to determine the physical impairments and the underlying causes of pain and to delineate the interrelationship among environmental and psychological strains and physical stresses (Fig. 7–2). A physical therapy evaluation should include: the history of the problem, a discussion of environmental and occupational strains, an appraisal of medical and psychological factors that may refer pain or alter the pain threshold, and an examination of the structures and functions of the physical systems that seem to relate to back activity. Even with a thorough evaluation, it may not be possible to distinguish between primary and secondary symptoms and in many instances the evaluation may not uncover the exact cause of the disability.

A careful **history** detailing the onset of the dysfunction will aid in localizing the cause of the problem. The most common precursors of LBP include falls and other accidents, faulty posture, and poor body mechanics during the performance of occupational or recreational tasks. For example:

▶ A fall on slippery ground or from a ladder may result in muscular or joint tissue stresses, in a compression fracture, or other internal derangements that may require a medical evaluation. The sacroiliac joint is often traumatized by a fall and should be assessed for malalignment.

▶ Lifting a heavy object or a twisting motion may result in muscle strain, "spasm," and sprain of the joint structures. Localized pain often accom-

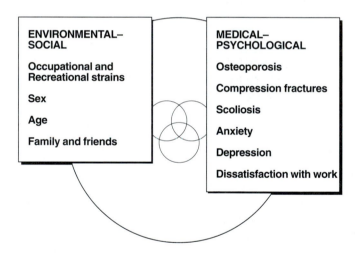

Figure 7–2. Examples of factors influencing physical function, categorized within the evaluation model.

panies such trauma. A description of "locking" or immediate and radiating pain may be indicative of damaged joint structures or discal involvement.

▶ The patient may have been involved in a motor vehicle accident (MVA). Knowledge of the angle of impact will help determine the segments and movements that need most careful evaluation.

▶ The patient may report chronic pain without any specific precipitating trauma.

The history should include a description of the patient's **environmental and social** condition as well as **occupational and recreational** activities. During this portion of the evaluation the therapist is trying to ascertain if external factors are related to the physical stress. Standing or sitting for prolonged periods and repetitive lifting or reaching with improper body mechanics can be expected to affect both joint and muscle tissue over time.[10] For example, if prolonged sitting is an issue, the therapist needs to ascertain the type of seat, the patient's posture, and the functional demands that occur while in this position. All of these can be determined either by conversation with the patient or inspection of the work environment.

Medical and psychological factors are screened to determine their association with the pain and whether referral to other practitioners is needed. A health-status questionnaire can provide the therapist with pertinent information relating to medical and surgical history, including a listing of all current medications and diagnostic tests, such as roentgenogram (x-ray), magnetic resonance imaging (MRI), and electromyogram (EMG).

The most common reason that the patient comes to physical therapy is for relief of pain. The therapist must try to differentiate pain of biomechanical origin, for example, from tissue compression, tension, or abnormal stress, from pain referred from internal organs, or from other pathological medical conditions. Pain that is relieved by rest, activity, or certain positions is most likely related to biomechanical factors that are amenable to physical therapy intervention. Patients with constant pain that does not vary with changes in movement, posture, or activity should be referred to a physician.[11]

Depression, anxiety, and other psychological states have been found to correlate with low back dysfunction.[12] Some patients may describe their pain using terms such as *strangling* or *torturing*. These patients may need care beyond that which physical therapy can provide. The therapist must ensure that the patient is properly referred to appropriate practitioners. In many of these cases, function may be improved by helping the patient regain movement capacity and reducing physical stress.

Physical Systems

The physical systems and functions that need to be assessed are the autonomic nervous system (ANS), the musculoskeletal system, movement control, and capacity.

Autonomic Nervous System

The physical examination begins with an assessment of the ANS (see Chapter 4). For many patients, physical therapy is the entry into the healthcare system, and base line measures of heart rate and blood pressure are needed. Cardiac function may be influenced by anxiety from adverse environmental or social conditions or deconditioning. The patient also may be anxious because of the pain or simply because it is the first experience with physical therapy. That anxiety may alter the intensity of pain symptoms and muscle tension. Vital functions need to be assessed before a lower- or upper-extremity bicycle or treadmill are used, either for warm-up or for conditioning.

The ANS influences the body's general reactions to stimuli as well as the reactivity of local tissues.[13] ANS imbalances, particularly increases in sympathetic functioning, can influence the patient's pain threshold and peripheral circulation. The variations in pain resulting from fluctuations in the ANS must be taken into account when evaluative and treatment decisions are made. For example, the assessment of skin temperature and administration of a scratch test may provide information regarding the local circulation. The scratch test should produce an evenly thin red line. The lumbar region may be normally cooler than the thoracic area but should be equal right to left. Decreased redness and temperature may indicate diminished circulation which occurs with a chronic condition; increased redness and temperature may accompany an acute problem. If these tests indicate that circulatory status is not normal, less intense heat or cold should be used in treatment. The patient's ability to relax and the responses to manual and other stimuli may also vary with an imbalance within the ANS.

Musculoskeletal System

An in-depth assessment of the structures of the musculoskeletal (MS) system is performed. Although the evaluation can take many forms and the sequences of evaluative measures may vary, the different tissues that influence low back function including skin, fascia, muscles, joints, ligaments, discs, and capsules need to be assessed. Abnormalities of these structures can affect mobility, alignment, stability and dynamic control, as well as contribute to complaints of pain.

The MS tissues must provide adequate flexibility and stability so that movement can be performed without a focal stress point and without fatigue of specific tissues. Such balance promotes proper trunk alignment during the performance of static and dynamic tasks to ensure equitable generation, transmission, and absorption of biomechanical forces.

Measures used to assess the MS system include observation, palpation, and measurement of joint and muscle range of motion (ROM). The therapist observes alignment and the ability to maintain static and dynamic postures, such as standing and sitting, without undue fatigue. Palpation of the low back area can detect imbalances in muscular tension, areas of tenderness, and painful trigger points. Observation and palpation of joint structures may indicate vertebral or other bony malalignment.

A **ROM** assessment, which includes general flexibility of the hips and trunk as well as movement of specific intervertebral segments, may help differentiate the involvement of joint from muscle and determine the relationship between range and functional limitations. For example, the patient's complaints of pain with prolonged sitting and the inability to maintain correct sitting posture may be related to stiffness of the posterior hip structures and decreased length of the low back extensors. In sitting or standing active ROM is performed with the upper trunk moving on the lower body. Flexion and extension, lateral bending, and rotational movements are included to determine limitations and those motions that reproduce symptoms. Movement within the spine, pelvis, and hips should be smooth throughout the range. Decreased movement in one segment may result in abnormal stress of other segments.[14] For example, during forward bending, excessive tightness in the hamstrings may restrict hip flexion and cause an increase in movement or stress in more proximal segments; tightness in the hip flexors may limit backward bending and focus movement in the lumbar spine near the proximal attachment of the hip flexors; tightness of the quadratus lumborum may contribute to an abnormal pelvic tilt and limited sidebending.[15]

The lower trunk can be moved on the upper trunk in supine, sidelying, or prone, where the compressive weight-bearing forces are minimized. The flexibility and bilateral symmetry of the back extensors, the quadratus, the hamstrings, hip flexors, extensors, rotators, and the tensor fascia lata are examined. For example, in supine, the assessment of trunk flexion with rotation can be performed by passively moving the lower trunk to both the left and right sides while observing the amount of pelvic elevation from the plinth. If the patient is not experiencing pain with these motions, a slight overpressure at end ranges will allow the therapist to feel the quality of the tissue resistance and distinguish among the more pliable feel of contractile tissue, the stiff feel of fascia, capsule, and ligament, and the hard feel of bony restrictions.[16] A small amount of range gained with the application of hold relax at the point of limitation may further implicate muscle as a contributing factor to the range limitation (Fig. 7–3). The performance of specific vertebral joint ROM assessments in sidelying or prone may indicate local areas of hyper- or hypomobility and may pinpoint any painful areas.

The muscular tightness commonly found in the one-joint neck extensors, anterior chest, low back extensors, and in all directions of hip motion can impact on postural alignment and function (Table 7–1). The combined tightness in the trunk extensors and anterior hip may contribute to an increased lordotic posture; reduced length of hip extensors and posterior capsule may limit movement into hip flexion and lead to excessive lumbar flexion, thoracic kyphosis, and cervical lordosis in sitting; hip-rotational tightness may result in an asymmetrical transmission of forces from the hips to the pelvis, sacrum, and lumbar spine during twisting motions in standing.

Straight leg raising (SLR) may be limited by hamstring tightness and has been a traditional means of assessing pressure or tension on the sciatic nerve. Neural tension may be increased by adding ankle dorsiflexion or neck and upper trunk flexion. The

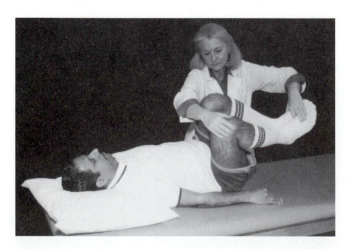

Figure 7–3. A: Supine; lower trunk flexion to the right. T: HR to the agonist.

TABLE 7–1. COMMON RANGE OF MOTION IMPAIRMENTS ALTERING POSTURAL ALIGNMENT

▶ Forward Head
  Shortened neck extensors
  Lengthened neck flexors

▶ Forward Shoulders
  Shortened pectoralis
  Lengthened trapezius, rhomboids, and upper-back extensors

▶ Tilted Pelvis or Lordosis
  Lengthened abdominals
  Shortened back extensors
  Shortened hip flexors and rotators

▶ Slumped Sitting Posture
  Lengthened back extensors
  Shortened hip extensors

▶ Specific Segmental Limitations

knee can be extended with the hip in flexion either in supine or sitting to compare consistency of reported limitations. Unilateral limitations in hamstrings or neural length may produce an unequal strain on the back, especially during forward flexion motions in standing.

Movement Control

Movement control encompasses the ability to dynamically stabilize the trunk in a variety of postures as the prerequisite to performing skilled movement. The assessment of strength by a manual muscle test (MMT) provides information regarding specific myotomal innervation and the ability to perform a one-repetition maximum contraction in one position. This type of strength assessment, however, does not provide information about interactive muscle function during maintenance of or movement in various postures. The attributes of movement categorized by the stages of control are assessed so that a specific intervention plan can be developed to achieve functional outcomes.

Mobility. This has been assessed during the evaluation of the MS system. The **initiation of active movement** is assessed during the myotomal evaluation to determine neural involvement. Patients exhibiting lower-extremity weakness corresponding to myotomal innervation should be referred to a physician.

Stability. Low back muscles, particularly the lumbar paravertebrals, appear to be dominated by type I, slow-twitch fibers with a large capacity for developing isometric endurance.[17] Holding of lumbar muscles enhances stability and decreases stress on surrounding joint structures. Therefore, the ability of these postural muscles to maintain an isometric contraction is critical and needs to be evaluated.

The two levels of stability, **muscular** and **postural,** are assessed by: (1) holding of the postural muscles against the resistance of gravity, and (2) maintaining postural alignment in various positions. The upper- and lower-trunk extensors, particularly the deep one-joint multifidi and rotatores, hip extensors, and the lower abdominals are the muscles which provide intersegmental and total trunk stability. The extensors are classically tested against gravity in prone. The abdominals can be tested in a hooklying position by asking the patient to flatten the lumbar spine or maintain a pelvic tilt. Deficits may be noted by a decreased ability to maintain the shortened range, oscillations in body segments observed as muscle "flickering," or an inability to move at a slow, controlled rate. Any of these deficits are an indication of muscle fatigue. Both the extensor and abdominal tests can be made more difficult by in-

creasing the body-weight resistance with the incorporation of extremity movements. For example, in prone, the upper extremities can be lifted overhead or, in supine, the lower extremities can be more extended. Diminished muscular stability, particularly of the extensors, may be the result of inhibition from painful or swollen joint structures.

Postural stability requires simultaneous contraction of the back extensors and abdominals.[18,19] Assessment includes observation and palpation of the alignment of cervical, thoracic, and lumbosacral regions in standing and sitting as well as in bridging, modified plantigrade, and quadruped. Curve deviations and asymmetries, and discrepancies in leg length and body landmarks may indicate malalignment of structural or muscular origin. The challenge can be increased by moving the arms or upper trunk while maintaining lumbopelvic alignment in sitting, standing, or in other postures. Maintenance of correct alignment in any posture may be difficult when both tightness and poor muscular stability exist.

Controlled Mobility. This is the ability to control alignment while moving in various postures. Dynamic stability is assessed by observing the quantity and quality of trunk movements during concentric and eccentric contractions or reversing of antagonists. Control can be observed in all postures, for example, as the upper body moves on the lower body when bending forward and backward in standing, as the lower body moves on the upper body during the performance of a pelvic tilt in sitting or standing (Fig. 7–4), or when rocking in quadruped. All movements can be combined in two or three planes to alter the stress on the tissues. Excessive, inadequate, or shaky movements may be due to deficits in the previous levels of mobility or stability as well as to a lack of dynamic control.

Static–Dynamic. These are intermediate movements between controlled mobility and skill. At this level, weight-bearing support is reduced, further challenging proximal dynamic stability of the trunk. For example, in quadruped, one limb is elevated from the surface, requiring the trunk to alter its stabilizing forces. Holding the limb at end ranges of flexion or extension will assess the isometric holding ability of the trunk muscles. Movements of the upper limb will challenge control in the thoracic spine; movement of the lower limb will test lumbar spine control. Movement of contralateral upper and lower extremities requires dynamic stability of the entire trunk. The therapist is observing the trunk for smooth, controlled movement. Abnormalities in the ability to stabilize dynamically may be noted as excessive lumbar ex-

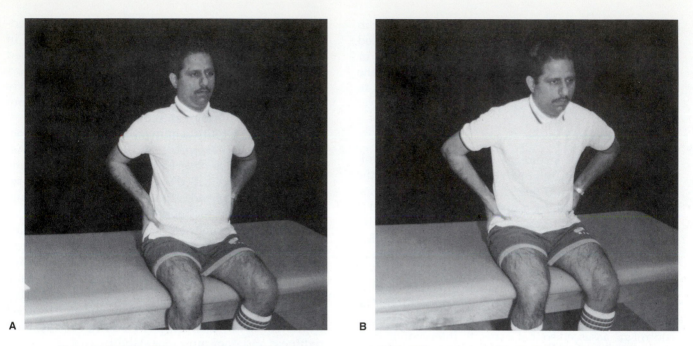

Figure 7–4. (A) A: Sitting; posterior pelvic tilt. T: Active movement. **(B)** A: Sitting; anterior pelvic tilt. T: Active movement.

tension during hip extension and increased lumbar flexion during hip flexion. Unilateral weight bearing in bridging will test the ability of the hip and lumbar extensors to stabilize dynamically in shortened ranges.

Skill. The skill stage implies trunk movement with sufficient timing, sequencing, and force to allow the performance of all ambulation and activities of daily living (ADL), including occupational and recreational tasks. A gait evaluation may reveal dynamic postural abnormalities such as reduced trunk counterrotation, short step length, and decreased heel strike. Whenever feasible, the evaluation and retraining of body mechanics during lifting, reaching, and movement should simulate the patient's ADL, employment, and recreational demands.

Sensory testing can be performed along the dermatomes of the lower trunk and lower extremities to determine nerve root involvement. Pain, paresthesias, or dysesthesias should be carefully noted including: type, location, occurrence, duration, and any predisposing postures or aggravating activities. Dermatomal numbness should be communicated to the physician. Proprioceptive sensation as measured by joint position sense is difficult to test in the trunk. Deficits can be inferred, however, from reports such as "I don't know where that part of my back is," or "it feels as if I am floating." These subjective comments may be related to decreased muscle stability and to an inability to maintain midline postures.

Movement Capacity

Both the patient's general exercise capacity and the muscle's capacity to contract for long durations may be limited. General aerobic capacity may be measured by resting heart rate and blood pressure and cardiac responses during ergonomic exercise tests.[20] Muscle fatigue, as noted as difficulty sustaining a low-intensity, long-duration contraction, may be due to poor muscle endurance. Patients may complain of "tiredness" or "aching" in the thoracic or lumbar region with prolonged activity. Improved endurance requires an enriched circulatory bed within the muscle as well as improved general aerobic capacity. Low-intensity, long-duration activities such as walking, swimming, or biking in addition to specific low-intensity, long-duration exercises to enhance muscle capacity should be incorporated into a daily routine.

Evaluation Summary

The objective and subjective information are compared to determine areas of consistency or discrepancy. Factors that do not cluster into categories of physical dysfunction may be indicative of a nonstructural cause of back pain requiring referral.[11]

The therapist at this point has developed a picture of: the patient's environmental and social conditions, including occupational or recreational strains that will require modification, the medical and psychological factors, and the physical impairments. The evaluation of the physical systems may have re-

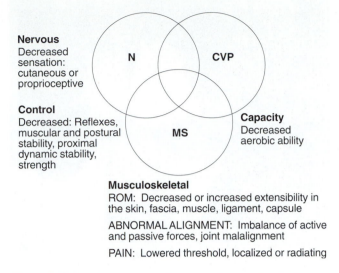

Nervous
Decreased sensation: cutaneous or proprioceptive

Control
Decreased: Reflexes, muscular and postural stability, proximal dynamic stability, strength

Capacity
Decreased aerobic ability

Musculoskeletal
ROM: Decreased or increased extensibility in the skin, fascia, muscle, ligament, capsule

ABNORMAL ALIGNMENT: Imbalance of active and passive forces, joint malalignment

PAIN: Lowered threshold, localized or radiating

Figure 7–5. Physical impairments categorized by physical systems.

vealed: an increased sympathetic level in the ANS, altered tissue density, decreased or excessive mobility, altered static or dynamic movement control, and decreased muscle or total body endurance (Fig. 7–5). These impairments are commonly associated with functional limitations such as decreased walking distance, limited sitting or standing tolerance, or the inability to lift or carry objects. Any of these limitations can impact on daily living, occupational, or recreational activities.

To develop a treatment plan, these findings are transposed into the classifications of the intervention model so that specific and appropriate treatment procedures can be developed and made progressively more challenging. To achieve the functional outcomes, the intervention should encompass alteration of the environmental and occupational strains, education in back care and compensatory strategies, as well as application of procedures to help the patient change the physical impairments.

INTERVENTION

The sequence of procedures presented in this section is designed to reduce anxiety and sympathetic responses, promote mobility, enhance stability of both upper and lower trunk, and to improve dynamic endurance and general movement capacity. The procedures designed to help the individual to change are integrated with those designed to alter external physical strains. These may include the addition of shoe lifts to correct a leg length discrepancy, improvement of body mechanics, and alteration of postural stresses by improving chair height or support. Even though

functional outcomes are as important for the patient with low-back dysfunction as for all other patients, intervention outcomes that primarily reflect a return to occupational tasks may not be as appropriate for this patient group.[21] Because numerous variables affect a return to employment, the outcomes of intervention can only reflect the physical gains in control and capacity that can be anticipated by physical therapy intervention. For example, "the patient can lift and move 40 pounds," "use the upper extremities while maintaining sitting for two hours," or "walk for two miles without pain."

Many controversies exist regarding the most beneficial treatments for patients with low back problems. The existence of many approaches can be attributed to the variable mechanisms of injury, multiple tissue involvement, and the variety of patient symptoms. In keeping with the general context of this book, the differences among the various treatment philosophies will not be addressed. Instead many of these approaches will be integrated into the intervention sequence, which is designed to alleviate the problems common to most patients with low back disability. Procedures include use of various physical agents to decrease pain, reduce muscle spasm, and increase local areas of circulation, as well as joint mobilization to increase mobility of restricted segments. The treatment presented in this chapter, however, focuses primarily on therapeutic exercise procedures. Depending on the extent of involvement and the goals of treatment, exercise may be only a portion of the total rehabilitation program.

Procedures to Balance the Autonomic Nervous System

Imbalances in the ANS may be noted either in patients in acute distress or in those with chronic pain. Appropriate goals should include:

▶ Promote homeostasis, balance, of the ANS.

▶ Promote generalized relaxation and reduce localized muscle spasm to allow movement of the involved area.

▶ Improve general body conditioning.

Pain, a generalized increase in tension, and an oversensitivity to stimuli may all be associated with predominance of the sympathetic function within the ANS. Treatment procedures should attempt to increase parasympathetic influences to balance the ANS. Techniques that may be considered parasympathetic in nature include deep breathing, maintained pressure over the abdomen, neutral warmth, slow stroking down the posterior primary rami (PPR) located deep to the paravertebral muscles, and a slightly inverted tilt position of the body to stimulate the carotid sinuses (see Chapter 3). Some of these techniques may be combined. For example, treatment frequently begins with the patient lying prone, covered with a blanket, with a pillow under the abdomen and a hot pack placed on the low back. The stimuli included in this procedure are a slightly head-down position, maintained pressure on the abdomen, and heat. While many patients respond favorably to the application of hot packs, others report increased pain a few hours after treatment. This increased discomfort may be a rebound effect within the ANS that results in intensification of the original pain. Prolonged applications of ice, although often effective in producing an initial analgesic relaxation response, may produce a similar rebound effect. When the patient reacts adversely to extremes of temperature, a modification of these thermal applications is indicated and more neutral temperatures should be applied.[22]

Massage often follows the application of thermal stimuli and appears to be an effective relaxant.[23] The generalized relaxation might be further enhanced by the inclusion of caudally directed effleurage strokes. If prone cannot be tolerated, sidelying or a supported forward-sitting posture are appropriate alternatives.

Jacobsen's relaxation exercises have been found empirically to be effective[24]; the gradual increase and relaxation of muscle tension can be incorporated into treatment both to promote general relaxation and to decrease localized muscle spasm. For patients with pain and spasm in a specific area, muscle contraction is sequenced to follow an indirect-to-direct approach. Isometric contractions followed by conscious relaxation, or a modified hold relax technique against minimal resistance, can be performed first by segments distal to the painful area before contracting the muscles of the involved area. A sequence of low-intensity isometric contractions can be combined with deep diaphragmatic breathing to further enhance relaxation.

As a means of illustrating the indirect-to-direct approach, a sequence of procedures is outlined for a patient with pain in the **left lumbar extensors.** With the patient supine, treatment begins on the pain-free right side with a contraction of the muscles in the upper trunk antagonistic to the painful area. The right upper abdominals are activated by resisting the D2E pattern of the right upper extremity in the shortened range (Fig. 7–6). If this procedure does not elicit pain, the next procedure can be directed at either the right upper-trunk extensors or the right lower abdominals. Right upper-trunk extensors may be activated with a D2F pattern of the right upper extremity (Fig. 7–7), the right lower abdominals with D1F (Fig. 7–8) of the right lower extremity, and the right lateral trunk flex-

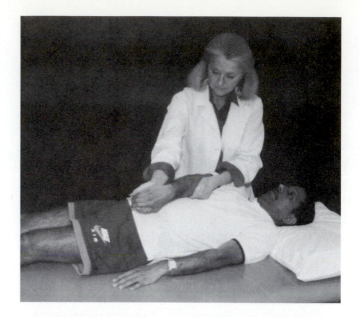

Figure 7–6. A: Supine; D2E right upper extremity. T: HR.

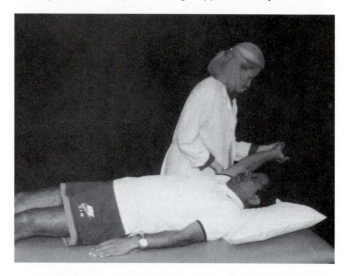

Figure 7–7. A: Supine; D2F right upper extremity. T: HR.

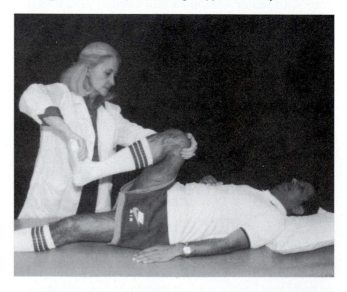

Figure 7–8. A: Supine; D1F right lower extremity. T: HR.

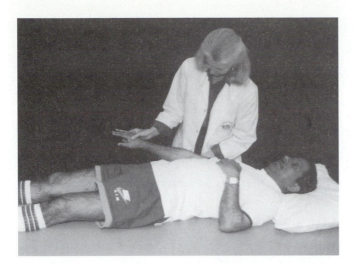

Figure 7–9. A: Supine; D1E right upper extremity. T: HR.

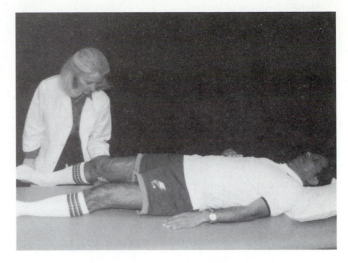

Figure 7–10. A: Supine; D1E right lower extremity. T: HR.

ors by D1E of the upper right extremity (Fig. 7–9). The last procedure directed toward the right side is to activate the right lower-back extensors with contraction of the D1E pattern of the right lower extremity (Fig. 7–10). Contractions of muscles on the involved side follow the same sequence just described for the uninvolved side. All these patterns are resisted in the shortened range. Direct contraction of the involved left low-back extensors with D1E of the left leg is the final activity of the sequence (Fig. 7–11). Incorporated into this program of isometric exercises are progressive movements of the extremities against minimal resistance. Like the isometric progression, the isotonic movements should begin with the contralateral upper extremity. Bilateral upper extremity patterns are followed by unilateral lower-extremity movements on the uninvolved and then on the involved

side. This gradual progression of procedures, from isometric to isotonic contractions of noninvolved to involved segments, is performed to teach the patient how to contract and relax and to gain some sense of control over the pain rather than being controlled by the pain.

Procedures to Improve Control and Capacity

Procedures at this stage of treatment are geared toward the patient who is not hampered by acute debilitating pain, even though discomfort may interfere with normal movement. The patient may have proceeded through the acute stage or, because of a less stressful injury, may begin treatment at this stage.

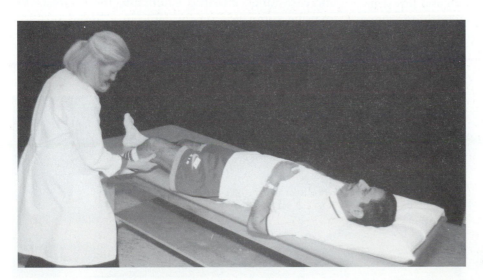

Figure 7–11. A: Supine; D1E left lower extremity. T: HR.

TABLE 7–2. TREATMENT GOALS AT EARLY STAGES OF REHABILITATION

Mobility–Range of Motion	Stability

• Increase extensibility of:
  Neck extensors
  Pectoralis minor
  Low-back extensors
  Hip motions
  Hamstrings—if asymmetrical
  Specific lumbar segments
	• Increase isometric holding of:
	  Scapula adductors
	  Upper- and lower-back
	   extensors
	  Lower abdominals
	  Gluteals
	• Increase endurance

The treatment goals are (Table 7–2):

▶ To increase ROM of the low back, upper trunk, and hips.

▶ To increase muscle stability and "strength" of back extensors, lower abdominals, and other weakened muscles.

▶ To improve static and dynamic stability of the trunk in various postures.

▶ To improve postural awareness and body mechanics and decrease environmental strains.

▶ To improve endurance of the postural extensors and increase general exercise capacity.

Increase ROM

A: Supine, sidelying, sitting, prone; lower- (LE) and upper-extremity (UE) motions, thoracic and lumbar segmental movements

T: Hold relax (HR), rhythmical rotation (RR), joint mobilization, massage, heat, ice, interferential, ultrasound (US), self-stretching

P: Low to moderate intensity, using pain as guide

ROM exercises (Fig. 7–12) are performed to increase tissue flexibility and to improve alignment before the application of procedures to improve control and capacity.[25] Mobility is initially increased in postures with a large base of support (BoS) and low center of gravity (CoG) to allow the patient more complete relaxation. Procedures to increase range in the hips and in the upper trunk may be included prior to

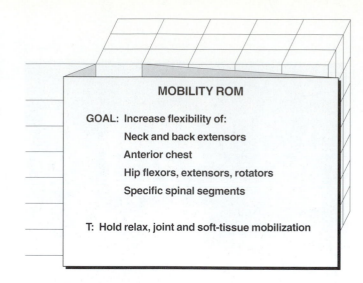

MOBILITY ROM

GOAL: Increase flexibility of:

Neck and back extensors

Anterior chest

Hip flexors, extensors, rotators

Specific spinal segments

T: Hold relax, joint and soft-tissue mobilization

Figure 7–12. Treatment goals and techniques appropriate when promoting Mobility–ROM.

procedures for the lower trunk to avoid the more painful area while teaching the patient how to relax.

Supine is an appropriate posture in which to increase hip and lower trunk motion. Range into **hip flexion** can be promoted by the D1F pattern, which combines hip flexion and rotation with the techniques of HR and RR (see Chapter 3). The isometric contraction of HR can be applied to the agonistic hip flexor or to the antagonist hip extensor. At least 110° of hip flexion is needed for functional activities, such as bending forward in sitting to assume standing, for dressing, or to move the legs while driving. However, stiffness in the hip structures or complaints of discomfort commonly occur earlier in the range. With the hip in approximately 90° of hip flexion, RR can be applied to increase **rotational range** as well as to increase movement into hip flexion. Rotation is required to allow an equal distribution of motion during twisting movements in sitting and standing. To increase range into **hip extension,** the opposite LE may be supported on the table in a flexed position while the iliopsoas, adductors, rotators, and anterior capsule are stretched in the shortened range of the D1

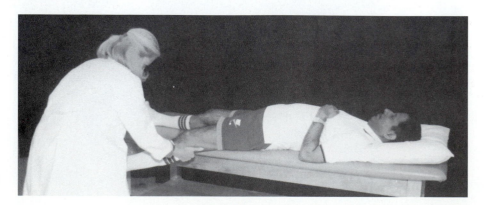

Figure 7–13. A: Supine; D1E lower extremity. T: HR into increasing ranges of hip extension.

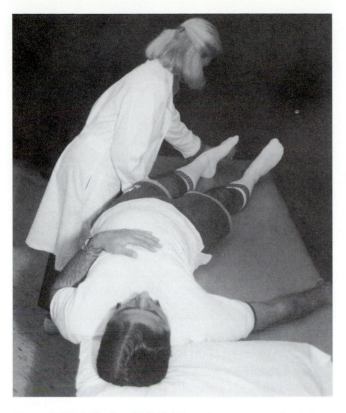

Figure 7–14. A: Supine; D2E. T: HR to elongate tensor fascia lata.

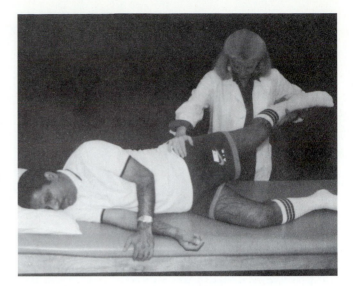

Figure 7–15. A: Sidelying; D1E. T: HR to increase range into hip extension.

extensor pattern (Fig. 7–13) and the tensor fascia lata is stretched in D2 extension (Fig. 7–14). HR to the agonistic hip extensor is the preferred technique if contraction of hip flexors in their lengthened range causes an anterior tilt of the pelvis, with a resulting increase in pain. The therapist needs to monitor the pelvic position by palpating the anterior superior iliac spine (ASIS) to ensure that hip movement rather than pelvic tilting is occurring. Range into hip extension can be promoted in supine with the limb off the edge of the table or in sidelying and in prone (Fig. 7–15). Adequate movement into hip extension is needed for erect standing and ambulation.

Extensibility of the low back extensors also can be increased in supine by combining lower trunk flexion with rotation patterns with the technique of HR. Because the knees are flexed, range in the low back can be promoted without the confounding effects of the hamstrings. The patient is passively moved to the shortened range of the lower trunk flexor pattern where HR to the agonist flexor pattern is performed. HR applied to the agonist has been empirically found to be more effective in increasing lumbar flexion range than contraction of the antagonistic back extensor muscles (Fig. 7–16). A disadvantage of this procedure is that the hip flexors, which may also be tight, are contracting in their shortened ranges. In a longsitting position, the relaxation techniques of

HR and rhythmic stabilization (RS) may be used to increase ROM in the low back area. Upper-trunk flexion patterns are effective movements to combine with longsitting to increase ROM of the hamstrings as well as the low back extensors (Fig. 7–17).

Joint mobilization can be performed to passively increase the extensibility of noncontractile tissues and thus improve the alignment of joint structures. Muscle energy techniques employ active isometric contractions to improve joint alignment. HR, which is also an isometric technique, is performed to increase muscle length, thereby altering forces and improving alignment around a joint. The following example illustrates how the three techniques may be performed

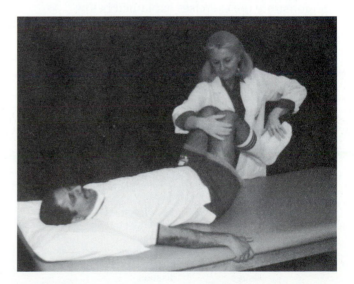

Figure 7–16. A: Lower-trunk flexion. T: HR to agonist.

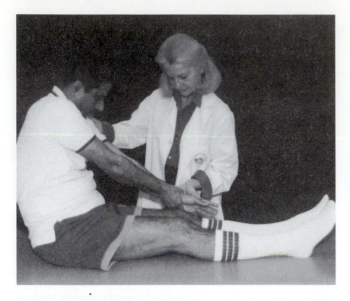

Figure 7–17. A: Longsitting. T: HR to increase extensibility of back extensors and hamstrings.

in combination to improve joint position. To increase hip extension, joint mobilization may be necessary to increase extensibility of the anterior capsule, HR may be performed to increase extensibility of the hip flexors, and muscle energy techniques can be performed using the hamstrings to tilt the pelvis posteriorly. The combination of these three techniques will improve the mobility and alignment of the lower trunk so that subsequent stability procedures can be effective (Table 7–3).

Home Program to Increase Mobility

The reader is referred to the visuals for the home exercises at the end of the chapter (pp. 185–193) to demonstrate the exercises explained below.

As part of the patient's home or independent program, range in the hip can be maintained by stretching the hip in supine and in standing with one

leg flexed on a chair or low table. The patient stands facing the table and rocks forward, stretching the posterior hip structures on the flexed limb and the anterior flexors and capsule of the extended limb. The patient sustains a gentle stretch about 5° from the fully lengthened position. When the knee of the anterior limb is extended, the hamstrings are also lengthened. To stretch tight adductors, the patient turns 90°, keeping one leg on the table. Another 90° turn, facing away from the chair or table, will put the hip flexors on stretch. In all of the positions, the patient is instructed to keep the pelvis level and equal, without allowing rotation or anterior tilt. In sitting, the patient can stretch the hip extensors by flexing one limb toward the chest while assisting the movement with the upper extremities. The hamstrings can be stretched in supine by flexing the hip then extending the knee or in sitting by positioning the foot on a stool or chair.

Improve Muscular and Postural Dynamic Stability

The main focus of this portion of the treatment is to develop proximal dynamic stability in various postures by improving control of the lower abdominals and the low back extensors and by enhancing the patient's proprioception and body awareness. ROM may continue to be a goal while more complex levels of control are being achieved. The treatment goals emphasized are:

▶ Increase muscle stability of back extensors, lower abdominals, and other weakened muscles in non–weight-bearing postures (Fig. 7–18).

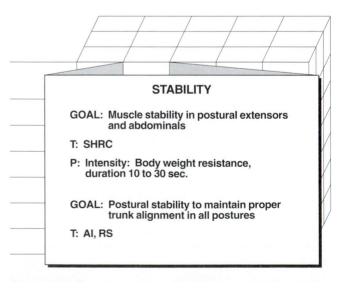

Figure 7–18. Treatment goals and techniques appropriate when promoting stability.

TABLE 7–3. RELATIONSHIP OF THREE MOBILITY TECHNIQUES

	Hold Relax	Joint Mobilization	Muscle Energy
Method	Active	Passive	Active
Purpose	Improve joint alignment by increasing extensibility of contractile tissues	Improve joint alignment by increasing extensibility of noncontractile tissues	Improve joint alignment by muscle contraction

▶ Improve static and dynamic postural stability.

▶ Improve endurance of specific trunk musculature and general exercise capacity.

The treatment outcomes encompass the physical functional needs of the patient, which commonly include dynamic control in sitting and standing, with sufficient capacity to sit for prolonged times, and to walk, lift, or move without undue fatigue.

The progression of the **activities,** the treatment postures and movements, takes into account the interrelationship of biomechanical, anatomical, and kinesiological factors and the patient's deficits. The difficulty of treatment activities can be increased by varying the BoS, the height of the CoG, the resistance of gravity, the muscle length, the number of segments to be controlled, and the compressive forces through the spine. Postures and movements should be varied to include diagonal and rotational components to optimally recruit all muscle fibers and to enhance stability responses.[18] Dynamic stability can be challenged further by positioning the patient on a ball or bolster.

The progression of the **techniques** follows the stages of control. In conjunction with increasing range in the trunk and hips, isometric contractions are performed in non–weight-bearing postures. The isometric contractions will improve muscle stability and the proprioceptive sense of correct postural alignment. Muscle stability is essential to protect the joint structures. Postural stability is promoted in weight-bearing postures before movement within and between postures is emphasized. Functional activities, including simulation of occupational tasks, can be emphasized when the patient has developed sufficient prerequisite control to focus on the normal timing and sequencing of movement.

The progression of the **parameters** first reflects the need for improved muscular control by keeping the intensity of effort at approximately 40% of maximum and the duration of the isometric contractions to approximately 10 seconds to optimize alpha–gamma coactivation.[26,27] Slow, deep breathing is encouraged during isometric contractions to promote aerobic activity and avoid a Valsalva maneuver. To increase endurance during static or dynamic postural exercises, the intensity remains constant but the duration needs to increase to achieve the patient's functional requirements. Improving the body's general aerobic capacity begins early in the program with progressive nonspecific exercises such as the treadmill, and upper- and lower-body ergometry. Home exercises are performed frequently throughout the day to improve endurance and carry-over. Certain environmental cues can be used to remind the pa-

	Mobility	Stability	Controlled Mobility	Static-Dynamic	Skill
SUPINE SIDELYING	X	X	X	X	
PRONE	X	X			
HOOKLYING BRIDGING	X	X	X	X	
QUADRUPED	X	X	X	X	
SITTING	X	X	X	X	X
MODIFIED PLANTIGRADE		X	X	X	
STANDING		X	X	X	X

Intensity *gradually increase*
Duration *X X*
Frequency *education*

Figure 7–19. Intervention model indicating procedures emphasized to promote movement control and capacity.

tient: for example, assumption of correct postural alignment during every TV commercial break, upon stopping at a red light, or saving a document on the computer.

Within each of the following postures the procedures are sequenced according to the stages of control. Many of the activities can be performed within the same treatment session, depending on the treatment goals and the patient's ability to cope with the progressive stresses of each procedure. For example, a treatment session may include procedures in supine, prone, and sitting to increase both mobility and stability. Advantages and disadvantages of treatment in each posture will be discussed (Fig. 7–19).

Supine

Mobility–ROM. Movements to promote mobility–ROM of the trunk and extremities (Table 7–4) can be performed as described earlier.

Stability. Stability of the trunk and hip extensors can be enhanced by holding in the shortened range. The therapist can manually resist the contraction with one

TABLE 7–4. PROCEDURES PERFORMED IN SUPINE TO IMPROVE MOBILITY AND STABILITY

Mobility	Stability
• Increase length of:	• Increase holding of:
Pectoralis minor	Scapula adductors
Long back extensors	Back and neck extensors
Quadratus lumborum	Gluteals and quadriceps
Hip extensors, flexors, rotators	
Hamstrings	

Figure 7–20. A: Supine; scapula adduction and trunk and hip extension. T: SHRC.

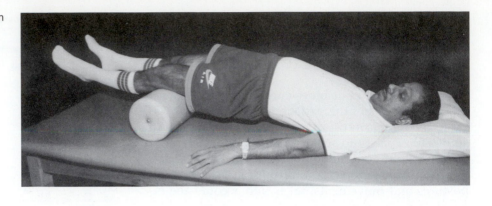

contact positioned under the knees and the other under the feet. For a home program, a pillow is placed under the knees and the patient pushes down with the quadriceps against the pillow and lifts the hips and lower trunk. To avoid pain, movement may be limited to about 1 inch from the surface. The upper trunk extensors and scapula adductors are resisted by pushing the elbows into the table, "pinching the shoulder blades together," and slightly arching the upper back (Fig. 7–20). To help ensure aerobic muscular activity, the duration of the contraction can be measured by the number of deep breaths the patient takes while maintaining the contraction. For example, patient instructions may be "tighten your knees and hips, breathe 3 times, then relax; progress to holding for 5, then 10 breaths."

Upper trunk flexion and extension patterns and extremity combinations can be performed to strengthen specific trunk muscles: the lower abdominals and the lower-back extensors are promoted with the lower trunk flexion and extension patterns respectively. The movement combinations should be restricted to mass flexor and mass extensor patterns to reduce the stress on the low back that may occur with straight leg patterns.

Advantages. Complete relaxation can be gained in supine.

Disadvantages. The hip flexors are lengthened, which may tilt the pelvis anteriorly and extend the lumbar spine.

Sidelying

Mobility. Range in the trunk and in specific vertebral segments can be performed with HR and joint mobilization. Manual contacts (MC) can be positioned progressively closer together to facilitate specific segmental movement.

Stability. A shortened held resisted contraction (SHRC) of the postural extensors and scapula adductors can be maintained by manual, elastic, or pulley resistance (Fig. 7–21). Alternating isometrics (AI) and RS are performed to alternately, then simultaneously activate the abdominals and extensors to further promote isometric stability. MC can be placed on the scapula and pelvis to facilitate the entire trunk or, as with mobility techniques, can be placed closer together for specific segmental emphasis (Figs. 7–22, 7–23).

Controlled Mobility. When pain does not limit movement, the techniques of slow reversal hold (SRH) and slow reversal (SR) are useful to promote isotonic ac-

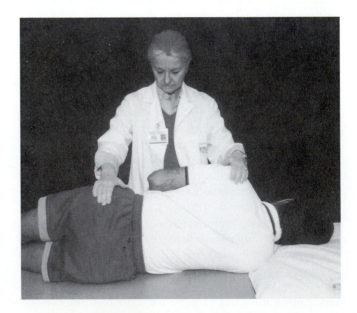

Figure 7–21. A: Sidelying. T: SHRC.

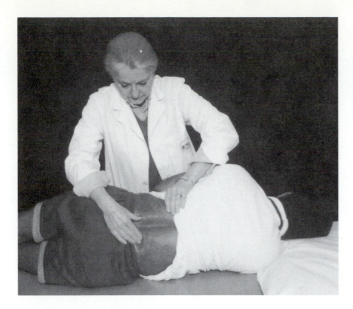

Figure 7–22. A: Sidelying. T: AI → RS. MC lumbar spine.

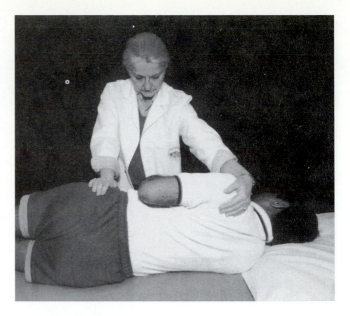

Figure 7–24. A: Sidelying; lower-trunk rotation. T: SRH.

tivity of the lower trunk muscles during lower trunk rotational movements (Figs. 7–24, 7–25).

Skill. Counterrotation can be performed with SR to enhance the sequencing of trunk movement that occurs during gait (Fig. 7–26).

Advantage. The lower extremities can be positioned in extension so that the shortened range of hip flexion will not be reinforced. This is one of the few postures in which the abdominals can be emphasized without activating the hip flexors in the shortened range. With the involved side uppermost, sidebending can

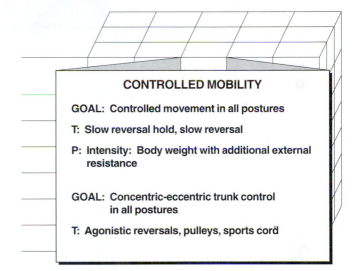

CONTROLLED MOBILITY

GOAL: Controlled movement in all postures

T: Slow reversal hold, slow reversal

P: Intensity: Body weight with additional external resistance

GOAL: Concentric-eccentric trunk control in all postures

T: Agonistic reversals, pulleys, sports cord

Figure 7–25. Treatment goals and techniques appropriate when promoting controlled mobility.

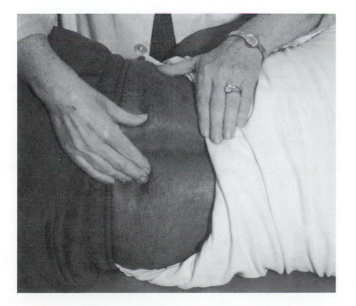

Figure 7–23. A: Sidelying. T: AI → RS. MC lumbar spine.

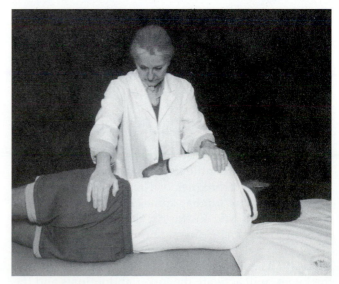

Figure 7–26. A: Sidelying; trunk counterrotation. T: RI → SR.

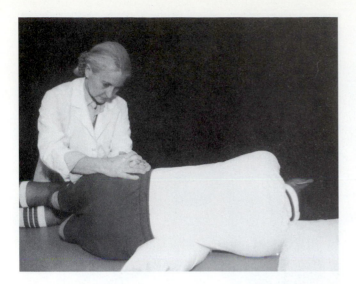

Figure 7–27. A: Sidelying; sidebending to the right.

are first applied with the knees together, a position that may lead to greater activity of the trunk musculature than when the knees are separated. AI will produce a greater amount of muscular activity on alternate sides of the trunk, whereas RS will facilitate simultaneous muscle contractions around the lower trunk. During these procedures, the patient's low back and pelvis are monitored to ensure that the lower abdominals are contracting and lumbar spine position is maintained in proper alignment. AI and RS can be applied to the entire trunk with one MC on the knees and the other on an upper-trunk pattern

Figure 7–28. A: Lower-trunk rotation. T: HR, MC knees, stabilizing thoracic spine.

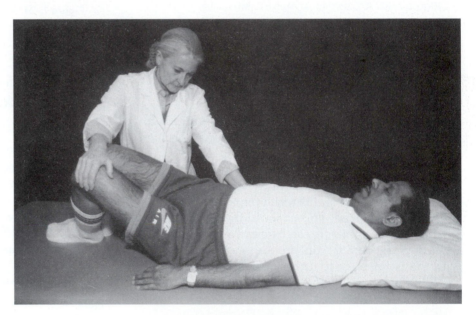

be promoted, followed by positional traction performed as part of a home program (Fig. 7–27).

Hooklying and Lower Trunk Rotation

Mobility. Mobility of lower trunk segments can be achieved by rotating the knees to either side in hooklying with the techniques of RR and HR. To ensure movement in the lumbar spine, the thoracic spine is stabilized by a MC on the rib cage or by UE movement in the opposite direction (Fig. 7–28).

Stability. The techniques of AI and RS, with MC on the knees, will activate the lower abdominals and the lumbar back extensors (Fig. 7–29). These techniques

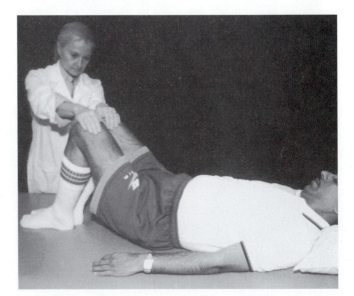

Figure 7–29. A: Hooklying. T: AI → RS, MC knees.

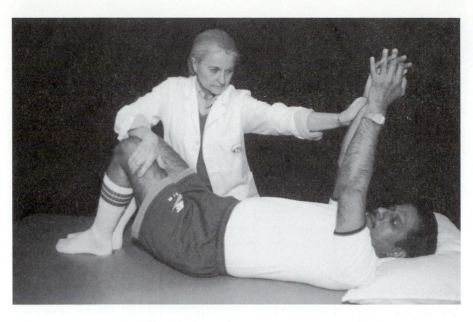

Figure 7–30. A: Hooklying with an upper-trunk pattern. T: AI → RS, MC wrists and knees.

(Fig. 7–30). As part of the home program, the lower abdominals are promoted by having the patient learn to flatten the back against the table. Additional resistance can be provided by sequentially flexing the legs while maintaining the lower abdominal contraction, then resuming the hooklying position. The challenge can be increased by beginning the leg flexion movement with the knees in more extension, which increases the length of the lever arm (Fig. 7–31). Performing UE movements dynamically alters the lever arm and further challenges the abdominals and extensors to maintain the lower-trunk position. Flexibil-

ity and stability around the hips and lower trunk is considered adequate to progress to bridging if a posterior pelvic tilt can be maintained when the hips are near full extension.

Controlled Mobility. Lower-trunk rotational movements through increments of range are performed as active movement to improve concentric–eccentric control in all of the lower-trunk muscles.[28] Strengthening techniques such as repeated contractions (RC) can be added to SRH to enhance the activity of the lower-trunk musculature when movement does not

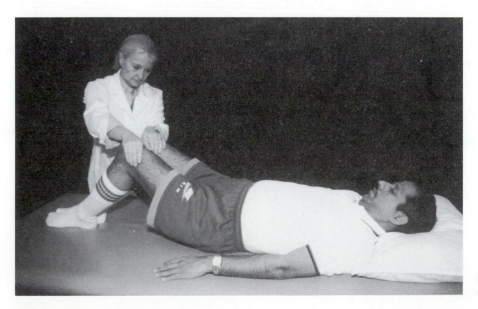

Figure 7–31. A: Hooklying; knees in more extension. T: AI → RS, MC knees.

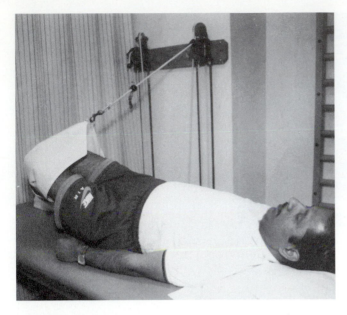

Figure 7–32. A: Lower-trunk rotation. T: AR, pulley resistance.

Advantages. No weight bearing occurs through the lumbar spine; torsional compression stress to the disc and facets is reduced during rotational movements, compared to other postures such as sitting or standing. The hip flexors are in mid range, not on stretch, reducing the tendency toward lumbar extension.

Disadvantage. The therapist cannot observe the alignment or movement in the trunk.

Bridging

Mobility. Hip flexor mobility first must be developed in other postures to allow achievement of a fully extended hip position. Discomfort in the lumbar or sacroiliac region may be due to the pull of the tight flexors.

Stability. The isometric activity of the low-back extensors can be combined with activation of the abdominals and hip musculature with the stability tech-

cause pain. Resistance provided by pulleys or an elastic can concentrically and eccentrically resist the movement (Fig. 7–32). The rotational movement should result in smooth, rhythmical contractions between lower trunk, pelvic, and hip musculature. In hooklying, controlled flexion and extension and lateral bending or sidebending of the lumbar spine can be actively performed.

Skill. Trunk counterrotation is accomplished by combining upper-trunk movement with lower-trunk rotation and the techniques of SR to promote the normal sequencing of the movement, followed by active movement when performed independently (Fig. 7–33).

TABLE 7–5. PROCEDURES IN HOOKLYING AND BRIDGING TO PROMOTE MOVEMENT CONTROL

Mobility	Stability	Controlled Mobility
Lower trunk rotation	Lower abdominals and low-back extensors in hooklying	Rotation and weight shifting in both postures
	Lower-back and hip extensors in bridging	
Advantage Minimal spine compression		Disadvantage Hip flexor stretch may extend spine

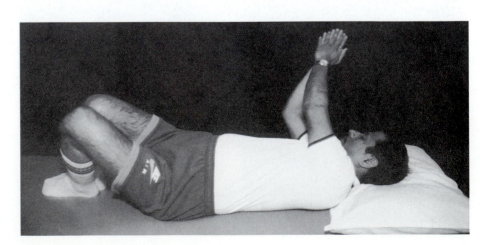

Figure 7–33. A: Hooklying; trunk counterrotation. T: Active movement.

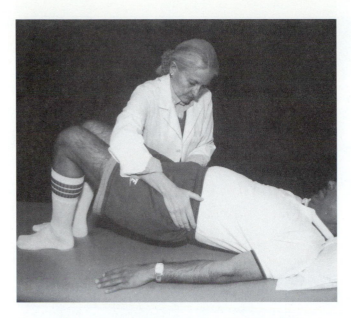

Figure 7–34. A: Bridging. T: AI → RS, MC pelvis.

niques of AI and RS (Table 7–5, Fig. 7–34).[29] Elastic or other weights placed on the pelvis or around the knees can be used to resist the position (Fig. 7–35). The patient's ability to maintain the lower trunk posture may be further challenged by performing upper limb movements.

Controlled Mobility. Rotation and lateral shifting of the lower trunk and pelvis needed during ambulation are promoted with the technique of SRH, then performed independently by the patient. Controlled raising and lowering of the pelvis, augmented by the technique of agonist reversals (AR) will improve concentric–eccentric control of the back and hip extensors (Fig. 7–36A). This motion can be performed

by first extending and then lowering the hips, or by posteriorly tilting the pelvis and segmentally following the movement in the lumbar spine.

Static–Dynamic. Lifting one limb while maintaining the pelvic position increases the level of difficulty for the back and hip extensors (Figs. 7–36, 7–37).

Skill. Marching in place, with the feet moving progressively further from the buttocks, can be performed slowly, then with increasing speed.

Advantage. The low back and hip extensors are contracting in their shortened ranges against body-weight resistance in a range similar to standing. Increased activity of the LE musculature occurs when the feet are positioned further away from the buttocks. The placement of MC or other resistive forces can be progressed from the pelvis, to the knees, to the ankles.

Disadvantage. If hip flexor tightness and abdominal weakness are still present, lumbar extension may occur, increasing the stress on the low back. If this is evident, the patient may not be ready to assume this posture.

Prone

Mobility. Lumbar extension can be increased by having the patient maintain a prone on elbows or prone on hands posture. Range into both hip and lumbar extension is promoted further by HR and joint mobilization techniques. Elderly patients may be limited in assuming prone by cardiopulmonary abnormalities; tight hip flexors may make prone difficult for some patients.

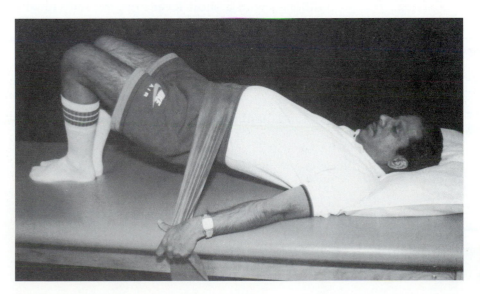

Figure 7–35. A: Bridging; pelvic elevation. T: Maintaining the posture, elastic resistance.

Figure 7–36. (A) A: Bridging. T: AR. **(B)** A: Bridging; lifting one lower extremity. T: Active movement.

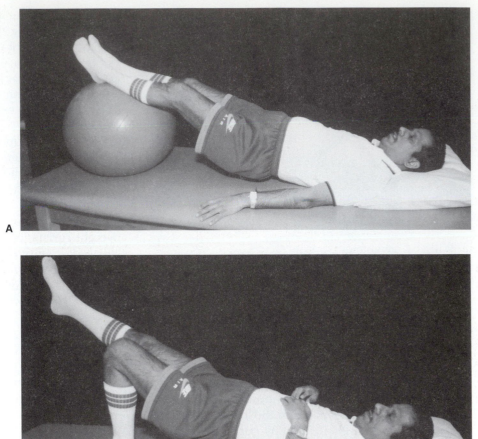

Stability. Muscular stability in the back and hip extensors can be emphasized in prone.[30] First the limbs, positioned with a short lever arm, are individually raised from the surface, holding the contraction for three breaths. The progression is to increase the duration of the contraction, and lengthen the lever arm, raise two, then all four limbs. A pillow under the abdomen may improve comfort.

Modified Plantigrade

Mobility. Unlike bridging, ROM of the low back or LE does not commonly restrict assumption of the posture.

Stability. Maintenance of the posture is not difficult for most patients because of the neutral position of the lumbar spine. No tissues are being passively stretched. AI or RS with MC on the pelvis or scapula

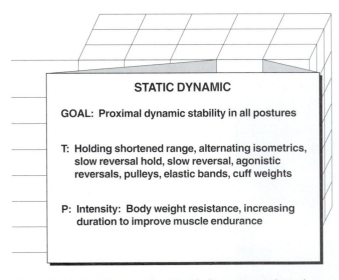

STATIC DYNAMIC

GOAL: Proximal dynamic stability in all postures

T: Holding shortened range, alternating isometrics, slow reversal hold, slow reversal, agonistic reversals, pulleys, elastic bands, cuff weights

P: Intensity: Body weight resistance, increasing duration to improve muscle endurance

Figure 7–37. Treatment goals and techniques appropriate when promoting static–dynamic control.

and pelvis can further enhance stability in the posture.

Controlled Mobility. Movement of the trunk can be performed in the anterior–posterior, lateral, and rotational directions with the techniques of SR or SRH or can be practiced independently as part of the home program.

Static–Dynamic. Movement of the limbs will emphasize trunk stability as one or contralateral limbs are lifted and maintained in extension. As in previous postures, dynamic trunk control can be promoted by movement of the limbs in various combinations and directions (Fig. 7–38). Resistance can be provided manually by free weights, pulleys, or elastic bands.

Advantages. In modified plantigrade, the hip is in some flexion, which reduces the stress on the lumbar spine. The abdominals support the viscera against the force of gravity and isometrically contract to produce a posterior pelvic tilt or neutral position. To reduce the stress on the lumbar spine, unilateral UE support in modified plantigrade is a position that should be encouraged when performing many ADL, for example, brushing teeth or shaving. Many of the controlled mobility and static–dynamic procedures are

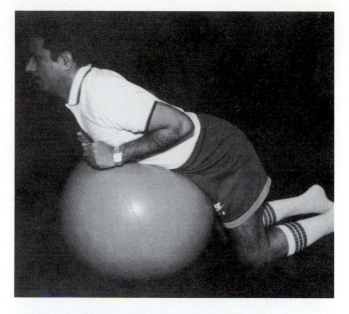

Figure 7–39. A: Quadruped. T: SHRC.

easily included in the home program, using the kitchen counter for support. For elderly patients with pain from arthritis or compression fractures, modified plantigrade is a posture in which muscle stability and endurance most easily can be enhanced.

Quadruped

Mobility. ROM restrictions do not commonly limit the assumption of quadruped.

Stability. Maintenance of the posture can be performed independently and enhanced with AI and RS with the pelvis in proper alignment. SHRC can be performed in a modified position to enhance contractions of trunk in shortened ranges (Fig. 7–39).

Controlled Mobility. Weight shifting is performed emphasizing proper control in the entire trunk and lumbar spine. Segmental vertebral movements can be encouraged in anterior–posterior, lateral, and rotational directions. Movement can first be performed in the thoracic spine before progressing to the involved area. MC are positioned as needed to apply resistance or to improve awareness (Fig. 7–40A–C).

Static–Dynamic. As in the movements performed in modified plantigrade, one or two limbs can be raised to promote trunk dynamic stability or they can be moved simultaneously to further promote dynamic trunk control (Fig. 7–40D,E).

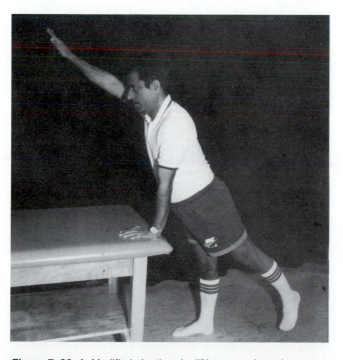

Figure 7–38. A: Modified plantigrade; lifting contralateral upper extremities. T: Active movement.

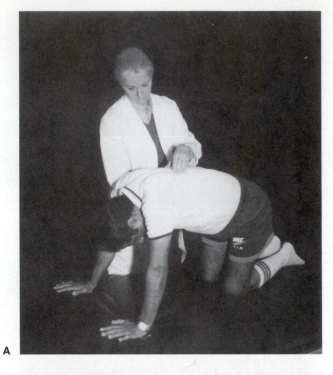

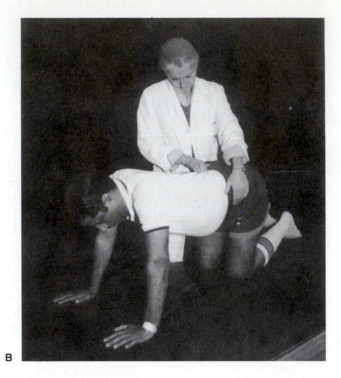

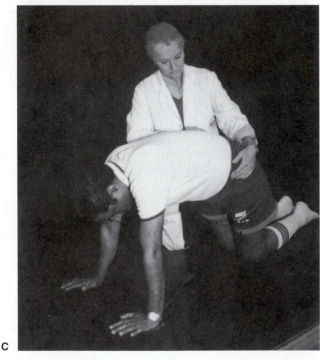

Figure 7–40. (A–C) A: Quadruped; thoracic and lumbar flexion and extension. T: Guided movement.

Advantages. The flexed-hip position reduces the passive stretch on the lumbar spine. The abdominals contract against gravity to maintain the lumbar spine position in conjunction with the lumbar extensors. Lowering the limbs slowly will improve the eccentric control of both trunk and extremity extensors. Procedures in quadruped usually provide more challenge than those in modified plantigrade because of the increased resistance of gravity and the greater excursions of the extremities.

Disadvantages. The flexed-hip position reinforces tight hip flexors and joint capsule. As the LE extends, the lumbar spine may extend or arch as a result of tightness in the hip flexors or weakness in the lower abdominals.

Sitting

Mobility. At least 90° of hip flexion is needed to maintain proper alignment of the pelvis and trunk, with greater range required while rocking forward to assume standing.

Stability. Stability in the trunk can be promoted with AI and RS with MC on the upper body. Holding, with the lower trunk in proper alignment, can be challenged while upper trunk and extremity movements are resisted manually by pulleys or elastic bands (Fig. 7–41). Resisted upper extremity D1F and D2F movements facilitate trunk extensors while resisted upper extremity D1F and D2E extension activate the abdominals.

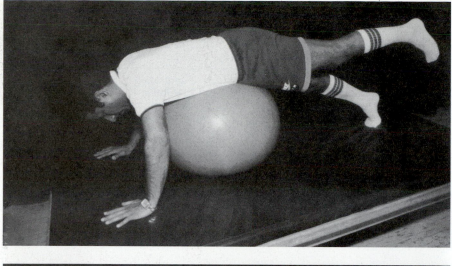

D

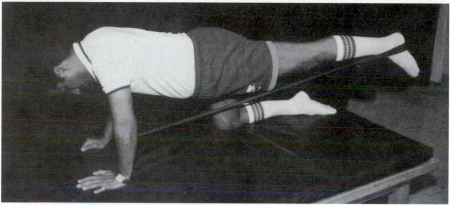

E

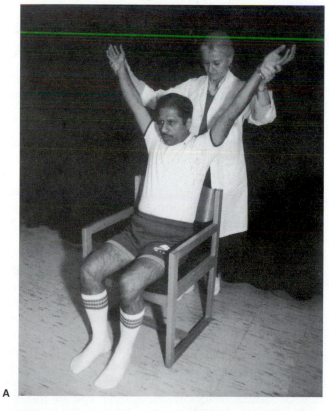

A

Figure 7–41. (A,B) A: Sitting. Bilateral symmetrical D2F. T: AR, manual and pulley resistance.

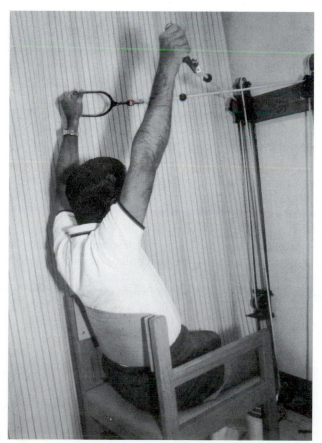

B

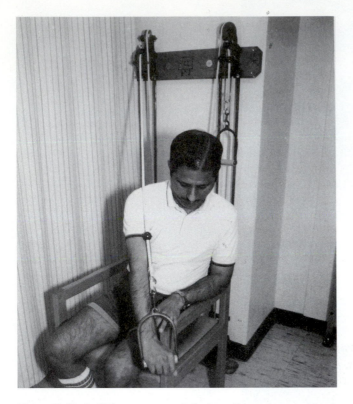

Figure 7–42. A: Sitting; upper-trunk flexion with rotation combined with D2E upper extremity. T: AR, pulley resistance.

TABLE 7–6. PROCEDURES IN SITTING TO PROMOTE MOVEMENT CONTROL

Stability	Controlled Mobility	Static–Dynamic
Isometric abdominals and extensors	Combined movements of the upper trunk Pelvic tilting	Increased range into combined movements of upper trunk
Problems Discal pressure Facet compression		Benefits Functional

Controlled Mobility. Controlled movement in the lower and upper trunk can be performed in three directions: flexion–extension by flattening the back and posteriorly tilting the pelvis, lateral flexion by hiking one hip or sidebending with the upper trunk, and rotation by twisting the upper body. Upper-trunk movements can be combined, for example, flexion with rotation to the left. This combined movement, if resisted, facilitates the oblique abdominals and stretches the right posterior tissues (Fig. 7–42). With the patient facing the pulleys, concentric–eccentric contractions of the trunk extensors can be performed. Static–dynamic lower abdominal strengthening can be performed by stabilizing the lumbar spine while flexing one lower extremity at the hip, then the other. This exercise simulates the control in the lower trunk needed for example, when driving a standard shift car. Opposite UE and LE movements can be performed sitting on a ball and stabilizing the trunk (Table 7–6).

Skill. When UE and LE movements can be performed with dynamic alignment, the skill stage has been achieved. Practicing daily living and occupational tasks can be performed to improve sitting tolerance and the sequencing of movements.

Advantages. Both UE and LE movements can be performed to challenge trunk control and to simulate functional activities. The lumbar spine position and the weight-bearing surfaces can be varied to reduce symptoms and redistribute compressive forces.[31]

Disadvantages. Weight bearing through the trunk can increase pain in some patients. The flexed hip position can reinforce the shortened range of hip flexors. For others, a limited range into hip flexion can result in posterior tilt and lumbar flexion. Abnormal movement in the lumbar spine can occur if muscular or postural stability is not sufficient.

Standing

The ability of the patient to stand and ambulate without pain and with good posture will indicate to the therapist the success of the previous procedures. A functional evaluation during active movements such as reaching, bending, and lifting should be conducted.

Stability. Holding of the lumbar position can be challenged by resisted UE movements (Fig. 7–43).

Controlled Mobility. Concentric–eccentric movements of the back extensors simulate the control needed while lifting or moving objects. Eccentric endurance can be promoted with free weights or pulleys.

Static–Dynamic. Lifting contralateral or ipsilateral extremities rhythmically or suddenly on a stable or moveable surface will simulate daily movements and improve the timing of movement.

As already mentioned, the patient must be educated in proper body mechanics and back care. ADL are modified to reduce back strain. Modifications may include rolling to sidelying during the assumption of sitting from supine, proper use of pillows while sleeping, alternating the lifting of feet onto a

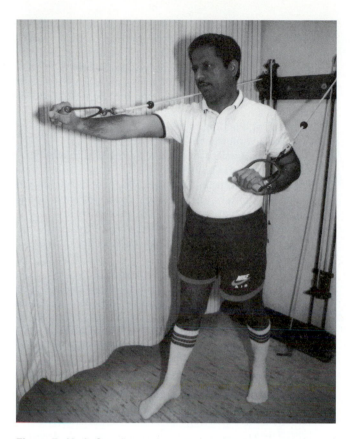

Figure 7–43. A: Standing; upper extremity movements. T: AR with pulley resistance.

low stool when standing for prolonged periods, and adequate support in sitting postures. Transfer of learning to every-day activities is essential and can be promoted with both instruction and practice in lifting, moving, and reaching for objects.

▶ SUMMARY

The progression of procedures in this chapter has been developed on the basis of the most common clinical findings among patients with low back disability: pain and tightness in the hip flexors and extensors and low back extensors, and decreased strength and stability of lower abdominals and low back extensors. Other therapeutic interventions will probably be indicated. These may include joint mobilization, external support, transcutaneous nerve stimulation (TNS), work conditioning, and behavior modification. The combination of therapeutic exercise procedures, carefully sequenced for each patient, coupled with other appropriate interventions should restore the patient to as functional a level as possible.

▶ REVIEW QUESTIONS

1. Your patient demonstrates decreased forward flexion during active movement in standing. What tissues could be restricting range? What treatments would be appropriate for each?

2. Your patient begins to experience fatigue after an hour of standing or while typing. What might be the causative factors and what treatments would be appropriate?

3. In quadruped your patient exhibits lordosis while performing static–dynamic leg movements. What are two possible causes and what treatments would remedy those problems?

4. Improving the control and endurance of the back extensors and abdominals is a goal for most patients with low back dysfunction. Describe a progression of activities for each of these muscle groups.

REFERENCES

1. North RB, Campbell JN, James CS, et al. Failed back surgery syndrome: 5 year follow-up in 102 patients undergoing repeated operation. *Neurosurgery.* 1991;28:685–691.
2. Turner JA, Ersek M, Herron L, et al. Patient outcomes after lumbar spinal fusions. *JAMA.* 1992;268:907–911.
3. Saal JA, Saal JS. Nonoperative treatment of herniated lumbar intervertebral disc with radiculopathy: an outcome study. *Spine.* 1989;14:431–437.
4. Deyo RA, Walsh NE, Martin DC, et al. A controlled trial of transcutaneous electrical nerve stimulation and exercise for chronic low back pain. *N Engl J Med.* 1990;322:1627–1634.
5. Spitzer WO: Diagnosis of the problem (the problem of diagnosis) *Spine.* 1987;12(suppl):516–521.
6. Deyo RA, Cherkin DC, Conrad D, et al: Cost, controversy, crisis: Low back pain and the public health. *Annual review of public health.* 1991;12:141–156.
7. Battle MC, Cherkin DC, Dunn R, et al: Managing low back pain: Attitudes and treatment preferences of physical therapists. *Phys Ther* 1994;74:219–226.
8. Waddell G. How patients react to low back pain. *Acta Orthop Scand Suppl.* 1993;251:21–24.
9. Roberts N, Smith R, Bennett J, et al. Health beliefs and rehabilitation after lumbar disc surgery. *J Psychosom Res.* 1984;28:139–144.
10. Woodward C. Repetitive strain injury: A diagnostic model and management guidelines. *Aust J Physiother.* 1987;33:96–99.
11. Boisonault WG. *Examination in physical therapy practice: Screening for medical disease.* New York, Churchill Livingstone, 1991.

12. Rachlin H. Pain and behavior. *Behav Brain Sci.* 1985; 8:43–83.

13. Selkowitz DM. The sympathetic nervous system in neuromotor function and dysfunction and pain: a brief review and discussion. *Funct Neurol.* 1992;7:89–95.

14. Demuth NJ, Gross BL. *The Relationship of Lumbar Mobility, Lumbar Angle, and Hip Flexibility to Low Back Pain in Female Ballet Dancers.* Boston, Mass: Boston University, Sargent College of Allied Health Professions; 1987. Thesis.

15. Kendall FP, McCreary EK, Provance PG. *Muscles: Testing and Function.* 4th ed. Baltimore, Md: Williams & Wilkins; 1993.

16. Cyriax J. *Text Book of Orthopedic Medicine,* 8th ed. London, England: Baillière Tindall Ltd; 1982.

17. Jorgensen K, Nicholaisen T, Kato M: Muscle fiber distribution, capillary density, and enzymatic activities in the lumbar paravertebral muscles of young men: significance for isometric endurance. *Spine.* 1993;18: 1439–1450.

18. Richardson C, Tupenberg R, Jull J. An initial evaluation of eight abdominal exercises for their ability to provide stabilization for the lumbar spine. *Aust J Physiother.* 1990;36:6–11.

19. Bogduk N, Twoomey LT. *Clinical Anatomy of the Lumbar Spine.* Edinburgh, Scotland: Churchill Livingstone; 1987.

20. Cohen M, Hoskins-Michel T. *Cardiopulmonary Symptoms in Physical Therapy Practice.* New York, NY: Churchill Livingstone; 1988.

21. Kellett KM, Kellett DA, Nordholm LA. Effects of an exercise program on sick leave due to back pain. *Phys Ther.* 1991;71:283–293.

22. Rood M. The use of sensory receptors to activate, facilitate and inhibit motor response, autonomic and somatic, in developmental sequence. In: Sattely C, ed. *Approaches to the Treatment of Patients with Neuromuscular Dysfunction.* Dubuque, Iowa: Wm C Brown Co Publishers; 1962.

23. Tappan FM. Healing massage techniques, 2nd ed. Norwalk, CT: Appleton and Lange; 1988.

24. Jacobsen E. *Anxiety and Tension Control.* Philadelphia, Pa: JB Lippincott Co; 1964.

25. Khalil TM, Asfour SS, Martinez LM, et al. Stretching in the rehabilitation of low back pain patients. *Spine.* 1992;17:311–317.

26. Astrand PO, Rodahl K. Applied Work Physiology. In: *Textbook of Work Physiology,* 3rd ed. New York, McGraw Hill; 1986.

27. Macefield G, Hagbarth KE, Gorman R, et al. Decline in spindle support to alpha motoneurons during sustained voluntary contractions. *J Physiol.* 1991;440: 497–512.

28. Konecky C. *An EMG Study of Abdominals and Back Extensors During Lower Trunk Rotation.* Boston, Mass: Boston University, Sargent College of Allied Health Professions; 1980. Thesis.

29. Rich C. *EMG Analysis of Trunk Musculature During Isometric Techniques in Bridging.* Boston, Mass: Boston University, Sargent College of Allied Health Professions, 1981. Thesis.

30. Haigh S. Training isometric endurance of the trunk extensors in a clinical environment. *Austr J Physiother.* 1993;39:99–103.

HIP AND TRUNK STRETCHING

Bring to the point of tightness, *not to the point of pain*. Keep in that range for about 10 to 20 seconds.

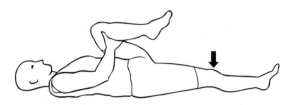

To stretch in front of your hip: Bring both knees toward your chest. Hold one in that position while you let the other lower down toward the surface.

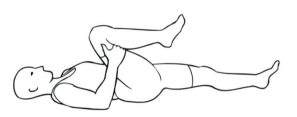

To stretch behind your hip: Bring thigh up toward your chest. You should feel the stretch behind your hip, not in your back.

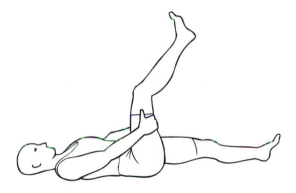

To stretch your hamstrings: Straighten your knee until you feel a pull in the back of your thigh.

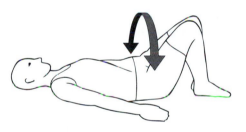

To twist your lower back: Turn or roll one hip up then turn in the other direction.

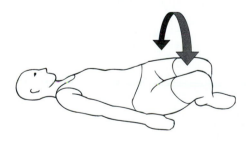

Let your knees turn in the same direction as your hips.

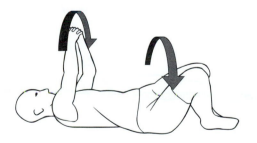

Turn your arms and your knees in opposite direction.

You may need to hold onto a chair or table while balancing on one leg.

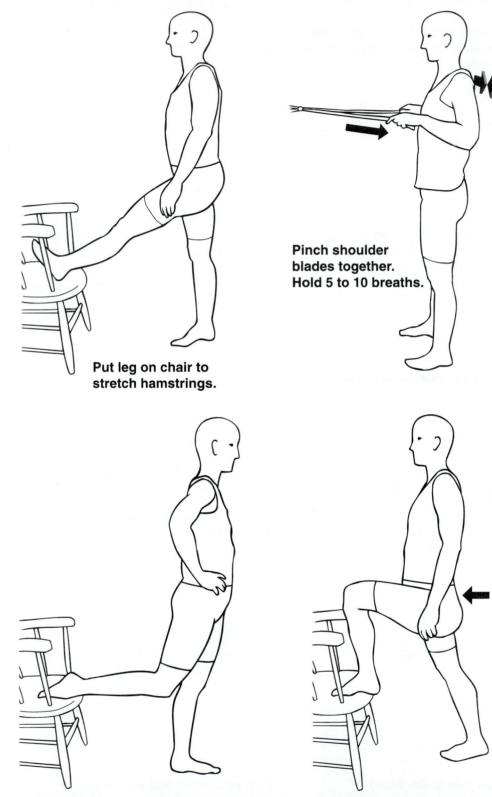

Put leg on chair to stretch hamstrings.

Pinch shoulder blades together. Hold 5 to 10 breaths.

Let the thigh go back to stretch in front of the hip. *Do not let hips twist.*

Rock forward to stretch behind your hip.

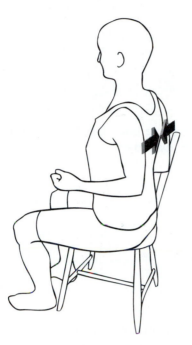

Pinch shoulder blades together, lift chest up. Hold position for 5 to 10 breaths.

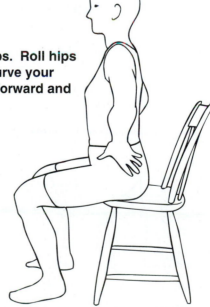

Keep back flat against the chair, bend knee up toward your chest.

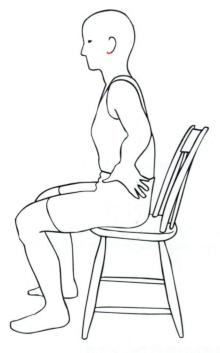

Put hands on hips. Roll hips backward and curve your back. Roll hips forward and arch your back.

ABDOMINAL STRENGTHENING

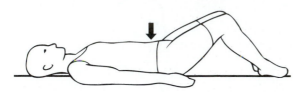

1. Flatten your back into surface.

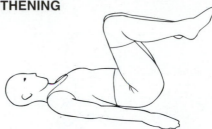

3. Keeping back flat, bring other knee toward chest.

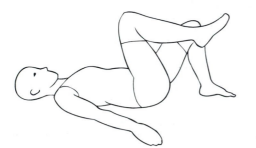

2. Keeping back flat, bring one knee toward chest.

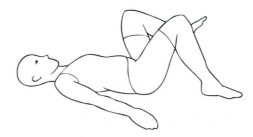

4. Keeping back flat, lower one leg to surface.

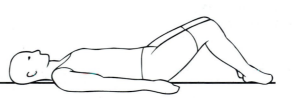

5. Keeping back flat, lower other leg to surface.

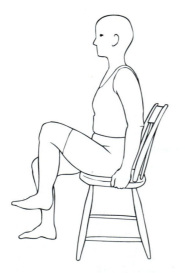

Flatten back against chair. Bring one knee toward chest.

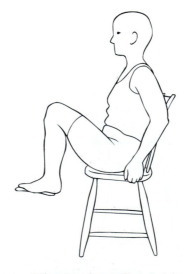

Keeping back flat, bring other leg toward chest.

BACK EXTENSOR STRENGTHENING

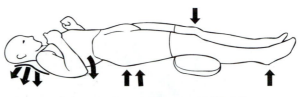

Push neck into surface, pinch shoulder blades together. Do not push with more than about 40% effort.

Also push knees into pillow and lift hips off the surface. If this hurts in your lower back, just tighten your buttock muscles and do not lift hips off surface.

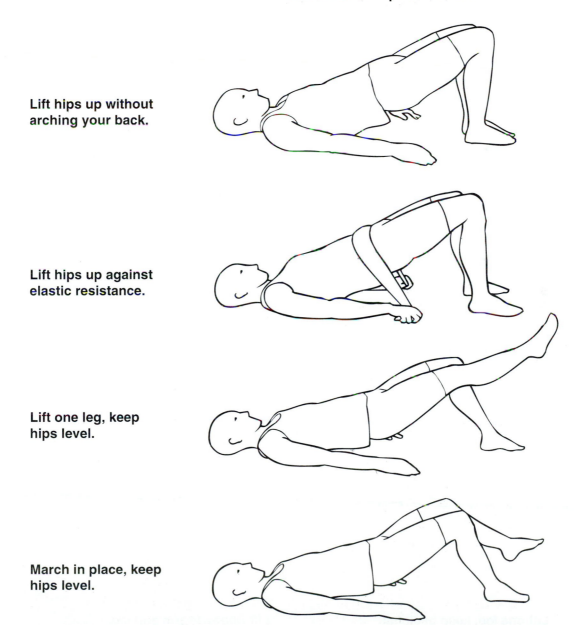

Lift hips up without arching your back.

Lift hips up against elastic resistance.

Lift one leg, keep hips level.

March in place, keep hips level.

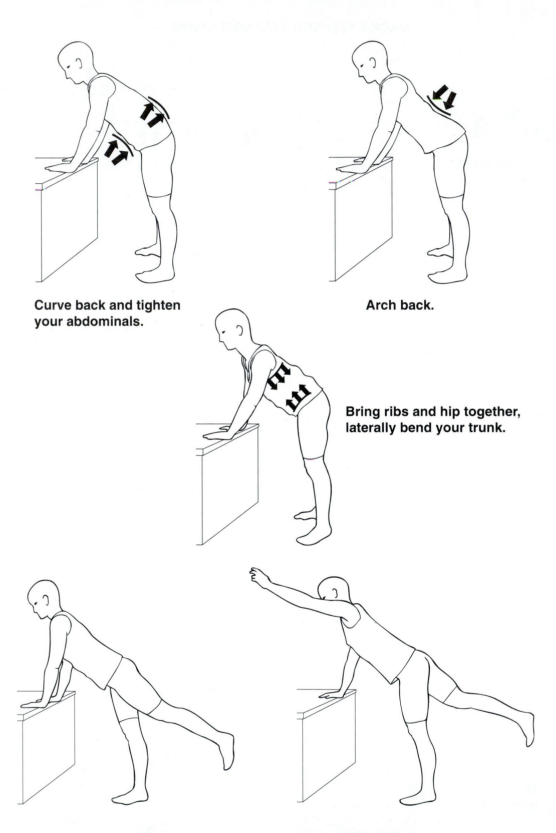

Curve back and tighten your abdominals.

Arch back.

Bring ribs and hip together, laterally bend your trunk.

Lift one leg, keep back flat.

Lift *opposite* arm and leg. Do not let back arch.

BACK EXTENSOR STRENGTHENING

Hold all positions for 5 to 10 breaths.

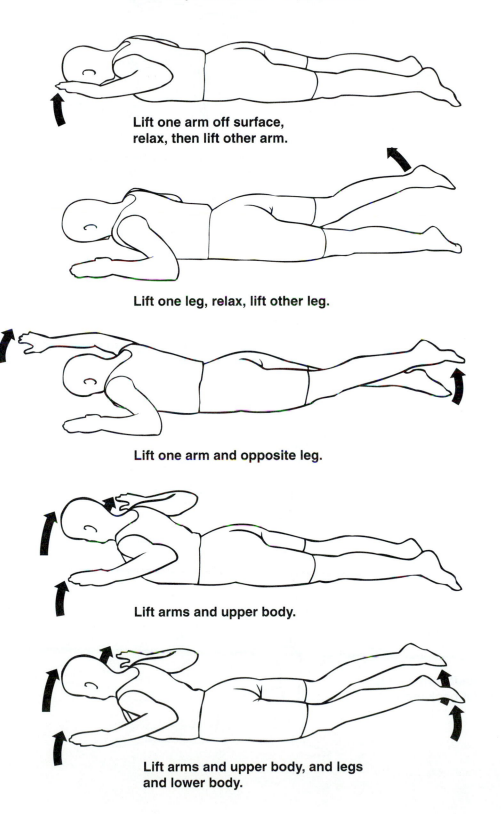

Lift one arm off surface,
relax, then lift other arm.

Lift one leg, relax, lift other leg.

Lift one arm and opposite leg.

Lift arms and upper body.

Lift arms and upper body, and legs
and lower body.

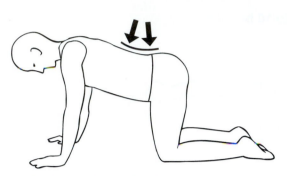

Arch your lower back.

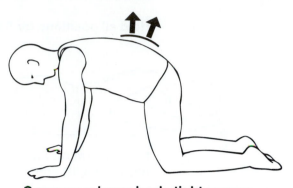

Curve your lower back, tighten your abdominals (your stomach muscles).

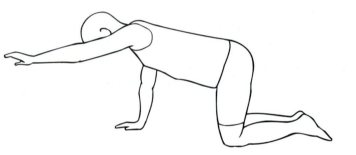

Lift one arm.

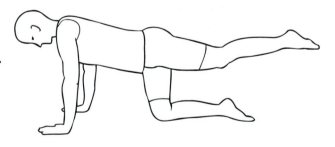

Lift one leg, keep back flat.

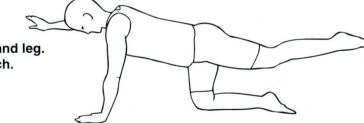

**Lift *opposite* arm and leg.
Do not let back arch.**

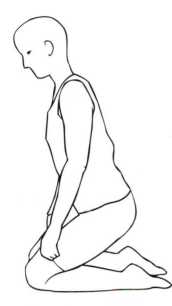

Move between kneeling and sitting on your heels, keep your back from arching.

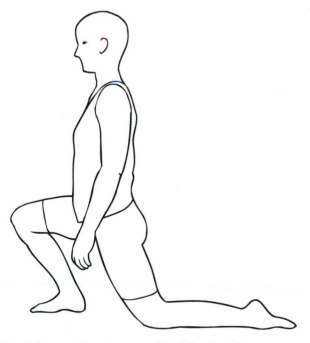

Rock forward onto your front foot and keep your back from arching.

CHAPTER 8

Spinal Cord Injury

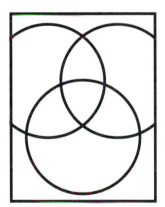

Spinal cord injuries (SCI) are most commonly a result of vehicular or sporting accidents and inflicted injuries such as gunshot or stab wounds. Such trauma primarily affects young people ranging in age from the late teens to the early twenties. Congenital deficits such as spina bifida and circulatory insufficiency, which usually occurs in an older age group, can also result in spinal cord dysfunction [1,2] (Fig. 8–1).

Physical therapy is a vital component of the rehabilitation process along with the other health care professions of medicine, occupational therapy, social work, nursing, vocational training, and psychiatry. The level and completeness of the lesion will largely determine the functional capabilities of the patient.

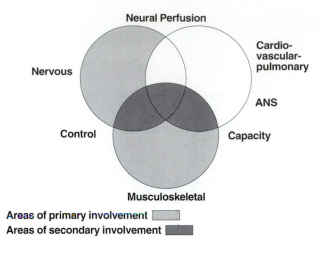

Figure 8–1. Primary and secondary involvement.

However, many other factors exclusive of the level of lesion are important determinants of the success of treatment. These variables include age, height and weight, the amount and pattern of spasticity, body image, motivation, family support, and prior occupational experience. Psychological acceptance of the injury may be the most difficult aspect of rehabilitation because the patient is continually confronted with the reality of functional limitations and compromises in life-style. The cooperation of health care professionals is essential to assist the patient in dealing with the many changes and adaptations that must occur.[3,4]

Improved emergency care and medical treatment have increased the likelihood of spinal nerve recovery and have permitted the earlier initiation of restorative procedures. Future advances in all aspects of treatment will lead to further improvement of patient care and enhancement of patient capabilities.

Although this chapter focuses on the treatment of patients with SCI, much of this information can be generalized to the treatment of other patients with quadrant or total-body involvement. For example, extremity strengthening procedures can be applied to patients with brachial plexus injury; mat procedures are appropriate for patients with Guillain-Barré syndrome or multiple sclerosis.

EVALUATION

Environmental and Social Factors

The length of stay in rehabilitation facilities has dramatically decreased in recent years. Inpatient treatment must focus on achieving optimal function within existing time constraints. Emphasis on compensatory aides, outpatient programs, consideration of independent living environments, and modification of existing architectural barriers will facilitate the patient's return to the community. Examination of the patient's living arrangement should begin early in the program and changes implemented before the patient is ready to return home either temporarily or permanently. Home adaptations and equipment needs such as a wheelchair and orthotic devices should be anticipated early in the rehabilitation process, especially if financial problems exist.

Vocational counseling will probably be indicated as rehabilitation progresses. The patient's occupational and educational history will affect long-term planning. The accessibility and feasibility of returning to previous positions must be evaluated and viable alternatives suggested.

Medical and Psychological Factors

Essential to the patient's acceptance of the present and future is the support given by family, friends, and professionals.[3,4] The SCI patient frequently passes through the stages of grief similar to those experienced by patients with other catastrophic illnesses. The achievement of functional potential is usually delayed until some level of acceptance is reached. Many patients maintain belief in full recovery but accept the fact that for the present they must learn how to overcome the limitations of their disability.

Depending on the trauma or the cause of the SCI, patients may have other medical or surgical complications that greatly influence the initial course of intervention. Because impairment of bowel and bladder control affects the patient's ability to function in society, a program to regulate these functions is an integral part of the rehabilitation process.[5] Skin integrity is extremely important and can be enhanced with good nutrition.[6,7] Pressure sores may affect the patient's long-term sitting tolerance and thus can severely limit or delay rehabilitation.[8] Bony prominences, such as the pelvic spines, greater trochanters, heels, and scapular spines require special attention. Particularly important are the ischial areas where skin breakdown may easily result from the pressure of prolonged sitting. Frequent relief of pressure by elevating the pelvis in sitting and turning in bed should become a habit. In addition, the use of special cushions or mattresses will help to decrease the occurrence of decubiti.

Physical Systems

Assessment of sensory and motor function and the status of the anal reflex provide early indication of the level and completeness of the lesion. As spinal shock subsides, innervation of sensory and motor segments below the level of the vertebral involvement may become evident.[9–11] Serial evaluations are a means of documenting the recovery pattern and of providing the therapist with the information necessary to plan an effective treatment. Although important, the initial evaluations are usually limited by bed positioning and external supportive devices used to immobilize the spinal column.

Cardiovascular–Pulmonary System

The respiratory functions of breathing and coughing may be severely impaired if the innervation to abdominal and intercostal muscles has been interrupted. Diaphragmatic involvement necessitates initial, if not long-term, mechanical assistance for respiratory support. Decreased forced expiration, occurring as a result of impairment to the accessory muscles of respiration, will require respiratory training and pulmonary care.[12]

Autonomic Nervous System

Disruption of autonomic functions can decrease the patient's ability to regulate blood pressure as upright postures are assumed. Medication, pressure wraps, and gradual postural changes may alleviate this problem. Changes in autonomic nervous system (ANS) responses such as increase in perspiration or headaches may indicate a full bladder or a need to defecate.[9–11] Some patients may have difficulty with peripheral circulation, which may be manifested as abnormal temperature control. Trophic changes occur when autonomic innervation is decreased, affecting skin integrity.

Nervous System

Sensation. The results of the sensory evaluation are important for treatment planning and patient education. Sensory testing is usually performed according to nerve root levels and may indicate the level of the spinal recovery. Exteroceptive superficial sensation is differentially evaluated from deep proprioceptive and visceral sensations. Because these sensations travel over different ascending pathways to higher centers of the central nervous system (CNS), they may be affected differently by injury. The patient may be able to detect deep-joint movement, for example, but not superficial touch. The patient may also be able to sense muscle contraction in areas where exteroceptive sensation is not present. Visceral sensations are monitored both through the ANS and cranial nerves and may be partially intact.

The sensory level of innervation does not always correspond to the level of motor function. Most fracture dislocations of the vertebral column cause damage to the adjacent anterior tracts in the spinal cord. If the posterior tracts are intact, as can occur with an incomplete lesion, the sensory functions may be partially spared.[10,11]

An incomplete lesion may result in a diffuse and spotty sensory and motor return; the condition of the patient may not stabilize for a long period of time. At the time of injury, a peripheral nerve root lesion may have occurred, especially if the direction of force was lateral or rotational. Regeneration along that nerve root may lead to return one level below the level of lesion.

Learning a movement and the execution of exercise procedures is always easier if the patient has sensation in that area. An intact body image, which depends partly on sensory feedback, may enhance the patient's functional ability.

If sensation in the lower extremities, especially the feet, is impaired, trauma or extremes of temperature must be avoided. Sensory deficits in the trunk or extremities suggest that attention to skin care be increased.

Musculoskeletal System

Range of Motion. Limb range of motion (ROM) and muscle extensibility should be normal during the initial posttrauma stage unless additional trauma has occurred. The role of the therapist at this stage is to maintain ROM of the extremities without compromising stabilization of the spinal column. However, limitations in range may eventually develop because of prolonged immobilization or imbalances of muscle tone. Limited passive movement is often found in the following ranges: shoulder extension, elbow, wrist, and finger extension, straight leg raise (SLR) and ankle dorsiflexion; toe touching in longsitting is frequently restricted. Although a certain amount of mobility is necessary, adaptive shortening in some muscles can be used to optimize function and is actually encouraged. Tightness of the finger flexors, for example, will improve the "strength" of a tenodesis grasp. The combined length of low-back extensors and hamstrings should be such to allow the patient to balance anteriorly in the longsitting position without upper-extremity support. Overstretching can result in excessive mobility and may decrease the support usually provided by the posterior structures. During early stages of treatment of a patient with a low thoracic or lumbar lesion, passive straight-leg or lower-trunk movements are usually contraindicated.

Movement Control

Strength. A specific muscle evaluation following myotomal levels will provide the therapist with an indication of the level of innervation. Although manual muscle testing (MMT) may not be the most valid method of testing strength,[13] it does provide the therapist with information to help determine the level of involvement with SCI patients. Based on findings, muscles can be grouped according to strengths and weaknesses. It is not uncommon to find asymmetries of motor innervation between limbs. Sparing of sacral motor tracts is a frequent finding, evidenced by minimal motoric ability in the feet. All muscles that are attached to the involved vertebrae should be tested carefully with minimal resistance. In most instances, testing of those muscles around the injured site is postponed until joint stabilization has been gained.

Muscle Tone. Deep-tendon reflexes and resistance to passive stretch are used as a subjective means of assessing variation in tone.[10] Severe hypertonia may greatly affect treatment. The ability to independently assume longsitting can be severely limited when spasticity in the pectoralis major or biceps prevents the patient from positioning his arms posteriorly; excessive tone or tightness in the lower trunk or hamstrings may limit the lower limb position in longsitting. A patient with minimal spasticity in the quadriceps may be able to use his spasticity advantageously during transfers, although excessive spasticity may interfere with mobility and dressing.

Functional Outcomes

The information gleaned from these assessments will help to determine the feasible functional outcomes. The outcomes may include: (1) locomotion, which may be limited to wheelchair mobility or ambulation with crutches and orthoses, and (2) performance of activities of daily living (ADL) skills such as feeding, dressing, personal hygiene, and vocationally directed activities. The treatment goals are adjusted periodically and should include the improvement of the patient's internal motivation.

To a large extent, the level of the lesion and result of the MMT will determine the projected functional outcome. However, many patients will not attain their potential, whereas others may greatly exceed expectations. Even when the level of innervation is similar, variations in function can occur among patients because of the numerous factors that contribute to the rehabilitative process.

THE TOTAL TREATMENT PLAN

The treatment planning process requires the interaction of the rehabilitation team. Continual communication among all the health care services is essential to provide the necessary continuity of treatment. Coordination of evaluation and treatment between physical and occupational therapies is always important but especially so when dealing with quadriplegic patients. Hand splints for positioning may be indicated initially and later, functional splints can be designed to assist with upper-extremity activities. The ADL abilities of feeding, dressing, and hygiene are usually emphasized by occupational therapists.[14] Depending on the availability of other personnel, the occupational therapist may be involved in vocational testing.

SPECIFIC TREATMENT PROCEDURES

The procedures presented in this chapter are designed to achieve specific treatment goals, which will be stated for each phase of treatment. The first sequence of procedures is designed for quadriplegic patients who have minimal or no triceps control. Patients with greater triceps strength should be able to progress through this sequence more quickly and may not need to perform all the intermediate steps. The second sequence is applicable to patients with paraplegia. The level of lesion and the extent of mus-

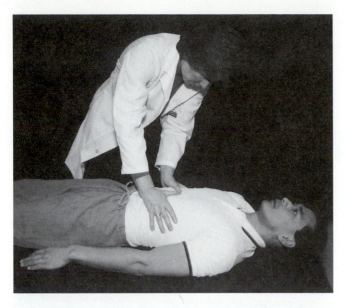

Figure 8–2. A: Supine; chest expansion. T: Guided movement.

cular innervation will determine the appropriateness of each procedure.

Treatment begins with procedures to strengthen the innervated muscles including the respiratory muscles (Fig. 8–2). Strengthening procedures are based on the principle that the activity of the weak muscles can be enhanced by promoting overflow from stronger musculature. Procedures are sequenced to progress in a proximal-to-distal direction. Overflow from stronger muscles to weaker groups can be facilitated within a limb or from one extremity to the other.[15,16] The activity of the strongest muscles should be maximized before they are used to enhance the weaker musculature through the effects of overflow. Following are typical examples of muscle grades obtained during an evaluation of a quadriplegic patient with a lesion at C5-6. Included in the subsequent discussion are the optimal patterns of movement for these muscles and suggestions for combining the activities and techniques to enhance function.

Muscle Grades:

Scapula

trapezius: G to N (4/5,5/5)

rhomboids: G (4/5)

serratus anterior: F +(3+/5)

lower trapezius and latissimus dorsi: P to F (2/5,3/5)

Shoulder

middle deltoid: G+ (4+/5)

posterior deltoid: G− (4−/5)

anterior deltoid: F+ (3+/5)

pectoralis major, clavicular portion: F+ (3+/5)

pectoralis major, sternal portion: T to P− (1/5,2−/5)

Elbow

biceps brachii: G to N (4/5,5/5)

triceps brachii: O to P (0/5,1/5)

Wrist

radial wrist extensors: G to N (4/5,5/5)

flexors: 0 (0/5)

The following indicates the patterns in which the muscles listed above can be facilitated optimally.

D2F:
trapezius: G to N (4/5,5/5)
middle deltoid: G+ (4+/5)
radial wrist extensors:
    G to N (4/5,5/5)

D1F:
serratus anterior: F+ (3+/5)
anterior deltoid: F+ (3+/5)
pectoralis major
    (clavicular): F+ (3+/5)
wrist flexors: 0 (0/5)

D1E:
rhomboids: G (4/5)
posterior deltoid: G− (4−/5)
latissimus dorsi: F (3/5)
radial wrist extensors:
    G to N (4/5,5/5)

D2E:
pectoralis major
    (sternal): P− (2−/5)
wrist flexors: 0 (0/5)

These patterns can be performed with the elbow remaining straight, flexing, or extending during the movement. On normal subjects the biceps have been shown to be active in all elbow-flexing patterns, particularly during D1F. As expected, the triceps are active in all elbow-extending patterns, but especially in D1E. The triceps are also highly active during D1E and D2F with the elbow straight.[17] The following paragraphs discuss how this knowledge can be specifically applied to activate weakened musculature.

The analysis of the MMT evaluation shows that D2F with elbow flexion is the strongest pattern for this patient. The muscles involved in this pattern, from proximal to distal, are the trapezius, middle deltoid, biceps, and the radial wrist extensors, all of which range from 4/5 to 5/5. Because the strength of all of these muscles is almost equal, the strengthening technique of repeated contractions (RC) is preferred over the technique of timing for emphasis (TE). The first procedure therefore is:

A: Supine; D2F, elbow F
T: RC

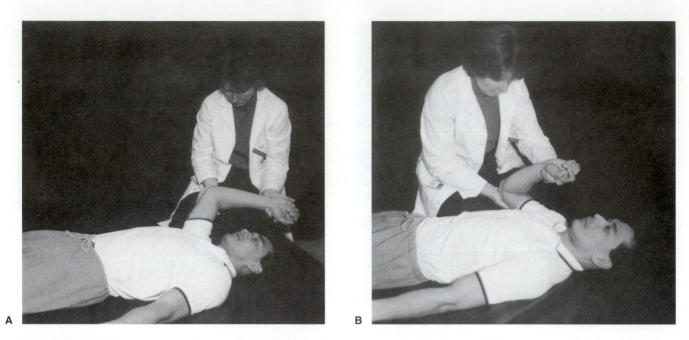

Figure 8–3. (A) A: Supine; unilateral D2F, elbow flexion. T: RC. **(B)** A: Supine; D1E, elbow flexing. T: TE on shoulder extension, scapular adduction.

This procedure will further strengthen the muscles as well as teach the patient how to move against resistance (Fig. 8–3A).

The second strongest group of proximal muscles (4⁻/5) are the rhomboids and the posterior deltoid, which are most active in the D1E pattern. By performing this pattern with the elbow flexing, overflow from the even stronger biceps is obtained. Because the biceps and wrist extensors are stronger than the proximal muscles, the technique of TE is indicated.

A: Supine, D1E, elbow flexing
T: TE on scapula adduction, shoulder extension

The stronger distal muscles are isometrically resisted in the range where they can hold best: the biceps at approximately 90° and the wrist extensors in the shortened range. While the isometric contraction of these stronger muscles is sustained, the weaker proximal muscles—the rhomboids, posterior deltoid, and latissimus dorsi—perform isotonic contractions against manual resistance with quick stretches superimposed. D1E is the pattern in which the ulnar and not the radial wrist extensors contract optimally in the normal condition. However, when the cord lesion is in the midcervical region the ulnar wrist extensors are not innervated. Therefore, patients are encouraged to extend their wrist with the innervated radial wrist extensor regardless of the pattern. Because the radial wrist extensors commonly are strong, they can elicit overflow effects in either D2F or D1E to the

weaker musculature. *Strengthening of scapular stabilizers and contracting into the range of shoulder extension is preliminary to independent assumption of supine on elbows and longsitting* (Fig. 8–3B).

The next group of muscles to be strengthened are the serratus anterior and the anterior deltoid (3⁺/5), which are most active in D1F. To promote overflow from the biceps, the pattern is performed with elbow flexion and with the technique of TE.

A: Supine, D1F, elbow flexing
T: TE to strengthen scapular abduction and shoulder flexion with adduction

The stronger biceps provides overflow to the weaker proximal muscles as they are resisted into their shortened range. Because the shoulder abductors are stronger than the adductors, the patient may have difficulty flexing in a D1 pattern, which requires movement toward the midline. Although always important, verbal cues and appropriate manual contacts are especially necessary in this instance to enhance the desired movement into D1F. *Strengthening of the serratus anterior and the anterior deltoid is needed for the assumption of prone on elbows and for lifting the pelvis from the mat in longsitting* (Fig. 8–4).

The sternal portion of the pectoralis major, usually only partially innervated in a midcervical lesion, is most active in D2E. Because of the decreased strength of the proximal muscles, this pattern is difficult for the quadriplegic patient. The technique of TE

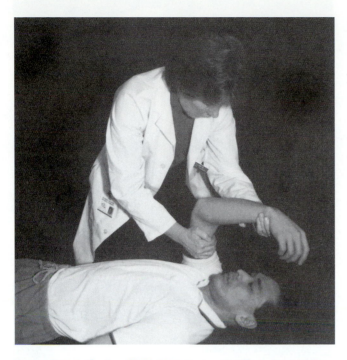

Figure 8–4. A: Supine; D1F, elbow flexing. T: TE on shoulder flexion with adduction.

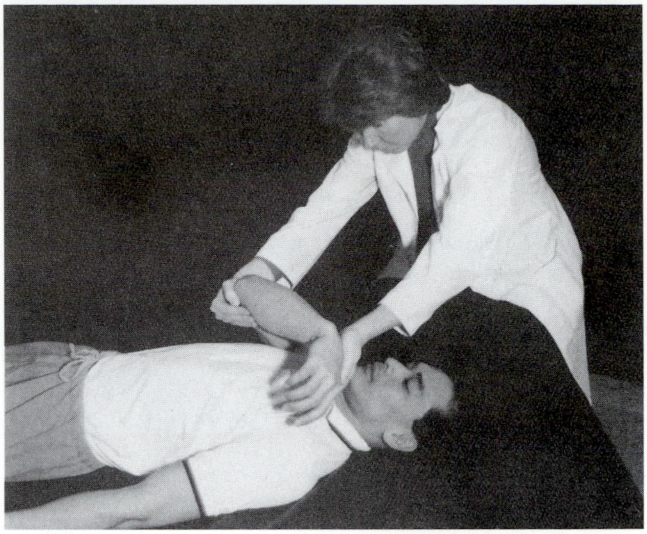

remains the most appropriate for increasing proximal activity through overflow from the stronger biceps.

> A: Supine, D2E, elbow flexing
> T: TE to shoulder extension and adduction

As with the D1F pattern, additional sensory input may be needed to promote the adduction component of the D2E pattern. *Strengthening of the adductors is important for shoulder stability during transfers and for movement of the upper extremities during dressing and other ADL* (Fig. 8–5).[14]

Progressing one joint more distally, focus in treatment is directed to strengthening of the triceps. Overflow into the triceps from the strongest shoulder musculature is obtained by performing the D2F pattern with TE.

> A: Supine; D2F, elbow straight or extending
> T: TE to the triceps

The stronger proximal muscles are resisted in the range where they can best perform an isometric contraction; for the shoulder flexors this range appears to be at or just beyond 90° of flexion. Initially the elbow is maintained in extension while approximation and resistance enhance tonic holding of elbow extensors. As strength increases, the triceps are resisted through gradual increments of range. Additional sensory input, such as icing or vibration, may prove effective in increasing the triceps response. *Holding of the triceps*

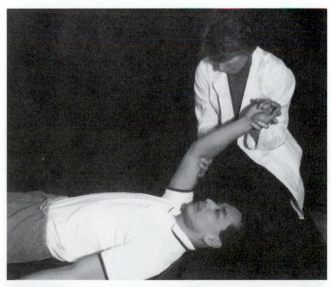

Figure 8–5. A: Supine; D2E, elbow flexing. T: TE shoulder extension with adduction.

in shortened ranges is important for the assumption of sitting and for transfers (Fig. 8–6).

Triceps activity also can be facilitated in D1E which is a movement incorporated into many functional mat activities. As with D2F, D1E can be performed with the elbow maintained in extension or extending through range, depending on the strength of the triceps.

> A: Supine; D1E elbow straight or extending
> T: TE on elbow extension

Figure 8–6. A: Supine; D2F, elbow straight or extending. T: TE on elbow extension.

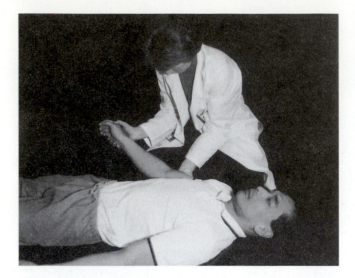

Figure 8–7. A: Supine; D1E, elbow straight or extending. T: TE elbow extension.

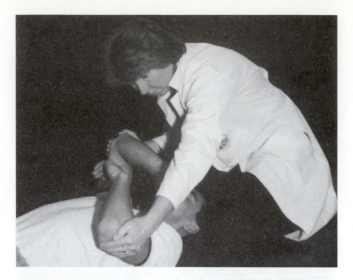

Figure 8–9. A: D2F right, D1E left. T: TE left shoulder extension with abduction.

Emphasis can be placed on holding in the extremely shortened range of the pattern to improve the ability to control elbow extension and to depress the scapula (Fig. 8–7).

Bilateral patterns will promote overflow between limbs if one upper extremity has more innervation. If the right arm is stronger, for example, isometric resistance is applied to the D2F pattern at approximately 90° of flexion to maximize overflow to the weaker left arm. While the right arm is isometrically resisted, the weaker extremity isotonically moves against manual resistance with repeated stretches superimposed to facilitate the contraction (TE). The sequence of patterns follows that already described for unilateral exercises (Figs. 8–8, 8–9, 8–10, 8–11).

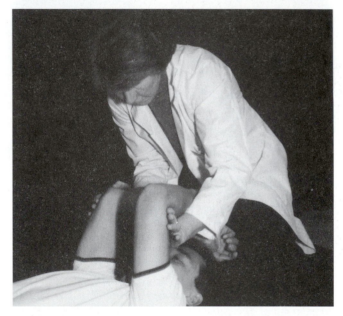

Figure 8–10. A: D2F right, D1F left. T: TE left shoulder flexion with adduction.

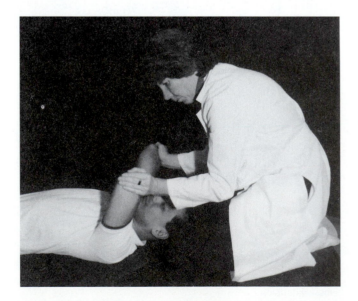

Figure 8–8. A: Bilateral symmetrical D2F. T: TE left shoulder flexion with abduction.

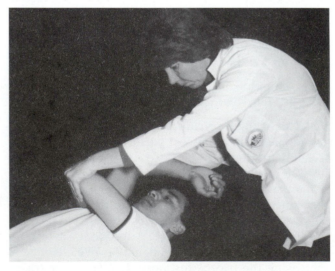

Figure 8–11. A: D2F right, D2E left. T:TE left shoulder extension with adduction.

Both unilateral and bilateral patterns are used to strengthen the weakened muscles of the quadriplegic patient and are designed to complement the mat program that is discussed in the following sections. If the patient has difficulty assuming supine on elbows, for example, strengthening of the scapula adductors and shoulder extensors in D1E needs to be emphasized.

MAT PROCEDURES FOR THE QUADRIPLEGIC PATIENT

The mat program for the quadriplegic patient is geared toward accomplishing the functional goals of wheelchair transfers and bed mobility. To reach this long-term functional stage, the levels of motor control in various postures must first be attained. The amount of innervated musculature will obviously affect the speed of progression and ability to accomplish all the procedures of the sequence.

The following procedures are divided into three progressions: those performed initially emphasize strengthening in functional patterns and stability and controlled mobility in the various postures; middle-stage procedures further enhance controlled mobility; advanced procedures promote skill.

Initial Progression

Supine. Manual resistance is applied to bilateral shoulder extension and scapula adduction necessary for the assumption and maintenance of supine on elbows. The elbows are positioned close to the trunk, with the forearms supinated and the hands near the shoulders. The patient pushes down with shoulder extension and attempts to elevate the chest with scapula adduction (Fig. 8–12). This motion promotes a shortened held resisted contraction (SHRC) in the rhomboids and posterior deltoid muscles. *Development of muscle stability is important for subsequent postural stability in weight-bearing activities.*

Assumption of supine on elbows may initially require assistance by the therapist. Some patients, because of tightness in the structures of the anterior shoulder, may experience pain when initial attempts are made to balance in this position. Although maintenance of supine on elbows may be difficult at first, alternating isometrics (AI) and rhythmic stabilization (RS) with manual contacts on the scapula can be used to improve stability in the posture (Fig. 8–13). *Holding of this supine-on-elbows position with the scapula adducted even further into shortened ranges will help to strengthen the proximal muscles isometrically.*

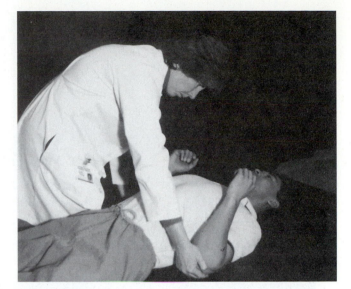

Figure 8–12. A: Supine; bilateral shoulder extension with elbow flexion. T: SHRC of shoulder extensors and scapula adductors.

Sidelying and Rolling. In sidelying, upper-trunk rotation is initiated with rhythmic initiation to teach the motion and reinforced with hold relax active motion. These movements are strengthened in both directions with the techniques of slow reversal hold (SRH) and RC. The trunk and scapula motions are combined with shoulder movements. Upper-trunk forward rotation and scapular protraction are combined with shoulder flexion to accomplish rolling from supine to prone (Fig. 8–14). The rolling movement proceeds through increments of range from sidelying until the patient can initiate rolling from supine. Exaggeration of the upper-trunk and upper-extremity movement causes the lower trunk to participate in the rolling movement. Rolling from supine is first practiced with a pillow under one side of the pelvis and the same lower extremity crossed over the other so that the patient has less body-weight resistance to overcome. The pillow may be removed and legs uncrossed as the patient becomes proficient in this activity. Cuff weights on the wrist can add momentum to the movement while simultaneously strengthening the shoulder muscles. Although the process is difficult, the patient must learn to disassociate the movements of elbow flexion and shoulder flexion in order to use the arms effectively to gain momentum in rolling. The arms should move with the shoulders in flexion and horizontal adduction and abduction with the elbows maintained in extension. To accomplish the disassociation of elbow and shoulder motion, the patient can practice shoulder flexion to approximately 45° in supine against the resistance of gravity or a cuff weight without allowing the elbow to flex.

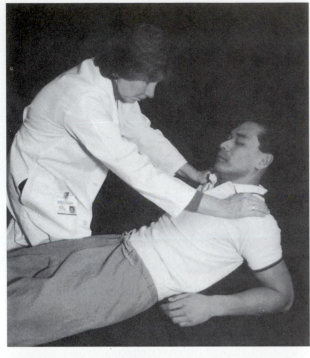

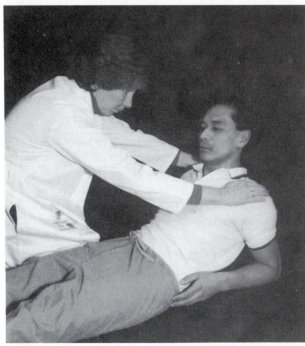

Figure 8–13. A: **(A)** Supine on elbows T: AI → **(B)** RS.

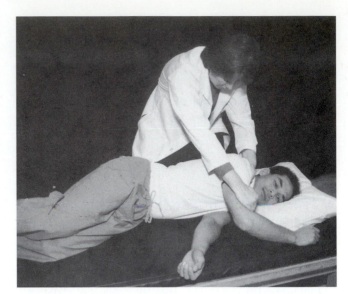

Figure 8–14. A: Sidelying, upper-trunk rotation with shoulder flexion. T: RC.

phasis is placed on arching the back and on abducting the scapula as much as possible to strengthen the serratus anterior (Fig. 8–15).

In the prone-on-elbows posture with manual contacts on the scapula, AI and RS will improve isometric strength and postural stability. Lateral weight shifting is promoted by the technique of SRH through increments of range, which will gradually increase the weight-bearing resistance and improve balance reactions. The anterior–posterior direction of weight shifting is practiced to strengthen the scapular and shoulder muscles needed for independent assumption of the posture. In the prone-on-elbows position, repeated arching of the upper trunk is emphasized for purposes of strengthening the muscles that will be used later to lift the pelvis in the longsitting position. Scapular abduction and shoulder flexion are coupled

Prone. *Quadriplegic push-ups are preliminary to assuming prone on elbows.* In prone, the patient's hands are positioned near the shoulders and the elbows are placed near the trunk. The patient abducts the scapula and flexes the shoulders in an attempt to lift the upper trunk off the mat. As with all activities, the patient may initially need assistance to push up. Em-

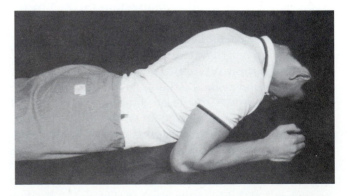

Figure 8–15. A: Prone, elbows flexed; quad push-ups. T: Active movement.

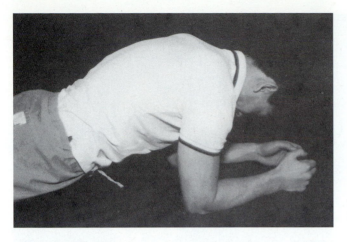

Figure 8–16. A: Prone on elbows, scapular abduction (arching upper back). T: Active movement.

with head and neck flexion to obtain maximum range in this lifting motion (Fig. 8–16). Upper-trunk arching should be practiced first in prone on elbows, where the base of support (BoS) is large and the center of gravity (CoG) low, before attempting this movement in the more difficult longsitting position.

Longsitting. Independent assumption and maintenance of longsitting is necessary for dressing activities. Maximal assistance will be needed to assume the longsitting posture during this initial stage because of decreased strength and flexibility. If triceps weakness is present, assistance also may be needed to maintain this position until the patient learns to externally rotate the shoulder and mechanically lock the elbow. Hypotension may be experienced until circulation is regulated. As indicated in the evaluation, mobility in the lower-trunk extensors and hamstrings must be sufficient to allow the patient to balance forward in the longsitting position without requiring upper extremity support. Unsupported balance in longsitting requires that the CoG of the upper trunk be anterior to the hips. Excessive tightness of posterior structures will limit this forward position. However, mobility must be gained with caution. As previously stated, overstretching can reduce the support provided by both the ligaments and the passive insufficiency of the back extensors and hamstrings and result in an unstable posture.

The position of the fingers is important if a tenodesis grasp is necessary for the patient's function. The distal finger joints should therefore remain in flexion to prevent overstretching of the flexor tendons when weight bearing occurs on the hands.

In the longsitting position, the upper extremities can be positioned posteriorly, anteriorly, and laterally to the trunk to assist with stability in the posture.

With the arms in these three different positions, stability can be promoted by the techniques of RS and AI and controlled mobility can be promoted through increments of range with SRH. These procedures should begin with the arms posterior to the trunk, a position that results in the largest BoS. When the arms are placed anteriorly, the patient can increase balance by hooking both hands under the knees. Balancing "erect" with the hands laterally placed at the level of the greater trochanter decreases the BoS and is therefore the most difficult of the three positions for the quadriplegic patient (Fig. 8–17). To enhance the patient's ability to maintain this posture, the upper trunk and head can be flexed to keep the CoG within the BoS. The techniques to promote stability and controlled mobility are appropriate in this posture but may be difficult for the patient to perform. Resistance is given in the rotary and lateral directions before being applied in the anterior and posterior plane, where the support is most compromised. During all these procedures in longsitting, the patient can learn to balance by substituting head, upper-trunk, and upper-extremity movements to compensate for the lack of lower-trunk control.

Middle Progression

At this point in treatment, the patient should no longer require external orthotic immobilization. No physical activities are contraindicated. Strengthening exercises are continued with the added resistance of pulleys or cuff weights. Endurance and proficiency in wheelchair propulsion and transfer activities should be increasing.

The major goal at this middle stage is to further increase controlled mobility and dynamic stability in the previously discussed postures. Controlled mobility is attained when the patient can both shift weight through full range and independently assume the various positions. Assisted or independent practice opportunities should be provided so the patient can learn the most efficient combinations of movements to assume and perform functional activities in these various postures.

Supine. Some patients may achieve the posture of supine on elbows by hooking wrists or thumbs under the hips or in the pants pockets and by flexing the elbows to raise the upper trunk from the mat. The position can be assumed by moving the elbows posteriorly. Stronger patients may be able to extend the shoulders and "walk" the elbows back without the assistance of the initial elbow flexion.

In supine on elbows, lateral weight shifting can be progressed to unilateral weight bearing. *Static–dy-*

Figure 8–17. A: Longsitting T: **(A)** AI → **(B)** RS; MC shoulders.

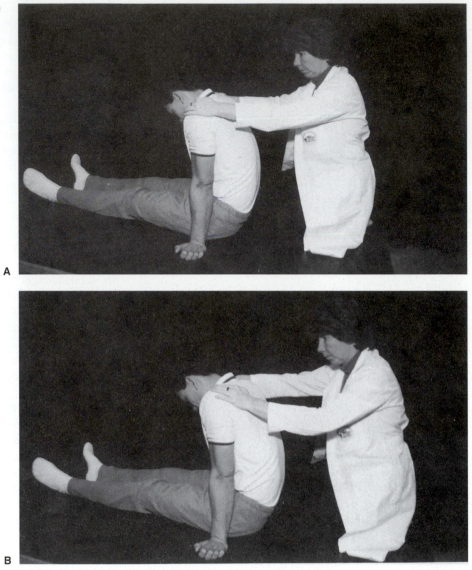

A

B

namic procedures are practiced to increase the dynamic stability of the static limb and to enable the patient to move into other postures from this position. Control in the static limb is further promoted by unilateral balancing in the posture. The weight-bearing arm must be positioned in shoulder extension and scapular abduction to move the BoS under the CoG. To enhance reactions in the supporting limb, the non–weight-bearing dynamic limb moves through increasingly larger ranges. These movements change the CoG and require proximal dynamic stability to counteract the weight shifting.

Both the prone-on-elbows and longsitting postures can be assumed from supine on elbows. Prone on elbows is gained by first moving into the unilateral supine-on-elbows position just described. The dynamic limb is brought forward across the body and the trunk is allowed to rotate until a midposition is reached. Abduction of the scapula on the supporting limb will promote upper body rolling to the prone-on-elbows position. The therapist can assist with this change in position by helping the patient assume the midline position and stabilize there with the techniques of AI and RS (Fig. 8–18). This is followed by slow reversal movements through increments of range. These activities are performed to improve the patient's upper trunk control and subsequent ability to assume prone on elbows independently.

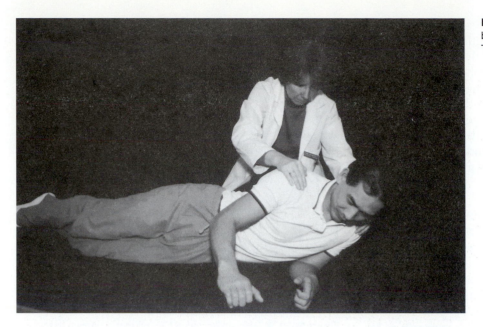

Figure 8–18. A: Sidelying; midposition between supine and prone on elbows. T: AI → RS.

As previously stated, the assumption of longsitting is extremely important. Many functional activities such as dressing and transfers are performed in the longsitting position. The ability to assume this posture unassisted will increase the patient's independence. The method of assuming longsitting can vary greatly among patients and is somewhat dependent on the flexibility of the shoulder and trunk, the strength of the triceps, and the amount of extensor spasticity in the lower extremities. Two means of assumption can be used as a guide but can be varied according to patient's needs. Both of these methods begin in supine on elbows:

1. Without rotating the lower trunk, the patient turns from a unilateral supine-on-elbows to a prone-on-elbows position and "walks" on elbows around toward the knees. One arm is then hooked under the knee, and by pulling with one arm and pushing with the other, longsitting can be assumed. This can be accomplished without triceps control but does require trunk mobility and some lower-extremity tone to keep the knee in extension (Fig. 8–19).

2. For the patients with triceps control and flexibility of the shoulders, longsitting may be achieved from a supine-on-elbows position by extending

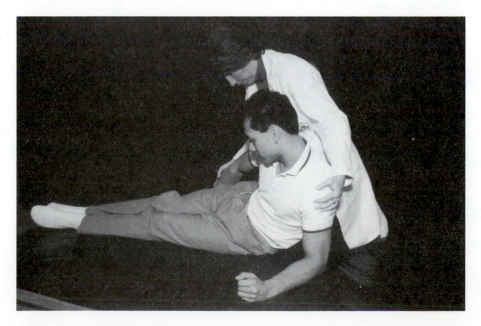

Figure 8–19. A: Longsitting. T: Assisted assumption from prone on elbows.

elbows and then walking forward on hands up to longsitting. If triceps strength is unequal, the weaker arm can be positioned posteriorly first so that the elbow can be mechanically locked. This is accomplished by swinging the weaker arm posteriorly from a static–dynamic supine-on-elbows position. The stronger upper extremity can then extend against the resistance of body weight. Patients may find that loops, bed rails, or other assistive devices may be needed to assume longsitting.

Longsitting. Wide-range weight shifting in longsitting is followed by static–dynamic activities. The postural control developed during these controlled mobility and static–dynamic activities can be challenged by the therapist by slowly disturbing balance, first with arm support, then without. Quick disturbances of balance in the unsupported position promote fast compensatory movements of the upper extremities to prevent falling. When trunk control is sufficient, one upper extremity can be freed from a supporting position to perform functional activities such as moving the lower extremities in preparation for transfers and dressing. By placing the extended wrist under the knee and flexing the elbow, the patient can reposition the leg.

Vertical elevation and control of the pelvis and lower trunk is important for independent transfers. With the hands positioned laterally beside the greater trochanters, the patient lifts the trunk by combining the motions of scapular abduction and depression, slight shoulder flexion, and head and upper-trunk flexion (Fig. 8–20). If necessary, the therapist can assist the assumption of the lift position by elevating the pelvis from the supporting surface. Stability in the lift position is first promoted by isometrically resisting at the shoulders, where the patient can feel the resistance applied, and later at the pelvis, where the manual contacts may not be felt. This progression of placement of manual contacts is an example of leading through the patient's strength. The goal of the procedure is for the patient to begin to maneuver the entire trunk, especially the lower trunk. Therefore, once the patient has experienced the sensory input and can adequately respond, the manual contacts are repositioned on the pelvis. Because the patient's trunk muscles may not be innervated, the minimally resistive forces provided by the therapist are compensated for by excessive upper-trunk motions. Because tactile sensation may be lacking, the therapist may have to emphasize verbal cues to assist the patient in responding to the resistance.

Controlled mobility or weight shifting follows the stability procedures. In the pelvic lift position, the pelvis is first moved laterally, then with rotation be-

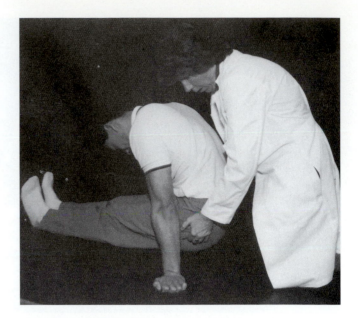

Figure 8–20. A: Longsitting; lifting hips off mat. T: Active assisted movement; MC pelvis.

fore movement in the more difficult anterior–posterior direction. The pelvic movement is assisted before resistance is provided.

Prone. Prone activities in this middle stage include weight shifting to unilateral weight bearing in prone on elbows. Isometric resistance to the static limb will improve control in that limb; resistance to the moving limb with reversal techniques will further improve the dynamic stability of the weight-bearing musculature (Fig. 8–21). By increasing the excursion of controlled mobility movements, especially in the anterior–posterior direction, the ability to assume prone on elbows is promoted. Arching of the upper trunk in

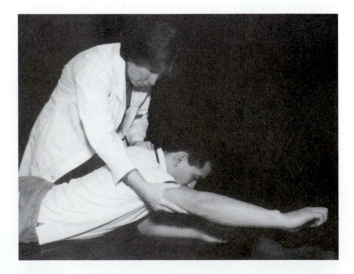

Figure 8–21. A: Prone on elbows; lifting one upper extremity. T: AI on weight-bearing limb → SRH dynamic limb.

prone on elbows is still incorporated into treatment procedures at this stage. This activity can be made more difficult by increasing the height of the lift, the number of repetitions, and the amount of resistance. *Emphasizing this activity and "quadriplegic push-ups" should improve the patient's endurance and ability to lift the pelvis in longsitting and ultimately to transfer.*

From a static–dynamic position in prone on elbows, the patient can move to supine on elbows. The dynamic limb pushes from the supporting surface as the upper trunk rotates until the midline position is reached. The dynamic limb is then extended to support the body in supine on elbows. If the upper-trunk rotational motion is exaggerated, the lower trunk will also turn to the supine position.

Advanced Progression

Wheelchair locomotion should be performed independently at this time, but transfers may still require minimal assistance. Transfer activities to the bed, wheelchair, toilet, and car seat should be practiced. Dressing and other ADL are also emphasized.

Longsitting. Procedures in longsitting will include added resistance to all pelvic motions while in a lift position. If these procedures are successful, the patient should be able to move on the mat in all directions by lifting and not sliding the pelvis and to transfer to surfaces of unequal heights. The transfer movement combines a lift, followed by a lateral and a posterior rotational motion. A wheelchair cushion

can be placed on the mat so that the patient can practice all the movement components of the transfer. In longsitting, the patient practices moving the lower extremities laterally with his arms and also practices crossing one leg over the other for dressing.

Prone. Prone procedures in this advanced stage include stability and controlled mobility techniques on elbows and knees, or quadruped if the patient has triceps control. Once the patient is assisted into the posture, AI, RS, and SRH through increments of range are performed with manual contacts on the scapulae, and then at the pelvis (Fig. 8–22). *The purpose of these procedures is not to make these postures functional, but rather to further stress the muscles of the arms and trunk and to use them to enhance the control of the lower-trunk movements. The lower-trunk motions promoted in these postures are necessary for transfers.* These motions have been previously enhanced during sidelying, longsitting, and movement from prone on elbows to supine on elbows. When manual contacts are positioned on the pelvis, the resistance provided is minimal, and additional sensory cues such as verbal input must be provided.

Sitting–Supine. Following a transfer from the wheelchair to a raised mat or to bed, the patient must be able to move from the shortsitting to the supine position. In shortsitting, stability and controlled mobility procedures are performed to enhance balance in the posture, and they follow a sequence that is similar to that performed in longsitting. To move to supine, the lower extremities must be lifted onto the mat. This

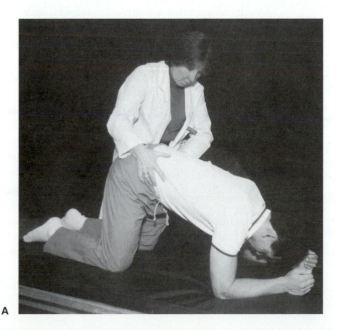 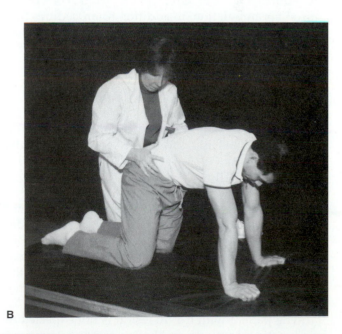

A   B

Figure 8–22. A: **(A)** Elbows and knees or **(B)** quadruped. T: AI → RS → SRH; MC pelvis. Increased hip and knee flexion may enhance independent maintenance of the posture.

may be accomplished by placing one arm under one or both lower extremities, followed by a pivoting motion on that elbow and rolling to supine. The patient flexes the lower extremities with the arm that is hooked under the thighs and rotates the trunk around to supine by swinging the dynamic limb.

The sequence of procedures presented in the initial, middle, and advanced progressions has been designed to enhance the patient's functional ability to transfer, dress, and perform other ADL. These functional outcomes have been achieved by progressing through stages of motor control in the sidelying, prone, supine, and sitting positions. Muscle and exercise endurance have been enhanced by increasing the intensity, frequency, and duration of the procedures.

MAT PROCEDURES FOR THE PARAPLEGIC PATIENT

Procedures for the patient with paraplegia are designed to reach more advanced goals, including increased mobility in and out of the wheelchair and, in some cases, ambulation.

As with the progression of procedures presented for the patient with quadriplegia, the procedures for the patient with paraplegia are divided into three levels, determined by level of lesion. Exercises appropriate for those with lesions at T-10, L1-2, and L4-5 are presented. The progressions are sequential. Many patients, however, are able to perform at more advanced levels than anticipated by the level of lesion. Patients with lower-level lesions benefit most from procedures that will develop the trunk control required for ambulation, in addition to procedures that will strengthen specific lower-extremity muscles. Some of the procedures may have to be modified if external trunk support limits trunk and hip flexibility.

The treatment goals are:

1. Increase the strength of the trunk musculature.
2. Improve stability and controlled mobility of the lower trunk.
3. Improve ADL.

To improve total-body endurance, the patient may perform low-intensity high repetitions on devices such as pulleys, upper-body ergometric (UBE) equipment, or a wheelchair treadmill. Practicing mat activities independently will help the patient find the combination of movements that makes functional tasks most efficient.

The patient with a T-10 lesion is not expected to be a functional ambulator. However, many young pa-

tients will want to attempt ambulation, and with adequate bracing it may be appropriate as a form of exercise. Highly motivated patients with good strength and appropriate body proportions may become semi-functional ambulators on flat surfaces.

Strengthening of the trunk musculature is promoted by using overflow from the stronger upper-extremity and upper-trunk musculature. Abdominals can be strengthened with an upper-trunk flexor pattern in supine, longsitting, or shortsitting with the technique of TE (Fig. 8–23). In longsitting, as the abdominals are resisted through range, the mobility in the low-back and hamstring muscles is maintained or increased. An upper-trunk extensor pattern performed in supine, sitting, and prone can strengthen the back extensors (Fig. 8–24). In addition, balance is promoted when trunk patterns are performed in sitting. Altering the posture in which the trunk patterns are performed will alter the amount of gravitational resistance. The greatest demands are placed on the trunk during flexion in supine and extension in prone.

The quadratus lumborum and latissimus dorsi can be strengthened by positioning one upper extremity in the shortened range of D1E and by resisting trunk extension, lateral flexion, and rotation. The technique of TE is performed by holding the arm and upper-trunk extensors in shortened ranges while isotonically contracting the lateral trunk movement (Fig. 8–25). The activity of the hip hikers is enhanced first in this reverse pattern for the quadratus, which leads from the patient's strength, before promoting isolated hip hiking in the supine, sitting, or standing position.

Sidelying is another posture in which stability and strengthening of the trunk musculature can be promoted. Overflow from the stronger upper-trunk musculature can be enhanced by the techniques of AI, RS, RC, and TE.

Prone procedures may begin with activities in prone on elbows to teach the patient how to stabilize and shift weight in a weight-bearing position. Because the upper extremities and upper trunk should be of good to normal strength, the patient should quickly progress to quadruped, where, after being assisted into the posture, stability and controlled mobility techniques can be applied. Weight shifting through increments of range may be performed in all directions. Lifting one upper extremity will help to improve the balance control in the static limbs and, most importantly, the trunk (Fig. 8–26). *Push-ups in quadruped or in prone will further strengthen the upper extremities that will be needed for ambulation and strenuous wheelchair activities.*

Sitting activities may begin with both upper ex-

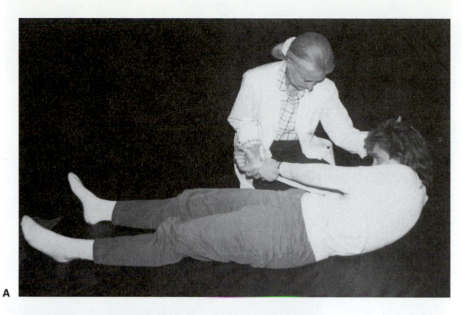

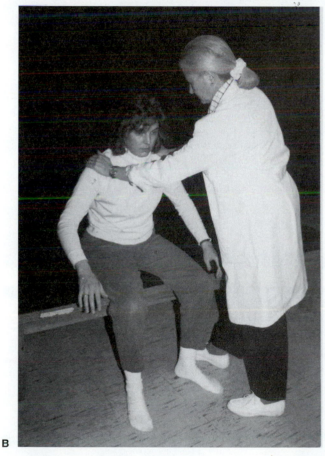

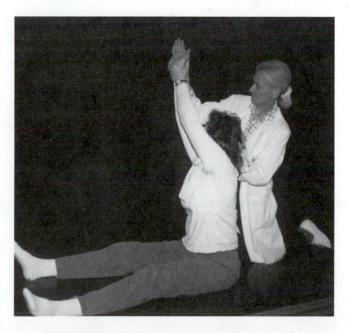

Figure 8–23. (A) A: Supine; upper trunk flexion. T: TE on abdominals. **(B)** A: Sitting; T: AI to abdominals.

Figure 8–24. A: Sitting; upper-trunk extension. T: RS.

Figure 8–25. A: Supine; D1E, quadratus pattern. T: TE on quadratus.

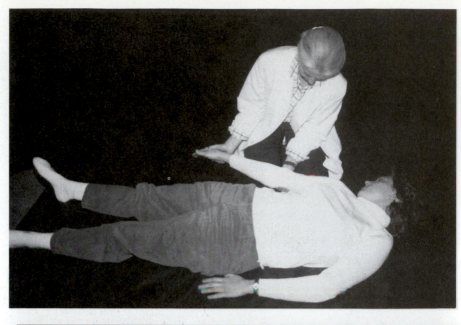

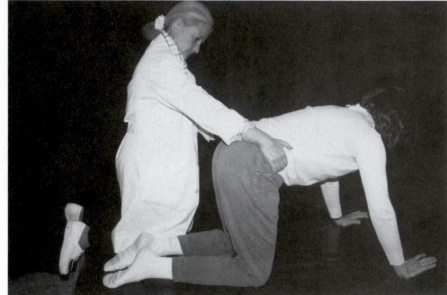

A

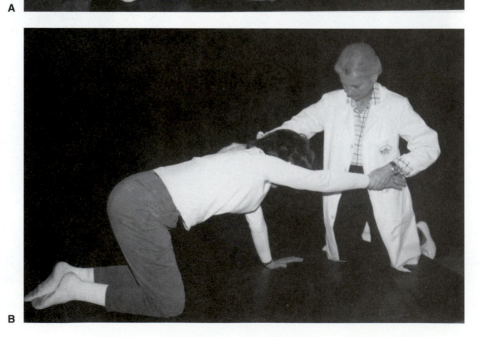

Figure 8–26. (A) A: Quadruped T: AI → SRH. **(B)** A: Quadruped; lifting one upper limb. T: AI on weight-bearing limb → SRH dynamic limb.

B

tremities providing trunk support. Arm support is gradually reduced until the patient can balance without upper-extremity assistance. Because of the larger BoS, longsitting should be easier for the patient than shortsitting. Therefore, balance should be improved in the less stressful longsitting position before progressing to shortsitting. As with all postures, the levels of motor control to be attained range from stability through skill. *Enhancement of trunk control for the paraplegic will allow use of arms to manipulate the environment and perform ADL.* As described in the quadriplegic section, pelvic lifts or elevation may be performed in long- or shortsitting to improve transfer ability.

Treatment of the paraplegic patient can include a greater amount of resistance and a wider range of weight shifting than can that for the quadriplegic patient. In addition to techniques applied to the pelvis, manual contacts can be positioned on the feet as the patient learns to balance and move the pelvis without the assistance of the proximal tactile input. The patient learns to move the lower extremities by moving the trunk. As the procedure is made more difficult by the distal placement of manual contacts, the stability and controlled mobility techniques may need to be repeated.

Standing procedures are initiated in the parallel bars with the arms supporting anteriorly, posteriorly, and then laterally to the hips. Stability techniques using manual contacts on the scapulae, scapula and pelvis, and pelvis will enhance maintenance of the standing posture. Weight shifting through increments of range in all directions will promote balance. One upper extremity can be lifted, then both can be raised as the patient attempts to maintain the balance point without assistance. With the upper extremities supporting on the parallel bars, stability and controlled mobility techniques are applied at the pelvis (Fig. 8–27). These techniques can be repeated with the lower extremities elevated from the floor. Once lower-trunk control is established by the preceding procedures, the focus is on improving the skill and endurance of walking. After ambulating with the support of parallel bars, the patient progresses to one forearm crutch and one parallel bar, then to both forearm crutches. After support from the assistive devices has been reduced, stability and controlled mobility procedures can be repeated to enhance balance and confidence. A patient with this level of lesion may be capable of performing a swing-to or swing-through gait. If ambulation is to be functional, falling and coming to standing from prone also are practiced.

Other functional activities that may be achieved at this level include transferring independently to a

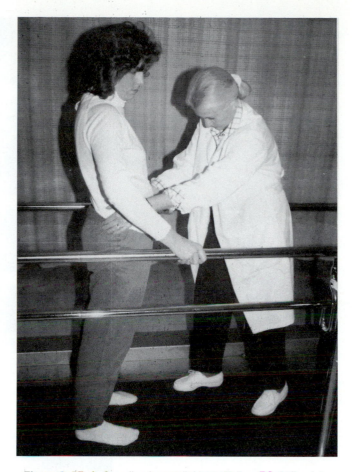

Figure 8–27. A: Standing in parallel bars. T:A → RS; MC pelvis.

car, maneuvering the wheelchair in and out of the car, and independent dressing.

Selected Procedures for a High Lumbar Lesion

The patient with an L1-2 level of injury should be able to perform all the procedures in the previous progressions. Most of the trunk muscles are innervated and partial innervation of the hip flexors and quadriceps is present. Additional procedures need to be performed to further strengthen the lower-trunk and innervated lower-extremity muscles. Ambulation should be more functional, and a four-point gait pattern may be possible.

In sidelying, lower-trunk rotation is performed with the strengthening technique of TE to increase the activity of the lower abdominals and back extensors. In this gravity-eliminated position, forward pelvic rotation is coupled with manually resisted hip flexion (Fig. 8–28).

In longsitting, lower-trunk control is further challenged by resisting isometric or isotonic move-

Figure 8–28. A: Sidelying; forward pelvic rotation with hip flexion. T: TE on pelvis, on hip.

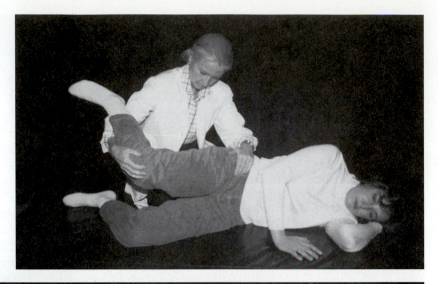

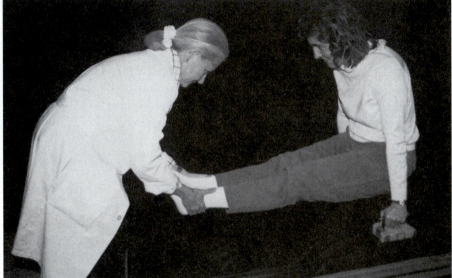

Figure 8–29. A: Longsitting; push-up on blocks. T: AI; MC pelvis → ankles.

ments with manual contacts on the pelvis or ankles. Lifting movements are practiced to assist the movement into the wheelchair. Push-up blocks may be used to simulate the upper-extremity control required during crutch walking (Fig. 8–29). The patient must develop sufficient strength to get into the wheelchair from the floor. This transfer can be performed from longsitting or quadruped. Lower-trunk stability and controlled mobility procedures performed in quadruped will improve abdominal and hip flexor control. If the patient can maintain a unilateral weight-bearing position, the hip flexors of the dynamic limb can be manually resisted in this gravity-assisted position (Fig. 8–30).

Ambulation activities in the parallel bars are performed to emphasize lower-trunk rotation and hip

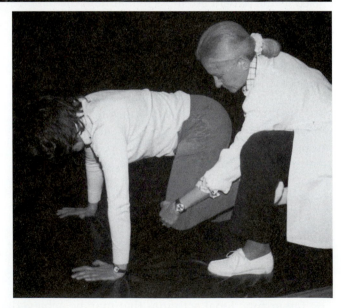

Figure 8–30. A: Quadruped; D1F lower extremity. T: TE on hip flexion.

flexion in preparation for a four-point gait. Because ambulation is a functional goal, more of the treatment session is now devoted to this activity.

Selected Procedures for a Low Lumbar Lesion

The patient with a low lumbar lesion, L4-5, will have innervation of more lower-extremity muscles than the previously described patients. The patient may have a combination of upper–motor-neuron and lower–motor-neuron dysfunction, depending on the site of the lesion. The evaluation may reveal motor and sensory loss that is indicative of a specific level of injury or of a spotty nerve lesion.

Specific patterns can be used to enhance overflow from stronger to weaker muscles. A treatment plan similar to that described at the beginning of this chapter for strengthening upper-extremity muscles for the quadriplegic patient can be designed. The innervated muscles and their grades of strength are first arranged into the patterns in which they function optimally. For example, the iliopsoas and anterior tibial muscles are most active in D1F, the gluteus maximus and posterior tibial muscles in D2E.

After assessing which muscles need to be strengthened and which are the strongest to be used for overflow, the therapist can design the treatment program. Because motor and sensory loss is so variable, general treatment guidelines rather than specific examples will be presented in this section.

GUIDELINES

Mobility: Initiation of Movement

Activities. The diagonal pattern in which the weakened muscle contracts optimally is determined. To optimize overflow from other muscles, resistance to trunk and bilateral patterns is appropriate. During unilateral patterns, overflow occurs primarily from within the limb. A mass movement pattern is usually chosen to enhance muscle responses, unless specific weaknesses indicate the use of another combination. If muscles are below a 3/5 gravity-assisted or eliminated postures may be necessary so that manual resistance can be applied. The range of initiation and of emphasis is determined by the muscle composition and its function. A primarily phasic muscle may respond favorably to repeated quick stretch in lengthened ranges. A weakened muscle that is primarily postural should be neither kept in the lengthened range for a prolonged period of time nor resisted maximally. For example, a weakened gluteus medius should be exercised initially in the supine position

where gravity is not a factor and manual resistance can be provided. A trunk extensor pattern or bilateral symmetrical (BS) D1E may be used to enhance overflow from the trunk muscles and from the contralateral limb to the weakened muscle. Application of a unilateral D1E with knee extension pattern may be appropriate if the quadriceps is of sufficient strength to increase gluteus medius activity.

Techniques. The techniques at the mobility stage should be chosen to emphasize the initiation of movement. Hold relax active movement (HRAM) or RC with repeated stretches in the lengthened range may accomplish that goal. As stated above, postural and phasic muscles may respond differently. The gluteus medius may respond best to HRAM because with this technique the muscle contraction is initiated in the shortened range and the lengthened range is not maintained or emphasized. However, if HRAM does not produce the desired initiation of movement, repeated stretches in the lengthened range may be effective if applied quickly and for short periods. Depending on the areas of intact sensory function, vibration, icing, tapping, and light touch may be indicated in addition to the quick stretch and resistance already mentioned.

Stability

Activities. The tonic holding stage of stability is most critical for those muscles acting as postural extensors. To accomplish tonic holding for a weak muscle, a posture is chosen so that gravity is eliminated or assists the contraction. The posture then may be altered to stretch the muscles and increase resistive forces. As previously stated, the shortened range of the D1E pattern, for example, places the gluteus medius in an optimal range to develop tonic holding. Once this occurs, postural stability may be promoted in the weight-bearing postures of bridging, quadruped, modified plantigrade, and standing.

Techniques. SHRC will best facilitate tonic holding and AI and RS can promote postural stability. SHRC can be facilitated by the use of joint approximation, vibration, and firm, maintained manual contacts.

Controlled Mobility

Activities. The same weight-bearing postures used to enhance the stability level of control may be appropriate to improve controlled mobility in the posture. Weight shifting occurs initially through a small arc that is gradually increased as balance and control are gained. Movements in the postures may be chosen to promote functional patterns, such as the pelvic motions needed during ambulation. During static–dynamic activities, one limb is lifted from the supporting surface and is free to move in any direction. The remaining weight-bearing limbs support the body weight and maintain the CoG within the BoS. As the dynamic limb moves through greater ranges and is resisted, the challenge to the static or stabilizing limbs is increased.

Techniques. Slow reversal (SR) or SRH through increments of range is most appropriate to enhance weight shifting. Eccentric control needed during ambulation may be promoted with agonistic reversals (AR). When static–dynamic activities are first performed, the focus of treatment may be on increasing the static control of the stabilizing limbs. Later, when proximal dynamic stability is the goal, the techniques of SR or SRH may be added to the dynamic limb.

In general, manual contacts should be placed directly on the segment that requires strengthening or control. For example, they may be applied to the dynamic limb to strengthen movement or to the stationary limb to enhance proximal dynamic stability.

Skill and Strengthening

Activities. Ambulation may be the functional outcome emphasized with these patients. The proper timing and sequencing of movement is essential. Unilateral leg patterns performed in sitting, supine, or prone may be used to improve the timing of movement. Control of advanced functional patterns is a goal at this stage. Deliberate ambulation can be practiced in all directions: forward, backward, sideways, and in a diagonal direction. Braiding, which combines all movement combinations of the lower extremity, can be used to enhance lower-trunk rotation. Ascending and descending stairs are also included.

The postures best used for strengthening are those with a large BoS and low CoG so that the patient's effort and attention can be focused on the movement. The combinations of patterns are selected to optimize overflow from stronger areas.

Techniques. Various techniques are used to promote strength at all levels of control. RC and HRAM can be used to initiate movement of phasic and tonic muscle groups respectively; SHRC, AI, and RS will increase isometric control and postural stability; AR, TE, RC, and SR will enhance concentric and eccentric control of a specific muscle or movement pattern; normal timing (NT) and resisted progression (RP) will promote timing and coordination of movements needed for gait.

SUMMARY

The need for specific strengthening procedures is determined by assessment of the patient's ability to perform certain movements and also by the results of a MMT and other evaluations of strength and function. Strengthening procedures are used throughout the course of rehabilitation to reinforce muscular control.

In conclusion, in addition to therapeutic exercise, the physical therapist may be called upon to order all necessary equipment, perform a home assessment, and to suggest appropriate environmental changes.

REVIEW QUESTIONS

1. A paraplegic patient has difficulty with trunk control during transfers. What procedures need to be incorporated into treatment to accomplish this functional goal?

2. Pressure relief in sitting is important for skin integrity. Which muscle groups need to be strengthened, and in which postures, to promote this ability?

3. Ambulation for a low-level paraplegic requires pelvic stability and the ability to accept weight onto each limb. What procedures can be incorporated into treatment to develop this control?

4. A patient has a C-5 brachial plexus nerve root injury of the right upper extremity. Which muscles would be weak and which would have normal innervation? In which patterns are the weak muscles primarily active? Which activities and techniques will maximize overflow from the strongest muscle groups to the weakest?

REFERENCES

1. Craigie EH. Vascular supply. In: Austin GM, ed. *The Spinal Cord.* 3rd ed. Tokyo, Japan: Igaku-Shoin Ltd., 1983.

2. Lee BY. Paralysis secondary to abdominal aortic aneurysm. In: Lee BY, Ostrander LE, Cochran GVB, eds. *The Spinal Cord Injured Patient: Comprehensive Management.* Philadelphia, Pa: WB Saunders Co; 1991.

3. Woodbury B, Redd C. Psychosocial issues and approaches. In: Buchanan LE, Nawoczenski DA, eds. *Spinal Cord Injury: Concepts and Management Approaches.* Baltimore, Md: Williams & Wilkins; 1987.

4. Pilsecker C. A changed world: socioeconomic problems of spinal cord injured patients. In: Lee BY, Ostrander LE, Cochran GVB, eds. *The Spinal Cord Injured Patient:*

Comprehensive Management. Philadelphia, Pa: WB Saunders Co; 1991.

5. Buchanan LE, Ditunno JF. Acute care: medical surgical management. In: Buchanan LE, Nawoczenski DA, eds. *Spinal Cord Injury: Concepts and Management Approaches.* Baltimore, Md: Williams & Wilkins; 1987.

6. Shils ME, Young VR, eds. *Modern Nutrition in Health and Disease.* 7th ed. Philadelphia, Pa: Lea and Febiger, 1980.

7. Agarwal N, Lee BY. Nutrition in spinal cord injured patients. In: Lee BY, Ostrander LE, Cochran GVB, eds. *The Spinal Cord Injured Patient: Comprehensive Management.* Philadelphia, Pa: WB Saunders Co; 1991.

8. Abruzzese RS. Pressure sores: nursing aspects and prevention. In: Lee BY, Ostrander LE, Cochran GVB, eds. *The Spinal Cord Injured Patient: Comprehensive Management.* Philadelphia, Pa: WB Saunders Co; 1991.

9. Pierce DS, Nickel VH. *The Total Care of Spinal Cord Injuries.* Boston, Mass: Little Brown and Co Inc; 1977.

10. Matthews PJ. The nervous system and spinal cord injury. In: Matthews PJ, Carlsop CE, eds. *Spinal Cord Injury: Rehabilitation Institute of Chicago Procedure Manual.* Rockville, Md: Aspen Publishing Co; 1987.

11. Stern J. Neurologic evaluation and neurologic sequelae of the spinal cord injured patient. In: Lee BY, Ostrander LE, Cochran GVB, eds. *The Spinal Cord Injured Patient: Comprehensive Management.* Philadelphia, Pa: WB Saunders Co; 1991.

12. Rinehart ME, Nawoczenski PA. Respiratory care. In: Buchanan LE, Nawoczenski DA, eds. *Spinal Cord Injury: Concepts and Management Approaches.* Baltimore, Md: Williams & Wilkins; 1987.

13. Hinderer KA, Hinderer SR. Quantitative methods of evaluation. In: DeLisa J, ed. *Rehabilitation Medicine: Principles and Practice.* 2nd ed. Philadelphia, Pa: JB Lippincott Co; 1993.

14. Trombly CA, Scott AD. *Occupational Therapy for Physical Dysfunction.* Baltimore, Md: Williams & Wilkins; 1977.

15. Knott M, Voss DE. *Proprioceptive Neuromuscular Facilitation.* 2nd ed. New York, NY: Harper & Row Publishers Inc; 1968.

16. Portney LG, Sullivan PE. *EMG Analysis of Ipsilateral and Contralateral Shoulder and Elbow Muscles During the Performance of PNF Patterns.* Read at the Annual Conference of the Society for Behavioral Kinesiology; Boston, Mass. 1979.

17. Sullivan PE, Portney LG. EMG of shoulder muscles during unilateral upper-extremity proprioceptive neuromuscular facilitation patterns. *Phys Ther.* 1980; 60:283–288.

CHAPTER 9

The Framework of Practice Applied to the Elderly Individual

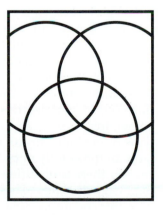

One of the primary purposes of physical therapy is to enhance the individual's physical ability to interact within the environment. Particularly important in the elderly is to improve, restore, or maintain the functional outcomes of ambulation and activities of daily living (ADL).

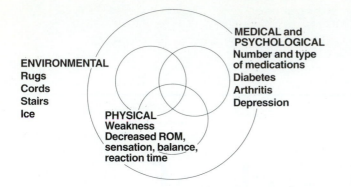

ENVIRONMENTAL
Rugs
Cords
Stairs
Ice

MEDICAL and PSYCHOLOGICAL
Number and type of medications
Diabetes
Arthritis
Depression

PHYSICAL
Weakness
Decreased ROM, sensation, balance, reaction time

Figure 9–1. Causes of falls in the elderly categorized within the evaluation model.

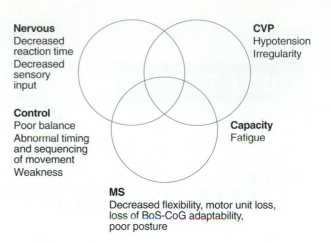

Nervous
Decreased reaction time
Decreased sensory input

CVP
Hypotension
Irregularity

Control
Poor balance
Abnormal timing and sequencing of movement
Weakness

Capacity
Fatigue

MS
Decreased flexibility, motor unit loss, loss of BoS-CoG adaptability, poor posture

Figure 9–2. Impairments associated with falls in the elderly categorized by physical system.

Figure 9–3. Examples of the many psychological and medical conditions that affect the elderly.

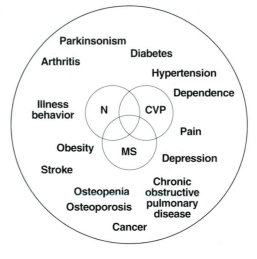

Parkinsonism
Arthritis
Diabetes
Hypertension
Dependence
Illness behavior
N
CVP
Pain
Obesity
MS
Depression
Stroke
Osteopenia
Osteoporosis
Chronic obstructive pulmonary disease
Cancer

The focus of this chapter is to describe the clinical decision-making process as it pertains to a population group. This differs from that of the other chapters, which have been organized by segmental or diagnostic groups. Much of the information presented in the other chapters pertains to the treatment of the elderly, for example, how to plan a program for an elderly patient with shoulder dysfunction. In contrast, this chapter takes a specific functional problem, reduced ambulatory ability, and moves in sequence through the framework. Dysfunctions of postural control and falling are also discussed because of their importance in the elderly population and their relationship to ambulation. Within the chapter there is no differentiation of the subgroupings of elderly, either according to age or ability. These need to be considered, however, as the therapist applies therapeutic exercise procedures.

Independent ambulation and walking at a functional speed are two of the most important factors in maintaining a self-reliant life-style for older individuals.[1] The ability to walk without undue fatigue at a functionally adequate speed for a reasonable time contributes to a comfortable and independent life.[2] Dependent ambulation and reduced safety during gait activities are common reasons for admission to nursing homes or other residential facilities. A large percentage of falls occur in elderly individuals while they are walking and may be attributed to various factors (Fig. 9–1, 9–2). Some falls result in injury; estimates suggest that as many as 25% of those who enter a hospital because of a hip fracture will die within 1 year. There is a societal need to decrease the number of falls, to reduce the need for nursing home placement, and to improve or maintain functional independence in the elderly.[3,4] Thus, the evaluation of ambulation and intervention to preserve or restore walking ability are critical.

Acute or chronic psychological and medical conditions and altered nutrition compound the changes in physical capability that occur as a result of both aging and diminished activity (Fig. 9–3).[5] A sedentary life-style for elderly people is not uncommon. It has been estimated that only 45% to 66% of older persons participate in regular exercise, even though activity seems to be critical to maintaining mental and physical function.[6] Despite their importance to physical therapy, however, many of the changes found in older persons have not been studied in relation to their functional ability and, particularly, to their ambulation.

The focus of this chapter is to analyze the physical impairments that seem to influence the function of ambulation in the aging population in general and to use this information as a basis for evaluation and intervention.

EVALUATION

The evaluation assesses the patient's capability to perform functional activities. In this section the commonly observed gait characteristics in the older individual are discussed, followed by findings within their physical and physiological systems. In addition to these factors, the environmental, social, psychological, and medical factors relative to the elderly require consideration.

Gait Characteristics

General changes in ambulation that are associated with aging are slower velocity and decreased stride length. During the stance phase of gait, elderly persons generally employ a wider base of support (BoS) and exhibit a shorter step length, thereby spending a longer time in double support. Less dorsiflexion is evident during the early swing phase and is compensated for by use of greater hip and knee flexion to accomplish toe clearance. At late swing, when the compensatory increase in knee flexion seen in early swing becomes impossible, toe clearance is minimized. Within the trunk and the proximal joints, there is less pelvic rotation and trunk counterrotation, increased shoulder extension and elbow flexion, increased hip abduction, greater toeing out, and less vertical projection of the trunk and pelvis at toe-off.[2,7,8]

Changes in the capacity to sustain movement for a given speed of ambulation, as measured by oxygen consumption, become more pronounced with advancing age. The energy expenditure in ambulation over level ground and in stair climbing is similar for many elder and younger persons because the elderly regulate their energy consumption by walking more

Table 9–1. Relation of Changes Found During Gait Analysis with Physical Impairments

Gait Analysis	Physical Impairments
• Slower velocity	• Decreased endurance
• Decreased stride length	• Decreased trunk and pelvic rotation
• Altered cadence	• Decreased ROM hips and ankles
• Shorter step length	• Decreased muscle and postural stability and strength
• Longer double stance	• Decreased sensory input

slowly.[2] Even when they perform more slowly, the energy cost of stair climbing can exceed the ability of some elderly persons. The association between changes during walking and various physical impairments has been noted but needs further assessment (Table 9–1). For example, decreased trunk counterrotation, decreased pelvic forward rotation, shorter step length, wider BoS, and decreased vertical projection at heel-off have been attributed to the attempt by the older individual to improve stabilization during ambulation.[8] However, these findings may be the secondary effects of decreased range in the trunk, hips, and ankles and decreased force production in the postural extensors and plantar flexors. Similarly, the altered speed of walking, especially during stair climbing, may be due to a decrease in the number of type II muscle fibers, a decreased ability to perform unilateral stance, or a decreased aerobic capacity. The

Loss of synapses and dendrites

Nerve conduction velocity slower

Threshold of H-reflex higher

Memory and learning changes

Reaction times in sedentary elderly
decreased more than in active elderly

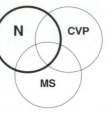

Figure 9–4. Changes in attributes of the nervous system occurring in the elderly.

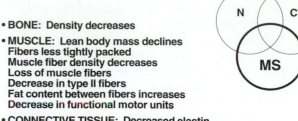

- **BONE:** Density decreases
- **MUSCLE:** Lean body mass declines
  Fibers less tightly packed
  Muscle fiber density decreases
  Loss of muscle fibers
  Decrease in type II fibers
  Fat content between fibers increases
  Decrease in functional motor units
- **CONNECTIVE TISSUE:** Decreased elastin
  Fibrin deposits occur, restricting movement
- **GENERAL** 20%-30% decrease in flexibility by 70 years

Figure 9–5. Changes in attributes of the musculoskeletal system occurring in the elderly.

increased shoulder extension noted during gait may be a mechanism to counterbalance the increased kyphosis and flexed hips that move the center of mass anteriorly.

During the evaluation, the impairments that lead to functional limitations with ambulation need to be identified so that an effective treatment plan can be developed. For example, decreased toe-off may be a clinical finding in the gait analysis. The therapist must determine whether this finding is due to a loss of range of motion (ROM) at the ankle, weak plantarflexors, poor motor control, limited capacity for movement, or any combination of these factors before an effective intervention can be designed. In addition to treatment of specific impairments, conscious changes in the gait pattern should be encouraged.

Variations in ambulation related to sex differences in the elderly have also been found. Women take shorter steps than men. To increase their speed, women take more steps, whereas men increase step length.[2,9] It is not clear whether these sex differences are related to variations in leg length, flexibility, strength, general physical condition, or some combination of these factors.

Physical Systems

Nervous System

Many changes in the nervous system may contribute to alterations in ambulation for the elderly (Fig. 9–4). Sensory input from proprioceptor, visual, and vestibular mechanisms are all generally reduced in the elderly.[10,11] The cutaneous and proprioceptive receptors have a longer latency and a higher threshold.[12] Other changes that may affect ambulation in the elderly include presence of fewer dendrites, reduced nerve conduction velocity, greater monosynaptic latency, decreased excitability at the myoneural junction, decreased numbers of functional motor units, decreased reaction time, and a higher threshold for the H-reflex. All these changes result in an increased sensorimotor loop time.[13–15] These neural changes slow the generation of automatic motor programs, increase the time required for peripheral feedback to be

received centrally, and delay the transmission of efferent responses.

Musculoskeletal System

Changes in the musculoskeletal system with aging that are relevant to ambulation include less tightly packed muscle fibers, an increase in fat content between muscle fibers, an increase in fibrin deposits, a decrease in the number of type II fibers and functional motor units, and loss of bone density (Fig. 9–5).[16] Clinically, a predominant finding in the elderly is a reduction in general flexibility. Any of these findings, as well as the changes that occur in the cartilage and joint surfaces, may lead to postural alterations.[17]

Cardiovascular–Pulmonary System

Elderly persons commonly exhibit an increased prevalence of coronary artery disease and hypertension (Fig. 9–6). Cardiac pathophysiology may be demonstrated by an increase in blood pressure, decreases in stroke volume, maximum heart rate, and coronary artery circulation, and narrowing of the

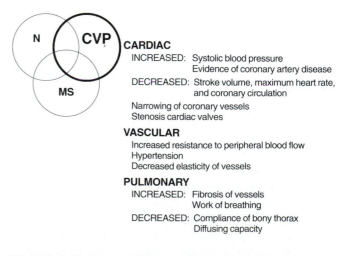

CARDIAC
INCREASED: Systolic blood pressure
Evidence of coronary artery disease
DECREASED: Stroke volume, maximum heart rate, and coronary circulation
Narrowing of coronary vessels
Stenosis cardiac valves

VASCULAR
Increased resistance to peripheral blood flow
Hypertension
Decreased elasticity of vessels

PULMONARY
INCREASED: Fibrosis of vessels
Work of breathing
DECREASED: Compliance of bony thorax
Diffusing capacity

Figure 9–6. Changes in attributes of the cardiovascular–pulmonary system occurring in the elderly.

coronary vessels and stenosis of the cardiac valves.[18]

The pulmonary system shows altered compliance of the bony thorax and in the lung tissue. There is a decrease in diffusing capacity and of efficiency in the work of breathing.

In the peripheral vessels, there is an increase in the resistance to peripheral blood flow and a decrease in the elasticity of vessels and of the number of capillary beds in the muscles. Clinically, cardiovascular–pulmonary (CVP) changes may be manifested in the elderly as lowered aerobic capacity, diminished exercise tolerance, and positional hypotension.

All these changes can lead to a reduced ability to respond to the aerobic demand of functional activities and thus promote further decline in aerobic capacity.[19] Elderly individuals may be forced to decrease the speed of walking and stair climbing because in a deconditioned state they are unable to sustain the output of energy required by the increased metabolic cost of these activities. The loss of speed, in turn, leads to an overall decrease in endurance for functional activities. For this reason, the 6-minute-walk test, which measures the distance walked in the designated time, is a common tool used to assess endurance.[20] In general, the ability of elderly people declines with advancing years, but the individual results seem more related to activity level rather than to age.

Movement Control and Capacity

The quality and quantity of ambulation are related to the interaction of the nervous, musculoskeletal, and CVP systems. Impairments in the nervous and musculoskeletal systems can lead to control alterations in the programming, planning, or execution of all movement including ambulation. Impairments within the CVP and musculoskeletal systems limit the individual's capacity to sustain movement and ambulation. In the following paragraphs, the effects of impairment on control and capacity are discussed.

Movement Control. The control of movement, postural responses, and ambulation are the results of complex interactions between the nervous and musculoskeletal systems (Fig. 9–7). Automatic, reflexive, and volitional levels of control may be influenced.[21,22] The automatic level of control relies on central mechanisms to interpret the position of body segments, implement common movements, judge disturbances accurately, and respond with the appropriate timing, sequencing, and force.[10] All of these are needed to maintain a posture and to respond to minor or previously encountered changes in the external environment. Automatic ambulatory patterns are generated from central feed-forward mechanisms and result in responses to known situations. These automatic pro-

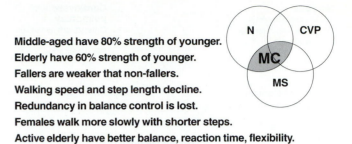

Middle-aged have 80% strength of younger.
Elderly have 60% strength of younger.
Fallers are weaker that non-fallers.
Walking speed and step length decline.
Redundancy in balance control is lost.
Females walk more slowly with shorter steps.
Active elderly have better balance, reaction time, flexibility.

Figure 9–7. Changes in attributes of movement control occurring in the elderly. *Data from Murray et al.[26]
*Murray, M.P. Age related differences in knee muscle strength in normal women. *J. Gerontology,* 1985;40:275-280.

grams may not be adequate in some elderly individuals because the total system for the control of movement may be slowed and the ability to detect novel environmental conditions impaired. The reflexive level of control involves peripheral sensorimotor links consisting of proprioceptive and stretch receptor mechanisms and higher-center reflexes such as the vestibulo-ocular reflex.[10,21,23,24] Volitional control requires conscious attention to the activity. Such attention is more important if the environmental conditions are unusual, such as walking in the dark, or if the ability to monitor conditions has been altered internally, as occurs with diminished distal sensation. The conscious effort usually results in a reduction of speed and an increase in the energy cost. The decreased sensory inputs coupled with the inability to vary motor strategies reduces the overlapping of sensory input and the adaptability of motor responses.[10]

Some of the motor control problems found in the elderly during ambulation can be analyzed by looking at three conditions inherent in purposeful movement: the position of the body must be known, the target position or goal to be achieved must be identified, and the correct combination of muscle forces in the correct sequence must be generated in order to move from the starting position to the goal position.

The combination of feedforward and feedback mechanisms and the sensory input contributing to movement control normally allow movement to occur from the existing body position toward a subsequent target position in a coordinated fashion. Programs within the central nervous system (CNS) underlying the automatic nature of ambulation are altered with aging through changes in both peripheral and central inputs. Visual, vestibular, and proprioceptive mechanisms that monitor conditions internal to the body, such as limb position and muscle length–tension relations, as well as the ability to monitor environmental conditions external to the individual, also change with aging.[10] If the sensitivity of these modalities is reduced, integration of the neces-

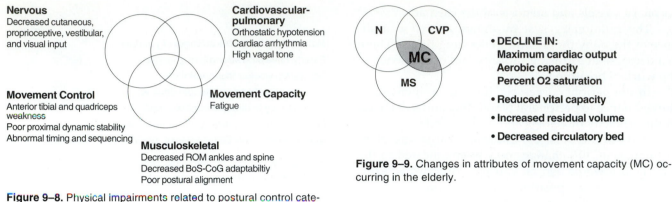

Nervous
Decreased cutaneous, proprioceptive, vestibular, and visual input

Cardiovascular-pulmonary
Orthostatic hypotension
Cardiac arrhythmia
High vagal tone

Movement Control
Anterior tibial and quadriceps weakness
Poor proximal dynamic stability
Abnormal timing and sequencing

Movement Capacity
Fatigue

Musculoskeletal
Decreased ROM ankles and spine
Decreased BoS-CoG adaptabiltiy
Poor postural alignment

Figure 9–8. Physical impairments related to postural control categorized by system.

• DECLINE IN:
Maximum cardiac output
Aerobic capacity
Percent O2 saturation

• Reduced vital capacity

• Increased residual volume

• Decreased circulatory bed

Figure 9–9. Changes in attributes of movement capacity (MC) occurring in the elderly.

sary afferent information into a motor plan can be difficult.

The speed of walking is influenced by the intensity of lower extremity muscle activation.[25] However, the ability to generate sufficient motor force in the proper sequence is diminished in the elderly.[26] Thus the decreased walking speed of elderly individuals may be an accommodation to the decreased ability to generate sufficient force in the required time.[27] The altered motor response may be due to delayed nerve conduction velocity, diminished sensory awareness, disuse atrophy, or a combination of all these factors. Any of these factors can create a cycle in which reduced ambulation leads to reduced capacity to sustain movement, which in turn further limits ambulation. In addition to the effect these impairments have on the function of ambulation, they also have been associated with abnormalities in static and dynamic postural control. These impairments can be categorized according to the physical systems (Fig. 9–8).

Movement Capacity. Functional limitations in ambulation can be due to changes in the CVP and musculoskeletal systems, which reduce the capacity for movement (Fig. 9–9). A decline in cardiac output, decreased maximum heart rate, reduced vital capacity, increased residual volume, decreased oxygen saturation, increased resistance to peripheral blood flow, diminished blood flow to the muscles, and decreased ability to extract oxygen from the blood[28] can all adversely affect the interdependent relationship between the CVP and musculoskeletal systems.

Clinical Impressions

It is difficult to differentiate impairments that result from aging from those that are due to diseases, such as diabetes, or to a sedentary life-style.[17] For example, persons who fall tend to be weaker than those who do not.[27] However, it is not always clear which of these problems has occurred first, the falling or the

weakness. What is evident is that if a fall occurs, many elderly persons, even those who have been quite active, may reduce their activity level because of anxiety or fear of falling.

Intervention has been shown to be effective in altering the changes that accompany aging and that may result from a sedentary existence. Therapeutic exercise programs administered to a wide range of elderly persons have resulted in improvements in their strength, flexibility, and exercise capacity.[5,19,29] To achieve the greatest functional gain, the impairments in all of the physical systems need to be considered (Fig. 9–10). For example, the inability to climb stairs after a hip fracture may be more related to decreased aerobic capacity than to diminished strength; poor balance may be the result of decreased ROM, proprioception, and stability in the ankles rather than more central neural impairments.

The most appropriate mode of intervention to remedy the impairments and maximize functional capability has not yet been determined. This clinical question is "should the intervention concentrate on changing the individual, on teaching compensatory strategies, or on decreasing the demand by modifying the environment?" (Fig. 9–11). Therapists can target interventions more specifically on the underlying cause when the relationships between pathology, impairments, functional limitation, and disability are

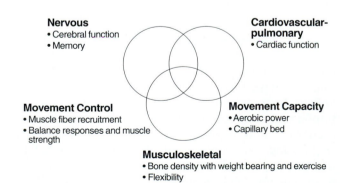

Nervous
• Cerebral function
• Memory

Cardiovascular-pulmonary
• Cardiac function

Movement Control
• Muscle fiber recruitment
• Balance responses and muscle strength

Movement Capacity
• Aerobic power
• Capillary bed

Musculoskeletal
• Bone density with weight bearing and exercise
• Flexibility

Figure 9–10. Beneficial changes in physical attributes resulting from exercise.

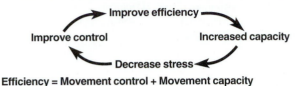

What are the impairments limiting progress?

How can intervention programs be modified for: home, nursing home, senior citizen's centers, for the individual or group?

What is the more effective or efficient mode of intervention – to change the patient or to modify the environment?

What is the relationship between improving control and capacity?

Efficiency = Movement control + Movement capacity

Figure 9–11. Questions regarding intervention choices.

better known as well as the influence of an active or sedentary life-style. The therapist's decision making will improve when more is known about the reversibility of the deficits and the ability of the individual to respond to the intervention in a realistic period of time.

In addition to assisting individuals in changing, the therapist can help to modify the environment. Environmental modifications may be a more efficient way to effect change and reach the functional outcomes when a number of individuals share common impairments, such as reduced speed of ambulation, decreased extremity ROM, and decreased postural stability. Interventions may include: decreasing step height, varying chair height, raising the height of toilet seats, prolonging the walk time at crossing lights, installing stall showers with grab bars and night-lights in the bathroom, and altering the size or shape of doorknobs.[30]

INTERVENTION

The physical therapy intervention is directed toward functional outcome desired by both the patient and the physical therapist. The outcome emphasized in the chapter is ambulation with sufficient control and capacity to be safe at a speed that allows independence with or without an assistive device on a variety of surfaces. Although this focus is toward improved ambulation, the person's ability to perform activities of daily living (ADL) and to communicate effectively also would be included in the complete rehabilitation plan.

The functional outcome can be characterized as being performed either with control or with compensatory strategies. Normal control assumes a standard timing and sequencing of movement with an amount of force appropriate to perform the task; normal movement is efficient and requires the least amount of energy. When normal control is not possible because of unalterable impairments, compensatory strategies

are indicated. However, compensatory movements commonly require more energy. Age-appropriate comparison movements must be kept in mind when determining functional outcomes and treatment goals for elderly patients.

As previously stated, the patient's functional capability, the impairments related to the limitations in ambulation, and the patient's potential for change are all determined during the evaluation. The next step in the clinical decision-making process is to translate these evaluative findings into an intervention plan. To do so, the impairments that limit function should be clustered into the classifications described in the intervention model. Realistic treatment goals can be prioritized according to the assessment of what changes are possible for the individual and which changes will have the greatest influence on improving the outcome of ambulation. The general goals could include: increasing ROM, increasing the time that standing can be maintained without assistance, and improving the ability to repeatedly assume standing from sitting. The goals also can include teaching the compensatory movements and the modification of the environment.

Units of the Procedure

Activities

The postures associated with ambulation include those that occur during the assumption of standing and those in which specific motor abilities can be practiced and achieved. To assume a standing position, the sequence of postures includes supine, side-lying, sitting, and standing. The control of the lower trunk and lower extremities required for the assumption of standing and for ambulation can be enhanced in hooklying, bridging, and modified plantigrade. These postures are included in treatment to improve ambulatory control, as well as to increase weight-bearing stress. For this reason, procedures in quadruped may be included in the treatment plan for some elderly patients, although for others quadruped may be too difficult.

Techniques

The treatment techniques employed may include those that increase ROM (*mobility*), improve the ability to maintain a posture (*stability*), enhance the ability to move within or between postures (*controlled mobility* and *static–dynamic* control), and improve the timing and sequencing of movement (*skill*).

Parameters

The exercise parameters are the frequency, duration, and intensity of each of the treatment procedures.

Intensity Duration Frequency	PHYSIOLOGICAL STRESS – Monitoring Heart rate, blood pressure, respiratory rate in different postures while varying the parameters of exercise.
	TISSUE HEALING – Adjusting the intensity of stretch, resistance, and force applied, and the duration of the exercise allowing for circulatory exchange.
	LEARNING VARIABLES – Alternating the intensity of stimuli, the task repetition, the components of the procedure, and the environmental conditions to improve generalization.

Figure 9–12. Considerations when choosing movement parameters.

These parameters are varied according to the patient's learning ability, CVP status, or the acuteness of the dysfunction (Fig. 9–12).

In patients who demonstrate difficulty with learning due to attention span deficits or decreased sensory-motor integration, the parameters can be altered to affect the practice schedule and the internal and external feedback. The duration of each treatment can be reduced and the frequency increased to distribute the repetition of the task; the intensity of patient effort can be altered to increase feedback and enhance the response of various peripheral receptors.[10,24,31]

Patients who are limited by exercise capacity deficits and involvement of the CVP system may require modifications in the exercise parameters so that appropriate physiological stress occurs during the procedures. Heart rate, blood pressure, and perceived exertion during the intervention program should be monitored in such circumstances.

If the patient is recovering from a musculoskeletal injury or surgery, exercise parameters should be adjusted according to the tissue's reactivity or ability to respond to varying amounts of intensity or frequency of exercise. Elderly patients may recover more slowly, manifest different responses to internal and external stress, and be more affected by the deleterious results of bed rest.

IMPAIRMENTS CLASSIFIED ACCORDING TO THE STAGES OF CONTROL

Examples of impairments related to the control of movement are classified within the model along the horizontal axis (Table 9–2). From these classifications, treatment goals and appropriate treatment techniques can be determined. For example, a patient you are treating is limited in moving from sitting to

TABLE 9–2 CHANGES WITH OLDER PERSONS

Mobility	Stability	Controlled Mobility	Skill
↓Flexibility Trunk Shoulders Hips Ankles	↓Balance ↑Sway ↓Strength Postural Muscles	↓Trunk Rotation ↓Dynamic Sway	↓Walking Speed
↓Strength			
↓Speed			

standing as a result of impairments that include tightness of the hip capsule and muscle. Limited range is classified within the mobility stage (see next section). To determine the treatment goal, the therapist considers the patient's range in comparison to that required for moving from sitting to standing,[32] the type of tissue involved, and the duration of involvement. If the limitation is in soft tissue and is of short duration, the assumption can be made that change can occur. If the impairment is chronic or if bone limits ROM, soft tissue changes are unlikely, necessitating treatment aimed at compensation, which might include raising seat height. Referral for surgical intervention might also be considered.

Mobility–Passive ROM

Impairment. ROM deficits that impede ambulation can be due to shortening or stiffness of the skin, connective tissue, muscle, ligament, and capsule in the trunk, hip, knee, or ankle (Fig. 9–13).

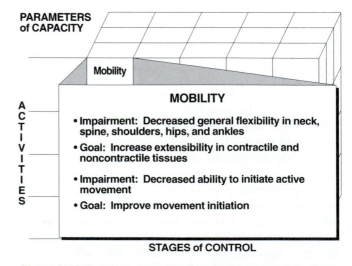

PARAMETERS of CAPACITY

ACTIVITIES

Mobility

MOBILITY

- Impairment: Decreased general flexibility in neck, spine, shoulders, hips, and ankles
- Goal: Increase extensibility in contractile and noncontractile tissues
- Impairment: Decreased ability to initiate active movement
- Goal: Improve movement initiation

STAGES of CONTROL

Figure 9–13. Impairments and treatment goals appropriate when promoting mobility.

Functional Implications. During stance and swing phases of gait, impairments of range may limit trunk counterrotation, pelvic rotation, step length, and both dorsiflexion and plantarflexion motions.[8] For example, decreased range into lumbar extension combined with tight hip flexors and plantarflexors may reduce terminal stance and step length. Patients with decreased range in the trunk and lower extremity may have difficulty moving from sitting to standing[32] and may be restricted to climbing stairs one step at a time. The first phase of assuming standing normally requires upper body and hip flexion and flexion of the knees and ankles as the feet move under the chair. If these joints or surrounding tissues are stiff, these initial flexion movements will be restricted. Another common finding is difficulty with erect standing following prolonged sitting, resulting from impairments including stiffness in the flexor muscles and decreased joint flexibility. Difficulty with stair climbing may be due in part to range deficits in the ankle, knee, or hip.

Abnormal range in the thoracic and cervical spine also can influence posture and gait. Typically, an elderly person will demonstrate thoracic and cervical changes that move the upper body's center of gravity anteriorly. To offset this change, the individual must alter muscular activity to maintain and move in sitting and standing and to control postural responses in these positions.

Treatment Goals. These include: improvement of trunk and limb ROM by decreasing tissue stiffness and improving length.

Techniques. If specific joint motions are limited by capsular or ligamentous tightness or by chronic joint effusion, joint mobilization and measures to reduce edema should be incorporated. If specific muscle tightness is noted, hold relax (HR) to increase contractile tissue extensibility is performed. Heat, superficial or deep, depending on the involved tissue, or active warm-up activities may be useful before these ROM procedures. Self-stretching has an advantage in that it can be performed independently, although it is not as specific to any one tissue. During self-stretching, the movements and instructions should be sufficiently specific to limit the stretch to the involved area. Whether individual or group exercise is performed, care must be taken with persons who have osteoporosis or whose bones are osteopenic.

Initiation of Active Movement

Impairment. The ability to initiate active movement is decreased and the speed with which movement is initiated may be delayed. The weakness that reduces the initiation of movement may be due to a combination of a decreased number of type II fibers, resistance from stiff antagonistic tissues, and a sedentary life-style.

Functional Implications. When initiation of movement is too slow or weak, postural reactions and automatic movements in standing or during ambulation may not occur with sufficient speed to compensate for environmental changes or to allow for an appropriate rate of walking. For example, if ankle proprioception is diminished or if the tissues around the ankle are stiff, activation of the dorsiflexors may be delayed. Difficulty overcoming internal resistance may impede ankle movements during postural disturbances,[23,27] ambulation, and stair climbing. A slowed postural response also can be due to inattention and decreased visual and vestibular acuity.

Treatment Goals. Goals are to improve initiation of active movement including the "strength" and the speed of recruitment.

Techniques. If the patient has difficulty initiating movement in the presence of increased tone as, for example, an individual with parkinsonism, rhythmic initiation (RI) is chosen to promote more normal tone while facilitating active movement (see Chapter 3). Because of the repetitive motion, RI is also appropriate for patients experiencing difficulty learning movements. If the patient has weakness in the postural extensors, hold relax active motion (HRAM) is performed to improve the holding ability in shortened ranges and the ability to initiate movement from the lengthened range. If weakness is primarily in the flexor muscles, the technique of repeated contractions (RC) may promote increased motor unit activation by superimposing a stretch reflex onto a voluntary contraction. By stimulating muscle spindle activity, these techniques also may enhance peripheral proprioceptive input. Electrical stimulation may augment voluntary contractions.

Stability

Muscle Stability

Impairment. The postural extensor muscles are weak, with decreased ability to contract isometrically in the

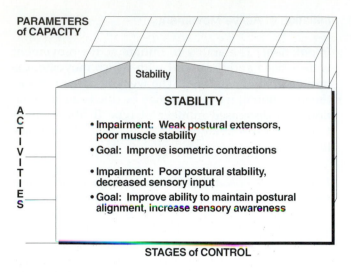

**PARAMETERS
of CAPACITY**

Stability

STABILITY

- Impairment: Weak postural extensors, poor muscle stability
- Goal: Improve isometric contractions

- Impairment: Poor postural stability, decreased sensory input
- Goal: Improve ability to maintain postural alignment, increase sensory awareness

A C T I V I T I E S

STAGES of CONTROL

Figure 9–14. Impairments and treatment goals appropriate when promoting stability.

shortened range against gravitational or manual resistance (Fig. 9–14).

Functional Implications. Maintenance of a contraction with resistance and approximately 40% effort is performed primarily by type I muscle fibers. In elderly patients with decreased strength and a decreased circulatory muscle bed, attempts at holding may require proportionally more effort, and muscular contractions may become anaerobic more rapidly. Another factor that may contribute to the weakness is a sedentary life-style, which causes the trunk and lower extremity postural extensors to be maintained in lengthened ranges. Although in elderly patients the loss of type II motor units appears to predominate, many clinical findings suggest a decreased holding ability. These findings include fatigue, reduced aerobic capacity, poor postural stability, and the decreased ability to maintain erect, upright postures. Promoting the tonic holding level of stability provides the prerequisite control in the postural muscles of the trunk, hips, knees, and ankles to maintain body weight in the upright position.

Treatment Goal. The goal is to improve isometric "strength" and improve the endurance of muscle contractions.

Technique. The technique of a shortened held resisted contraction (SHRC) can be used to facilitate an isometric contraction of the trunk, hip, knee, and ankle extensors in their shortened ranges.

With this technique, the extensor muscle maintains an isometric contraction for approximately 10 or more seconds in or near its shortened range. Increas-

ing the duration of the contraction is one means of progressing the challenge and is essential to reduce muscle fatigue. Also altered is the type and amount of resistive force applied by gravity or manual and mechanical forces. The contractions should be graded to approximately 40% to foster contraction of primarily slow-twitch fibers. The duration of the contraction is gradually increased while maintaining this intensity level. The individual should be able to breath comfortably during the exercise. Heart rate and blood pressure may need to be monitored. The duration of the contraction can be progressed by the number of breaths. For example, hold the position for three breaths and progress to five. The intensity of this isometric contraction may need to be even less if the CVP system is involved.

Postural Stability

This is also termed static postural control, maintenance of weight-bearing postures, static balance, and static stability.

Impairment. The ability to maintain midline or weight-bearing postures is decreased.

Functional Implications. A posture must be maintained before functional activities can be performed in the posture. Maintaining the upright postures of sitting and standing is prerequisite to ambulation, although some of the muscular activity and kinetics differ. Postural stability, particularly in the lower body extensors can be emphasized in other positions such as bridging and modified plantigrade.

Treatment Goal. The goal is to increase the length of time the patient is able to maintain postures such as sitting and standing.

Techniques. Alternating isometrics (AI) and rhythmic stabilization (RS) can be applied to the shoulders or hips in upright postures. Resistance is applied slowly, consistent with the patient's ability. The speed of resistance is gradually increased and the intensity reduced to improve the rate of response time. Initially, the resistance is rhythmic and anticipated to assist the patient in learning the responses. These parameters are gradually altered and the sensory stimuli changed by asking the patient to maintain postures and balance without vision or to stand on foam. During these more difficult conditions the patient may be cued to focus on foot and ankle sensations as the techniques are applied. Resistance also can be applied with weights or elastic. In other postures, for example, modified plantigrade or bridging, AI and

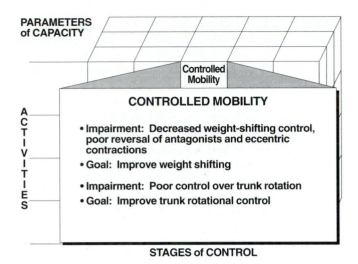

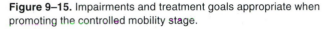

Figure 9–15. Impairments and treatment goals appropriate when promoting the controlled mobility stage.

RS can be applied to promote specific hip or knee control.

Controlled Mobility

Impairments. Many of the impairments classified at this stage result from deficits in the mobility and stability stages (Fig. 9–15). However, studies have noted that during weight shifting within a posture, older persons have less ability to control the outer limits of sway, even though they may be able to maintain a static posture.[10] It is not clear whether this weight-shifting difficulty is related to the range required during movement, to the decreased sensory awareness, or to the diminished motor ability to modify and increase force production as the center of mass moves.[33] Eccentric contractions, although requiring less capacity and force, may require more control than concentric contractions and are essential to self-controlled weight-shifting activities. In addition to promoting control, weight shifting over a limb increases the muscular and weight-bearing forces on bones.

Pelvic rotation during gait is commonly limited in the elderly. Analyses of trunk motion, however, have not differentiated between the available passive movement and the active ability to control that movement. Functionally, older persons tend to rotate the body less and have difficulty isolating neck rotation.

Techniques. Weight shifting can be performed either as a concentric–eccentric reversal of one muscle group, termed agonist reversal (AR), or as a reversal of antagonists, termed slow reversal hold (SRH) or slow reversal (SR). In either condition, resistance can be applied manually or with weights. Progres-

sion is achieved by: (1) increasing the range of movement, which in turn requires an increase in the ability to control the excursion of the center of gravity; (2) moving the center of gravity over a fixed base of support, then moving the base of support under the center of gravity; (3) performing movements on a stable surface, then on an unstable base; and (4) altering the sensory conditions. For example, in standing, weight shifting or swaying over the feet is performed before raising on the toes or heels, which decreases the size of the base. On a balance board a similar sequence is to maintain the position, then shift the position of the board. In both conditions, the weight-shifting motion is encouraged at the ankle to promote a more normal ankle strategy.[10] Vision can be obscured; standing on foam will challenge vestibular and proprioceptive mechanisms.

A deficit in eccentric control in the quadriceps and gluteals may be evaluated during the functional activities of descending stairs and moving from standing to sitting. To rectify this impairment, eccentric control of the quadriceps in the modified plantigrade position and the gluteals in bridging can be emphasized. Proprioceptive feedback and motor unit activity are increased with body weight or additional resistance.

Static–Dynamic

Impairment. The ability to maintain unilateral stance and perform transitional movements between postures is limited. The static control required for unilateral stance and the dynamic simulation of one step of the gait cycle is promoted at this level (Fig. 9–16).

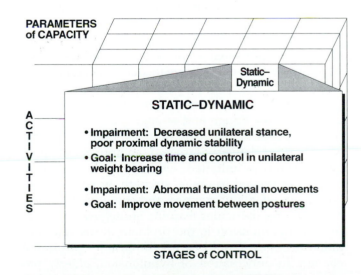

Figure 9–16. Impairments and treatment goals appropriate when promoting static–dynamic control.

Segmental trunk rotation and the ability to perform transitional movements between postures, such as from supine to sidelying, then to sitting, and to standing is included at this stage.

Unilateral stance is important for many functional activities, such as climbing stairs and dressing. Elderly persons have a great deal of difficulty with both unilateral weight bearing in standing and transitional movements. Winter et al, in their assessment of ambulation in elite elderly, described a poor relationship between static balance and ambulation. They found that during the unilateral stance phase of gait, the center of pressure did not laterally shift as wide as the unilateral base of support (BoS) but rather stayed more central.[34] However, while unilateral standing is maintained, the center of pressure must shift over the BoS. In contrast to the findings with elite elderly patients, the gait pattern of less active elderly subjects demonstrates a slower ambulatory speed, longer stance time, and increased lateral sway in the upper body.[8,9] These conditions may alter the center of mass–BoS relationship and muscular responses. For example, in younger persons and in the fit elderly, the muscular responses that control the mass of the upper body during ambulation occur primarily in the hip and back extensors and hip abductors. In some elderly persons the wider BoS may alter the amount of abductor control required and, as well, increase the similarity between unilateral stance and gait.

Another variable affecting unilateral stance is the distribution of medial–lateral forces at the ankle and hip. To balance unilaterally requires sufficient range, position sense, and muscular control in the subtalar and hip joints. Because of the difficulty in obtaining objective measures, sensation and motor control of these joints are not commonly documented in elderly populations.

Many older people are reported to fall during transitional movements from supine to sitting and to standing[35] which may be due to: decreased range and weakness in the quadriceps and gluteals, difficulty executing the movement, and postural hypotension and dizziness. Range and strength of the lower extremity postural extensor muscles need to be assessed and if they are impaired, an appropriate program should be initiated. Difficulty with execution that is not related to range, strength, or control may be due to deficits in memory and cognitive function, necessitating particular learning strategies. To determine if hypotension is the problem, heart rate and blood pressure should be measured after positional change. In anticipation of hypotension, elderly patients should be encouraged to maintain the new position for a few seconds before continuing with an activity.

Techniques. Weight-bearing procedures can be performed independently with or without resistance. AI and RS can be used to enhance the stability control of the supporting segments; SRH and SR can be added to improve the dynamic control of the moving limbs. Segmental upper and lower trunk motions can be initiated, either in the upper or the lower body. For example, while sitting, trunk segmental movements can first be performed with the upper body moving on a fixed lower trunk; this is followed by lower trunk movement under a stabilized upper body.

Skill

Locomotion, Manipulation, and Communication

Impairment. Normal proximal to distal timing, sequencing, and speed of movement may be lacking. The functional outcome of intervention, ambulation, occurs at the skill stage of control (Fig. 9–17). At this stage the normal timing and sequencing of movement are promoted to achieve a normal quality of ambulation. Some patients appear to have no physical impairments yet have difficulty ambulating within their environment. In these cases the deficit may be due to decreased automatic movement, difficulty learning and transferring functional abilities to other environmental conditions, or reduced exercise capacity for movement. For example, some elderly patients with primarily cognitive deficits may have difficulty walking in a new environment, particu-

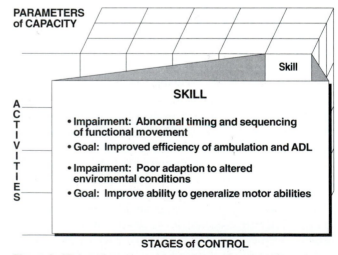

Figure 9–17. Impairments and treatment goals appropriate when promoting skill.

larly because they cannot remember directions.[31] The problem may be one of motor learning, of adapting to the environment, or of understanding the task, rather than of deficits of motor control or exercise capacity.

Practicing the functional task—whether it be walking, dressing, or feeding—under a variety of environmental conditions is emphasized at this skill stage. When the patient has difficulty performing the functional movement, the therapist determines the underlying impairments and develops a program to rectify those components, as has been described.

Techniques. The techniques at the skill stage promote the timing and sequencing of responses. Resisted progression (RP) is used to improve the sequencing of body segments during gait. Manual contacts are commonly positioned on the pelvis to guide and direct the proper progression. Additional support may be provided by the parallel bars, an assistive device, or having the patient hold the therapist's shoulders. If the patient has difficulty activating the distal musculature at the initiation of movement, the technique of normal timing (NT) may be indicated. For example, at the beginning of the swing phase, a patient may have difficulty initiating dorsiflexion, even though there is sufficient strength at other points in the range. At the initiation of the limb movement, the speed of dorsiflexion is facilitated by repeated stretches added to the voluntary attempt. For patients who have more difficulty with the timing and control of proximal segments, the techniques of SR, SRH, and AR are used in less challenging postures, such as supine or sitting.

Strength and Endurance

Impairment. Power and endurance of responses are decreased. Strengthening is an inherent aspect of each stage of control and of movement capacity. Strength impairments may be a result of delayed or improper neural messages, leading to activation of an insufficient number of motor units in an inappropriate sequence; reduced aerobic capacity can result in inadequate power, speed, or endurance to produce an effective response. The performance of many functional activities, including walking and stair climbing, can be limited by both these factors. While increasing strength in elderly patients, the frequency, duration, and intensity of the procedures must be carefully monitored to work within and improve the patient's movement capacity without overtaxing the physiological capability.

Techniques. RC and timing for emphasis (TE) are performed to enhance motor responses and to promote overflow from stronger segments. Techniques such as AI, SRH, and AR used to promote specific stages can be performed with increased resistance to enhance isometric, isotonic, or eccentric responses and with additional repetitions to improve endurance. In addition, endurance can be promoted by having the patient increase the frequency of the task as part of a supervised program using elastic or weight resistance. Pulleys, weights, or isokinetic devices provide a useful adjunct to the strengthening and endurance program.

▶ CASE STUDY

Mrs. J is a 79-year-old who comes to your facility with increasing difficulty walking on uneven surfaces and complaints of unsteady gait and an increased frequency of falling. To evaluate her status, the environmental, social, and psychological factors that may be influencing her ambulation are explored. The impairments related to the functional outcome of ambulation are determined by assessing the physical systems. These impairments are then sequenced within the stages of control with consideration of her exercise capacity. In the clinical decision-making process the next step is to develop the intervention plan and to determine specific treatment procedures leading toward the anticipated outcome.

Mrs. J's functional limitations are decreased walking speed and poor ability to climb stairs; she must use a banister and descend stairs one at a time (Fig. 9–18). Many environmental, psychological, and medical factors may positively or negatively influence her

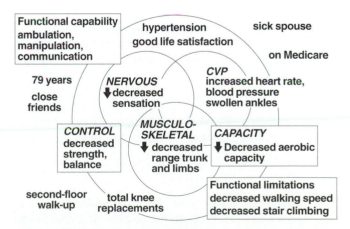

Figure 9–18. Evaluative findings categorized within the evaluation model.

physical functioning: she lives in a second-floor walk-up, enjoys a close friendship circle with the local church and volunteer group, has medical costs paid by Medicare, has slight hypertension, and has bilateral total knee replacements. At present she is satisfied with life but is concerned about a sick spouse. Measurements of the physical systems have noted reduced range in the trunk into extension and rotation, stiffness near the ends of range in the lower extremities, diminished sensation, including position sense, in the feet and toes, minimal swelling around the ankles, decreased muscle strength in the lower extremity extensors and dorsiflexors, and decreased ability to maintain standing without vision. Her aerobic capacity is reduced as shown by increased heart rate, respiratory rate, and blood pressure while climbing one flight of stairs. Differentiating the findings within the evaluation model will help the therapist determine if the functional limitations can most easily be rectified by modifying the environment, by teaching compensatory strategies, or by helping to remedy the impairments.

The evaluated impairments are classified into the intervention model according to their control or capacity characteristics. For example, the decreased trunk and limb range is listed under mobility–ROM; the decreased ability to maintain standing is listed under stability. Diminished aerobic capacity affects the parameters influencing the ability to perform each stage of control.

The functional outcome desired by the patient is to maintain independent community living, to ambulate on all surfaces and stairs with improved safety, and to increase walking speed. The therapist determines whether these are achievable outcomes. Also determined are the most effective means of accomplishing the outcomes and prerequisite treatment goals, including estimates of the frequency and number of treatments.

The treatment goals sequenced within the model are stated as positive changes in the impairments. The goals that anticipate change in the individual may include:

▶ Increasing ROM in the hips, knees, ankles, spine, and proximal upper extremities;

▶ improving the speed, frequency, and intensity of movement initiation;

▶ improving static and dynamic stability of the postural muscles with the sequencing and duration needed for postural responses and for ambulation;

▶ improving strength in the postural muscles during weight-bearing activities, including concentric and eccentric contractions with appropriate intensity, duration, and frequency for functional activities.

If change in the person is not a realistic expectation, compensatory strategies and environmental change may be needed and may include:

▶ Adding a half stair to reduce the ROM requirements of stair climbing; adding a raised toilet seat and bars and adjustable chair if decreased lower extremity range or strength requires this modification;

▶ additional assistive devices to improve stability and speed when ambulating out of the house or on uneven surfaces;

▶ adding an additional banister to provide external support while stair climbing;

▶ improving patient shoe support and augmenting education regarding foot care.

Intervention Plan

The procedures are sequenced according to the difficulty of treatment activities: the postures and movement patterns. This progression is chosen to minimize the need to move Mrs. J between postures to decrease patient stress and increase treatment effectiveness. Within each activity, the stages of control are progressed. These treatment suggestions, which focus on balance impairments and common gait deviations, represent general principles that may need to be modified for individual patients. Depending on the treatment setting, many of these procedures can be performed as group activities. This works well with persons functioning at high levels or with those who have similar impairments. Group activities, in addition to improving the physical attributes, may enhance socialization and discussion about creative ways to overcome physical impairments.

The parameters of duration, frequency, and intensity may need to be individually adapted. If the program is too vigorous, the individual may complain of tissue soreness and be discouraged from participating; more importantly, the program may overly stress cardiopulmonary structures and result in excessive fatigue or other signs of distress. The impairments of many elderly persons are the results of tissue changes that have occurred over time and consequently will take time to reverse. The intervention outlined in this section presents a number of varied and alternative procedures that address many of the existing and anticipated problems.

Specific Treatment Procedures

Procedures in the Supine Posture

In supine, upper trunk extension can be combined with scapula adduction and shoulder flexion or extension. In the lower body, various combinations of trunk and lower extremity movements can be performed.

Mobility–ROM
Goals include improving or maintaining range and decreasing tissue stiffness, particularly in the trunk, hips, knees, and ankles (Fig. 9–19). Techniques to achieve these goals include heat, massage, HR, and joint mobilization.

Mobility–Initiation of Movement
Goals include improving the ability to initiate and move through the range. Although Mrs. J is ambulatory and can initiate all movements, her ankle musculature is weak and the timing of the contraction is slowed; thus the initiation of ankle dorsiflexion, plantarflexion, and eversion is emphasized. HRAM, RC, and electrical stimulation are techniques that may achieve these goals.

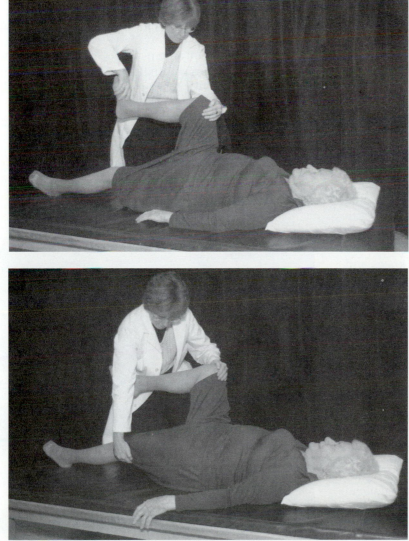

A

B

Figure 9–19. A: Supine; increasing range into **(A)** D1F, **(B)** D1E; T: HR.

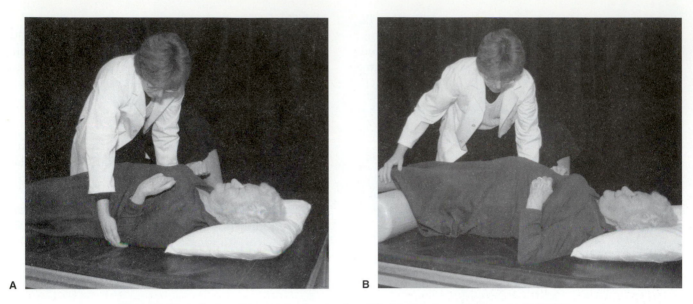

Figure 9–20. A: Supine; **(A)** upper trunk extension, **(B)** gluteal and quadriceps sets; T: SHRC.

Stability–Muscle

Goals include holding of low-intensity isometric contractions of postural extensors in the shortened range. The duration of the contraction is gradually increased from 5 to 30 to 60 seconds to increase Mrs. J's endurance and decrease complaints of fatigue. The intensity level begins with body-weight resistance with the gradual addition of external resistance as tolerated.

In supine, the upper body extensors and scapula adductors can be resisted by pushing the elbows into the surface and "pinching the shoulder blades together" (Fig. 9–20A). The lower body extensors can be resisted by placing a pillow under the knees and having Mrs. J perform quadriceps and gluteal sets against the resistance of the pillow (Fig. 9–20B).

Home Exercise Program

The reader is referred to the visuals demonstrating the program of home exercises located at the end of this chapter (pp. 245–252).

At home, Mrs. J can increase the duration of these supine and other activities, being careful to breathe evenly during the exercise. The difficulty can be increased by having Mrs. J roll into the prone position, which alters the gravitational resistance to the postural extensors. The prone position also is beneficial to stretch her tight hip flexors. By stretching hip flexors and strengthening trunk and hip extensors, a more erect posture, improved standing balance, and increased range into hip extension during gait can be

achieved. If CVP problems occur in prone, upper trunk extensors can be resisted in sitting and hip flexors can be stretched in supine or supported standing.

Procedures in the Hooklying Posture

Mobility–ROM

Increasing range of lumbar rotation is important for improved stride length during gait. Hooklying is an

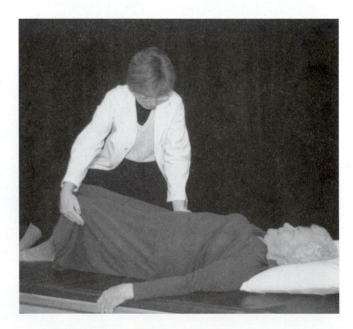

Figure 9–21. A: Hooklying; lower trunk rotation; T: HR.

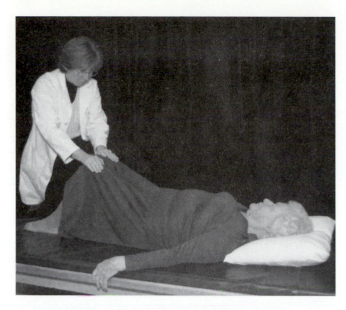

Figure 9–22. A: Hooklying; T: AI → RS, MC knees.

appropriate posture in which to promote this rotation; no weight bearing occurs through the spine, an important consideration for those with osteopenia. In such cases, the torquing motion combined with weight-bearing compression may be contraindicated. To increase range of lower trunk rotation the technique of HR or RI is suitable (Fig. 9–21). Once range is gained, the patient can maintain mobility by performing rhythmic rotational movements as part of the home program.

Stability

Maintaining hooklying and improving isometric ability of the lower abdominals and back extensors can

be enhanced by AI with manual contacts on the knees (Fig. 9–22). Mrs. J can perform lower abdominal exercises independently by first flattening her back, tilting the pelvis, and then bringing one knee toward her chest (Fig. 9–23). An elastic strapping can be placed around her knees to begin to resist hip abduction, which can be better emphasized in bridging.

Procedures in the Bridging Posture

In bridging, the lower trunk and hip extensors, and the hip abductors can be strengthened in the ranges needed for gait.

Mobility

The patient needs to have sufficient extensibility in the hip flexors and strength in the trunk and hip extensors (3/5) to achieve the hip extended or bridging position. Mobility of the hip flexors can be gained in the non–weight-bearing postures of supine or prone as described; the strength of the hip extensors can be initially promoted in supine.

Stability

As Mrs. J maintains bridging for an increasing length of time, the endurance of the back and hip extensors increases. The techniques of AI and RS with resistance provided at the hips, knees, or ankles progressively increases the difficulty of the procedure (Fig. 9–24). These procedures achieve the treatment goal of improving lower-trunk and hip stability which is needed for the stance phase of gait and to increase the

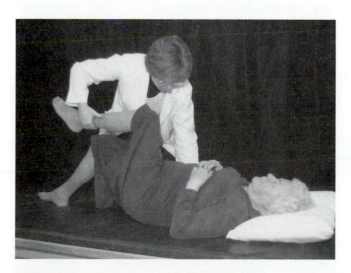

Figure 9–23. A: Hooklying; lumbar flexion combined with unilateral hip flexion; T: SHRC for lower abdominals.

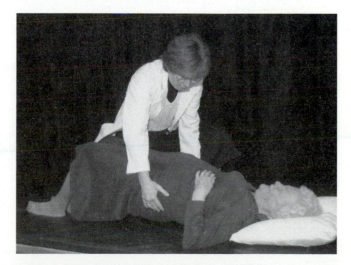

Figure 9–24. A: Bridging; T: AI → RS, MC pelvis.

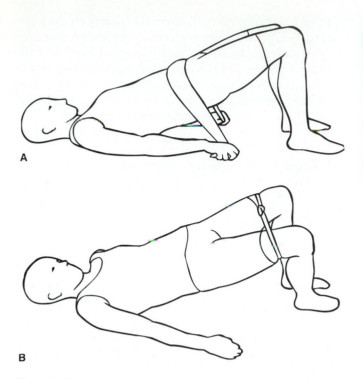

Figure 9–25. A: Bridging; hip extension and abduction; T: SHRC; **(A)** elastic over pelvis; **(B)** elastic around knees.

time of unilateral stance required for stair climbing. As part of her home program, elastic can be placed over the pelvis or at the knees to resist and emphasize hip and lumbar extensor or hip abductor control (Fig. 9–25).

Controlled Mobility

Pelvic lateral shifting and rotation can be emphasized by the therapist with SRH and can be performed independently by Mrs. J as part of her home program. Weight shifting increases the weight-bearing control on each leg. The concentric–eccentric reversal of moving into and out of bridging is performed to enhance her control while raising and lowering herself from a supporting surface.

Static–Dynamic

Lifting one leg from the supporting surface increases the resistance to the supporting limb and focuses on the control needed for unilateral stance and single-limb support while descending stairs.

Procedures in the Sitting Posture

The movements that can be performed in sitting include upper trunk extension combined with rotation and various upper extremity motions, lumbar spine flexion and extension, hip flexion, knee flexion and extension, and all ankle motions.

Many elderly persons may lose their balance backward when reaching overhead or looking up because of many factors, including decreased ROM in shoulders and upper trunk. Improving mobility in these segments, which can be accomplished in sitting, may improve postural control. Postural instability may result from poor dorsiflexor and quadriceps control which can also be emphasized by procedures performed in sitting.

Mobility

Increasing the range of trunk rotation, thoracic extension, and scapula adduction is particularly important for improved postural alignment (Fig. 9–26A–C). The range gained in the upper trunk and upper extremities, and in hip flexion with the techniques of HR and joint mobilization can be maintained by self-stretching movements.

Stability

Holding in the shortened range of the upper trunk extensors and scapular retractors can be performed with resistance provided manually, by pulleys, or by elastic bands (Fig. 9–26D,E). Isometric holding of knee extensors, flexors, and of the foot musculature may improve muscle stability and proprioceptive feedback (Fig. 9–26F–H).

Controlled Mobility

Weight shifting of the trunk on the hips is performed to improve the trunk balance needed during dressing. Moving the pelvis on the hips may improve the ability to assume standing from sitting.

Skill

Lower extremity movements are performed in sitting to emphasize the quadriceps and dorsiflexor activity that is required for postural responses in standing and during the gait sequence. For many elderly patients, weak quadriceps may limit stair climbing and the ability to move between standing and sitting. The techniques of SRH and TE may be used to improve the reversal of antagonists and the strength of knee and ankle musculature; NT may improve the sequencing of dorsiflexor–quadriceps activation. An elastic band, isotonic, or isokinetic resistance also may be appropriate to increase concentric and eccentric quadriceps strength.

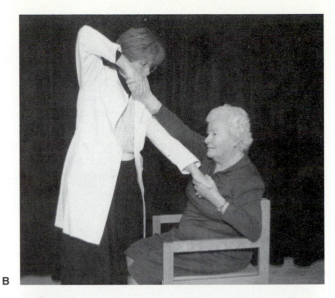

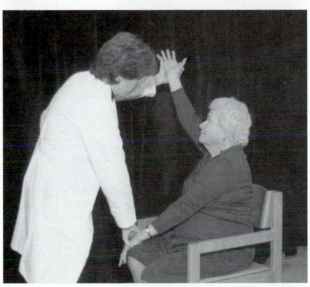

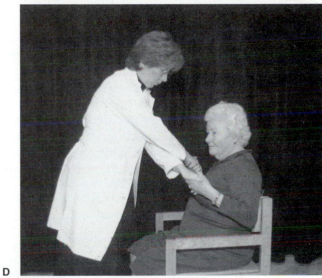

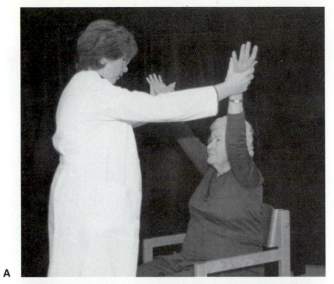

Figure 9–26. A: Sitting; **(A)** BS D2F; **(B)** BR D1 thrust; **(C)** BR D2; T: HR to increase passive range, RI to improve active range. **(D)** D1E (withdrawal); manual resistance; **(E)** D1E (withdrawal); pulley resistance; T: AR and SHRC A: (continued)

Procedures in the Modified Plantigrade Posture

Treatment in modified plantigrade includes exercises for the lower trunk, knee extensors, and ankle. Control around these joints can be emphasized in this posture, which is also easily incorporated into the home program. Modified plantigrade also increases weight bearing through the upper extremities, which can help reduce bone loss in segments that usually perform only open-chain movements.

Stability

AI and RS can be performed to improve postural stability and the timing of muscle contractions in the trunk and lower extremities (Fig. 9–27A).

Controlled Mobility

Weight shifting and small-range, knee-extensor, eccentric exercises are performed to improve Mrs. J's ability to reproduce the movements required when posture is challenged and to improve the control needed to descend stairs. By positioning an elastic band around her knee and attaching it to an immovable object, such as the leg of a table, concentric–eccentric resistance can be provided to quadriceps or to hamstring contractions (Fig. 9–27B,C).

Static–Dynamic

Lifting and holding one upper extremity or lower extremity, then contralateral limbs simultaneously will increase her trunk and hip extensor stability, challenge the postural responses of the supporting limbs, and increase weight-bearing forces on supporting bony structures (Fig. 9–28).[36]

Procedures in the Standing Posture

In standing, trunk, hip, knee, and ankle control can be enhanced further. As more difficult procedures are attempted, Mrs. J may require support provided by parallel bars or she can perform these procedures while standing next to a stable surface.

Stability

AI and RS can be applied to the pelvis or trunk to improve the ability to maintain upright postural alignment. Pulley resistance to the upper extremities can challenge Mrs. J's ability to maintain the posture. Resistance while facing the pulleys requires her to "balance" with her toe flexors, plantarflexors, hamstrings, and hip and trunk extensors (Fig. 9–29A).

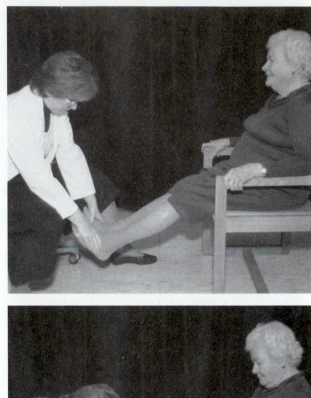

F

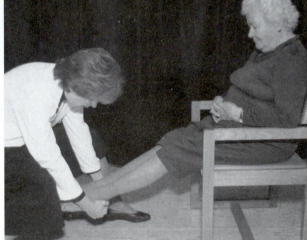

G

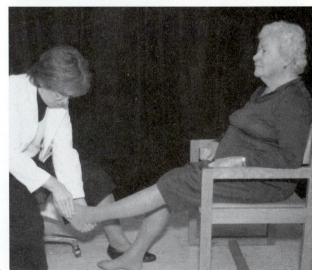

H

Figure 9–26. (continued) (F) BS knee extension; **(G)** BS knee flexion; **(H)** unilateral ankle motions; T: SCHRC → AI → NT.

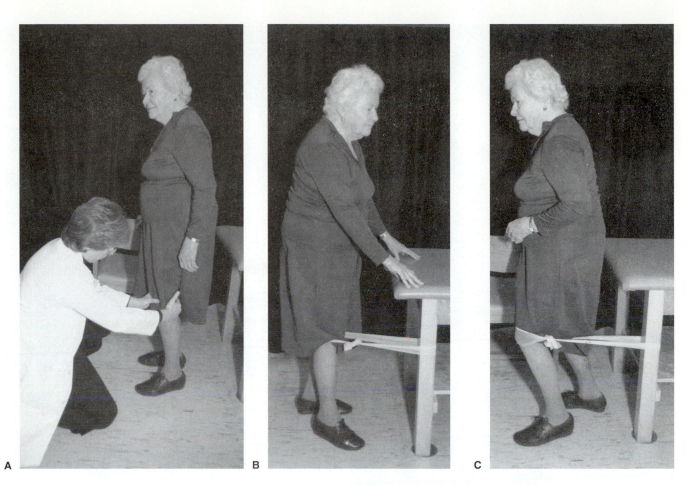

A   B   C

Figure 9–27. A: Modified plantigrade or supported standing; short-arc squats; **(A)** manual resistance to antagonists; **(B)** resistance to knee extensors; **(C)** resistance to knee flexors; T: AI → AR.

When facing away from the pulleys anterior tibials, quadriceps, and abdominals are more activated (Fig. 9–29B).

Because the goal of this procedure is to improve postural control, not to strengthen her muscles, the amount of weight is minimized.

Controlled Mobility and Static–Dynamic

Weight shifting can be performed both in bilateral and unilateral standing. As the body rocks in various directions postural control strategies are performed (Fig. 9–30A). The activity is made more difficult by rocking up on toes and heels which reduces the size of the BoS or by balancing on a moveable surface. On a balance board ankle motions occur independent of other segmental movements (Fig. 9–30B). These balance tasks are performed with eyes closed to enhance Mrs. J's proprioceptive feedback to improve aware-

ness while walking on uneven surfaces or when walking to the bathroom at night. Measuring balance responses can help determine the extent of weight shifting and monitor change (Fig. 9–30C).

Skill

Resisting the walking progression can emphasize the sequencing of pelvic motions during gait. At this stage, walking may be practiced on a treadmill to enhance learning and improve muscular endurance (Fig. 9–31). Upper and lower body ergometers may be appropriate to improve CVP endurance.

The quadruped posture was not included in Mrs. J's treatment program because of her age, cardiac status, and knee replacements. However, for others it may be very appropriate to increase upper-extremity weight bearing and improve trunk stability.[36]

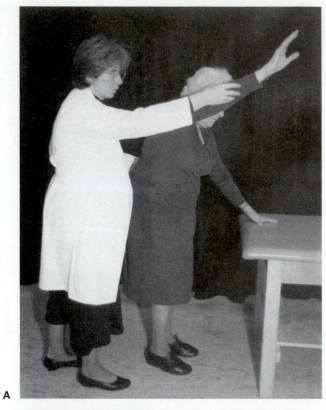

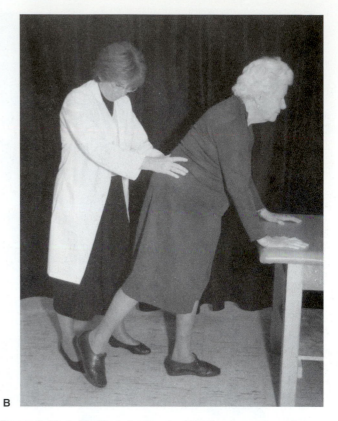

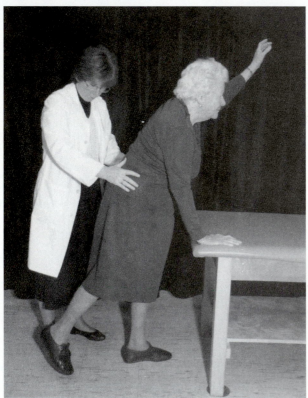

Figure 9–28. A: Modified plantigrade; **(A)** lifting one upper extremity; **(B)** lifting one lower extremity; **(C)** contralateral limbs; T: Active Movement.

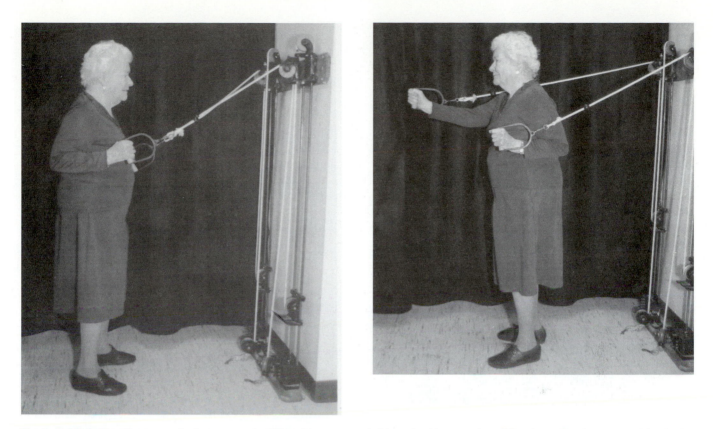

Figure 9–29. A: Standing; upper body movements; **(A)** resistance to trunk, hip and ankle extension; **(B)** reciprocal resistance to abdominals, knee extensors and ankle dorsiflexors; T: AR, pulley resistance.

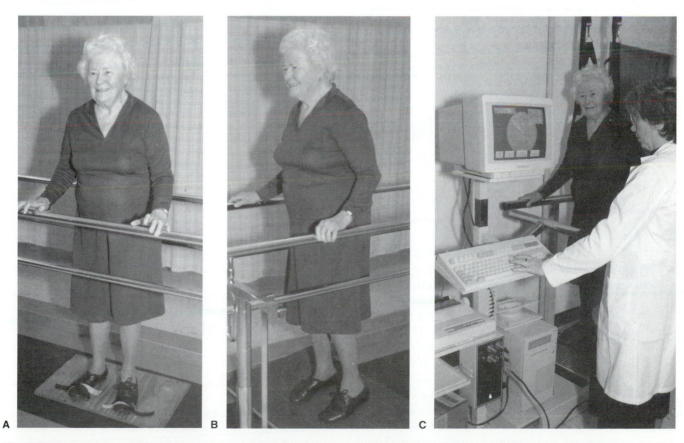

Figure 9–30. A: Standing balance system: **(A)** controlled mobility board to improve dorsiflexor control of backward sway; **(B)** balance board anterior–posterior ankle motions; **(C)** measuring and providing feedback for balance tasks; T: Active movement.

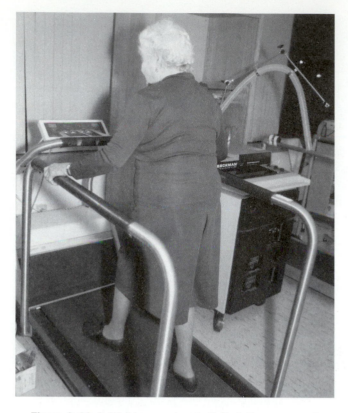

Figure 9–31. A: Walking on a treadmill; T: Active movement.

Intensity	Body weight or slightly greater			
Duration	Varied according to tissue healing			
Frequency	and learning needs			
ACTIVITIES	**Mobility**	**Stability**	**Controlled Mobility**	**Skill**
SUPINE	T: HR, RI, HRAM, RC	T: SHRC AI, RS	T: SRH	
HOOKLYING, LOWER TRUNK ROTATION	T: HR, RI HRAM	T: AI, RS	T: SRH	
BRIDGING		T: AI, RS	T: SRH, AR	
SITTING	T: HR, RI	T: SHRC, AI, RS	T: SRH	T: SRH, SR
MODIFIED PLANTIGRADE		T: AI, RS	T: SRH, AR, active mov't	
STANDING		T: AI, RS	T: SRH, AR, active mov't	T: RP, active mov't

Figure 9–32. Intervention model sequencing treatment procedures.

SUMMARY

A primary functional goal of physical therapy with the elderly population is to maintain or improve walking speed and to ensure safety while walking and moving between postures. This general therapeutic program and specific example have been designed to improve the components of movement associated with these functional activities.

The process of interconnecting physical impairments with functional limitations and developing an intervention program designed to rectify the impairments to achieve the functional outcome has been illustrated by the program for Mrs. J. Her functional capability was evaluated, considering environmental, social, and medical factors as they might influence physical functioning. The physical systems were assessed, comparing her findings to changes expected as part of the aging process and the physical requirements needed for functional activities. The impairments were evaluated as to her (1) ability to change, (2) the need to develop compensatory strategies, or (3) the need to make environmental modification. The treatment plan was developed by categorizing the physical impairments within the intervention model and determining the functional outcome that could be achieved and treatment goals required to at-

tain that ability. The specific treatment procedures incorporated appropriate postures and movements and techniques to achieve the stages of control and were developed with consideration of the parameters of movement appropriate to Mrs. J's physiological status and learning needs (Fig. 9–32). A group and home program can be designed to complement the individual therapy plan.

REVIEW QUESTIONS

1. An elderly patient demonstrates poor postural control, which appears to be primarily due to an abnormal ankle strategy. What impairments can contribute to this abnormal response? What sequence of procedures would you use to remedy these deficits?

2. You are treating an elderly patient who has a Colles fracture as a result of a fall. What secondary factors need to be addressed in the total treatment plan?

3. Osteoporosis is a common complication of aging. What procedures can be incorporated into a home or group exercise class to help reduce bone loss?

4. You are a consultant to the development of elderly community housing; what suggestions might you make to the architect to minimize environmental barriers?

REFERENCES

1. Tynnetti ME. Factors associated with serious injury during falls by ambulatory nursing home residents. *J Am Geriatr Soc.* 1987;35:644–648.

2. Bendall MJ, Bassey EJ, Pearson MB. Factors affecting walking speed of elderly people. *Age Ageing.* 1989; 18:327–332.

3. Alexander BH, Rivera FP, Wolf ME. The cost and frequency of hospitalization for fall-related injuries in older adults. *Am J Public Health.* 1992;7:1020–1023.

4. Kelly-Hayes M, Jette AM, Wolf PA, et al. Functional limitations and disability among elders in the Framingham study. *Am J Public Health.* 1992;82:841–845.

5. Fiatarone MA, Evans WJ. Exercise in the oldest old. *Top Geriatr Rehabil.* 1990;5:63–77.

6. Smith EL, DiFabio RP, Gilligan C. Exercise intervention and physiologic function in the elderly. *Top Geriatr Rehab.* 1990;6:57–68.

7. Brownlee MC, et al. Considerations of spacial orientation mechanisms as related to elderly fallers. *Gerontology.* 1989;35:323–331.

8. Murray MP, Kory RC, Clarkson BH. Walking patterns in healthy old men. *J Gerontol.* 1969;24:169–178.

9. Himann JE, Cunningham DA, Rechnitzer PA: Age related changes in speed of walking. *Med Sci Sports Exerc.* 1988;20:161–166.

10. Woolacott MH, Shumway-Cook A, Nashner LM. Aging and postural control: changes in sensory organization and muscular coordination. *Int J Aging Hum Dev.* 1986;23:97–114.

11. Sorock GS, Labiner DM. Peripheral neuromuscular dysfunction and falls in an elderly cohort. *Am J Epidemiol.* 1992;136:584–591.

12. Spirduso WW. Reaction and movement times as a function of age and physical activity level. *J Gerontol.* 1975; 30:435–440.

13. Sabbahi MA, Sedgwick EM. Age-related changes in monosynaptic reflex activity. *J Gerontol.* 1982;37:24–32.

14. Hart BA. Fractionated myotatic reflex times in women by activity level and age. *Gerontology.* 1986;41:361–365.

15. Lexell J, Taylor C, Sjostrumm M. What is the cause of the aging atrophy? *J Neurosci.* 1988;84:275–294.

16. Thompson LV. Effects of age and training on skeletal muscle physiology and performance. *Phys Ther.* 1994; 74:71–80.

17. Kauffman T. Posture and age. *Top Geriatr Rehabil.* 1987;2:13–28.

18. Peel C. Cardiopulmonary changes with aging. In: Irwin S, Tecklin JS, eds. *Cardiopulmonary Physical Therapy.* 2nd ed. St. Louis, Mo: CV Mosby Co, 1990.

19. Ades PA, Hanson JS, Gunther PG, et al. Exercise conditioning in the elderly coronary patient. *J Am Geriatr Soc.* 1987;35:121–124.

20. McGavin CR, Artvinli M, Naoe H, et al. Dyspnea, disability, and distance walked: comparison of estimates of exercise performance in respiratory disease. *Br Med J.* 1978;2:241–243.

21. Lord SR, Clark RD, Webster IW. Postural stability and associated physiological factors in a population of aged persons. *J Gerontol Med Sci.* 1991;46:M69–M76.

22. Shenkman M, Butler RB. A model for multisystem evaluation, interpretation and treatment of individuals with neurologic dysfunction. *Phys Ther.* 1989;69:538–547.

23. Anacker SL, DiFabio RP. Influence of sensory inputs on standing balance in community-dwelling elders with a recent history of falling. *Phys Ther.* 1992;72:575–584.

24. Manchester D, Woolacott M, Zederbauer-Hylton N, et al. Visual, vestibular and somatosensory contributions to balance control in the older adult. *J Gerontol.* 1989; 44:M118–M127.

25. Brooks VB. *The Neural Basis of Motor Control.* New York, NY: Oxford University Press; 1986.

26. Murray MP, Duthie EH, Gambert SR, et al. Age-related differences in knee muscle strength in normal women. *J Gerontol.* 1985;40:275–280.

27. Whipple RH, Wolfson LI, Ameiman PM. The relationship of knee and ankle weakness to falls in nursing home residents: an isokinetic study. *J Am Geriatr Soc.* 1987;35:13–20.

28. Astrand I, Astrand PO, Hallback I, et al. Reduction in maximal oxygen uptake with age. *J Appl Physiol.* 1973; 35:649–654.

29. Judge JO, Lindsey C, Underwood M, et al. Balance improvements in older women: effects of exercise training. *Phys Ther.* 1993;73:254–265.

30. Tideiksaar R. Falls among the elderly: community prevention program. *Am J Public Health.* 1992;6:892–893.

31. Drachman DA. Memory and cognitive function in normal aging. *Dev Neuropsychol.* 1986;2:277–285.

32. Ikeda ER, Schenkman ML, Riley PO, et al. Influence of age and dynamics of rising from a chair. *Phys Ther.* 1991;71:473–481.

33. Wolfson L, Whipple RH, Derby CA, et al. A dynamic posturographic study of balance in healthy elderly. *Neurology.* 1992;42:2069–2075.

34. Winter DA, Patia AE, Frank JS, et al. Biomechanical walking pattern changes in the fit and healthy elderly. *Phys Ther.* 1990;70:340–347.

35. Rubenstein LZ, Robbins AS, Schulman BL, et al. Falls and instability in the elderly. *J Am Geriatr Soc.* 1988; 36:266–278.

36. Marcus R, Drinkwater B, Dalsky G, et al. Osteoporosis and exercise in women. *Med Sci Sports Exer.* 1992; 24(suppl):S301–S306.

Pinch shoulder blades together and push elbows down into surface.

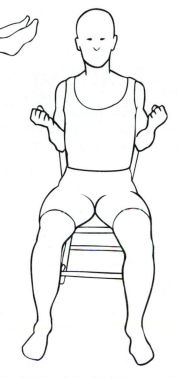

Pinch shoulder blades together.

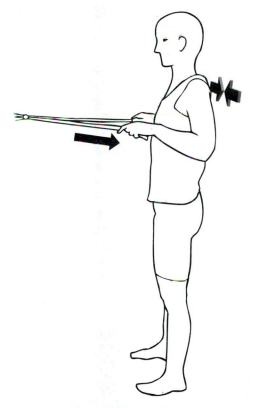

Pull back against the resistance and pinch shoulder blades together. Release slowly.

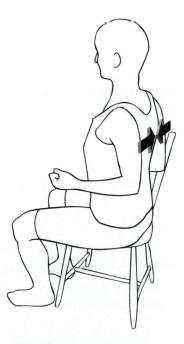

The arrows show you what your shoulder blades should be doing.

BACK EXTENSOR HOLDING

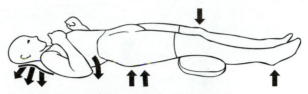

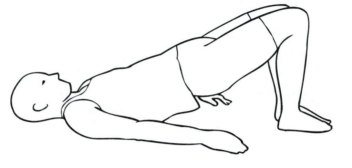

Push into pillow, pinch shoulder blades together and push elbows into the surface. Hold while you take 3 to 5 breaths.

Push knees into a pillow and lift hips slightly off the surface. Hold while you take 3 to 5 breaths.

Lift hips up.

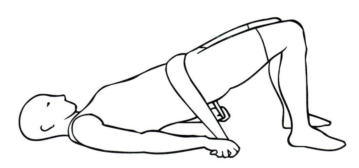

Lift hips up against the elastic resistance. Lower slowly.

Push knees apart against the elastic resistance.

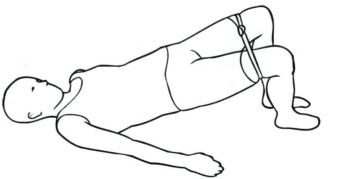

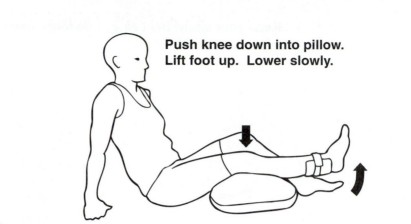

**Push knee down into pillow.
Lift foot up. Lower slowly.**

**Lift one foot up against the band.
Hold back with the other. Lower slowly.**

Hold onto a table while you do these standing exercises.

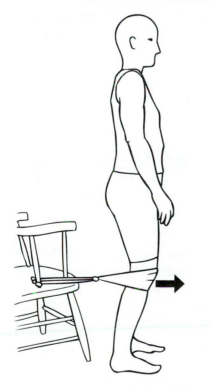

**Bend knee slightly forward and
control your knee as it goes back.
Do not let it snap backwards.**

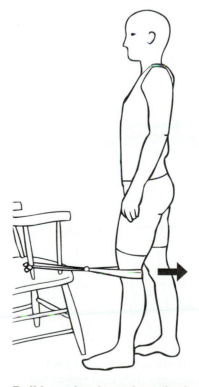

**Pull knee back against the band and
then let it bend slightly forward.**

Keep your elbow bent as you do these exercises.

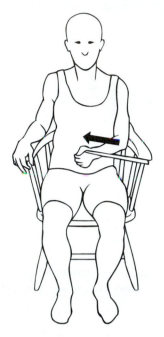

Pull hand in toward stomach and slowly release back to mid position.

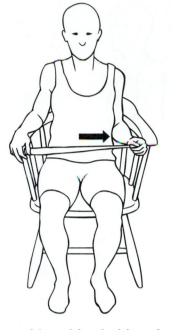

From mid position hold against resistance. Push hand out away from your stomach. Slowly release back to mid position.

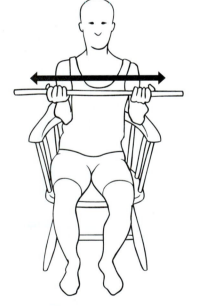

Pull, then push with your stronger arm and resist the motion with your weaken arm.

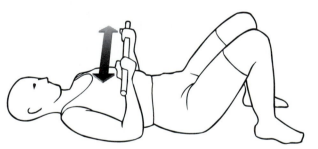

Pull, then push with your stronger arm. Resist the motion with your weaker arm.

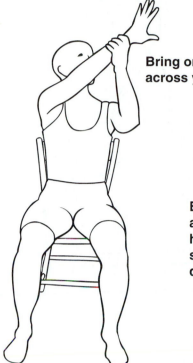

Bring one hand up and across your face.

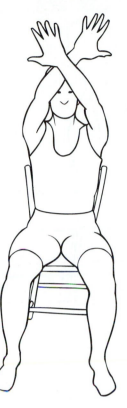

Bring both hands up and across your face. Bring hands back toward your shoulders and elbows down toward your waist.

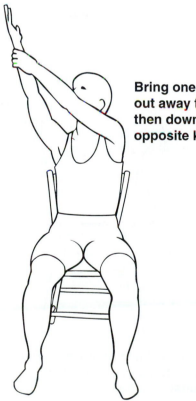

Bring one hand up and out away from your body then down toward your opposite knee.

Bring both hands up and away from your body then down toward the opposite knees.

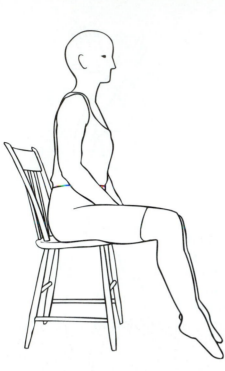 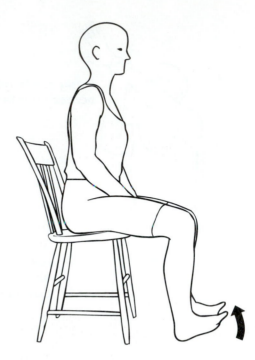

**Point toes down then bring toes up. Do both
together then opposite (one up and one down).**

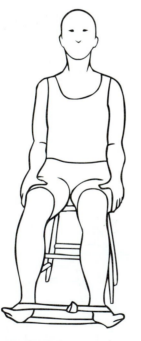 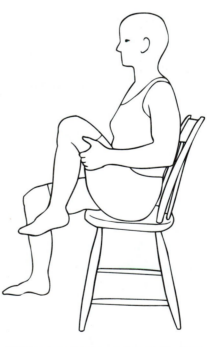

**Bring front part of your foot
out against the elastic band.
Try to keep your knees together.
Release tension slowly.**

**Bring one knee up toward your
chest. Keep your back flat
against the chair.**

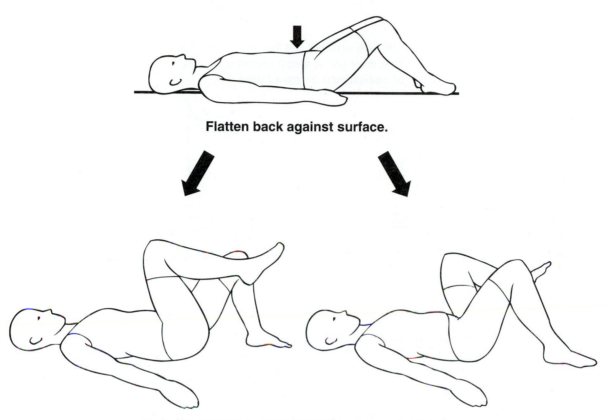

Flatten back against surface.

Keeping back flat, lift one leg toward your chest.

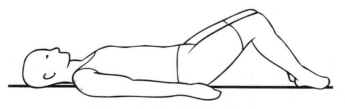

Return to starting position.

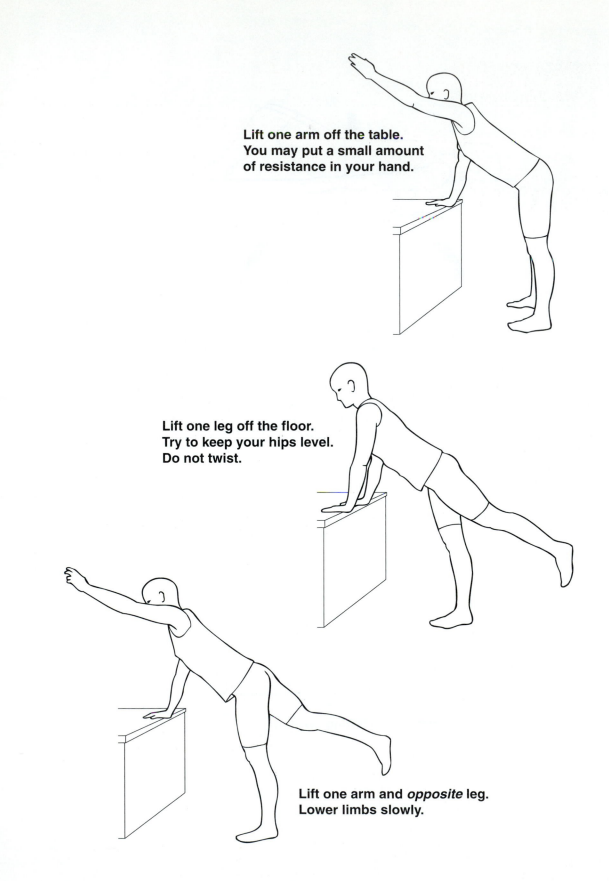

Lift one arm off the table. You may put a small amount of resistance in your hand.

Lift one leg off the floor. Try to keep your hips level. Do not twist.

Lift one arm and _opposite_ leg. Lower limbs slowly.

Hemiplegia

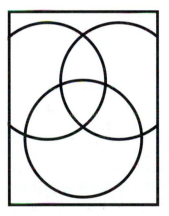

This chapter focuses on the evaluation and treatment of the hemiplegic patient. Although insults can occur in any of the vascular structures of the brain, many cerebral vascular accidents (CVAs) affect the middle cerebral artery and result in common physical findings.[1] Impairments of right or left sides of the body may be combined with visual field deficits. The upper extremity is usually more affected than the lower extremity and the symptoms, which include diminished sensation and decreased motor control, are usually more evident distally. The extent of language or perceptual deficit is influenced by the hemisphere in which the insult occurs: language problems are most prevalent with left hemispheric lesions and perceptual deficits with right hemispheric lesions. When blood vessels other than the middle cerebral artery are involved, problems such as ataxia, memory impairment, and cranial nerve damage may result.

Although many patients exhibit similar deficits, enough variation exists to make the treatment of each hemiplegic patient a unique experience. In addition to the area and extent of the lesion, these variables may include the time elapsed since the insult, the etiology, extent of neurological recovery, the ability to learn or relearn motor skills, and medical complications. The patient's age, premorbid personality, adjustment to the disability, and amount of family support can also influence the outcome of treatment. Because of these variables, it is difficult to generalize about rehabilitation potential. The evaluation and intervention procedures presented in this chapter focus on alleviating the most commonly found impairments. Treatment has been divided into initial, middle, and advanced stages to correspond with the most typical recovery pattern exhibited by the hemiplegic patient. The goals indicated at the beginning of each of the three divisions have been established according to the patient functional limitations and physical impairments.

Many unanswered questions exist concerning brain function, particularly in relation to plasticity, the interdependence of the cortical and brain-stem areas, the interaction of sensory, perceptual, and motor functioning, the mechanisms of learning and relearning, and hemispheric specialization. Increased knowledge in these and other areas will undoubtedly improve our treatments in the future. The evaluation and treatment described in this chapter is specifically designed for the patient with hemiplegia, but many aspects are appropriate for patients with other central nervous system (CNS) dysfunction.

EVALUATION

The initial evaluation of the hemiplegic patient is performed to assess the current level of functioning. The functional limitations and findings are translated into the classifications of the intervention model, from which treatment goals and functional outcomes can be developed. Equally important, although frequently ignored, is the evaluation of the patient's assets or abilities. To most easily attain the established goals, treatment should maximize the patient's attributes rather than focusing only on the patient's impairments. This concept of working through strength is most applicable to hemiplegic patients for whom relearning of functional movements may have to be reorganized in other areas of the brain and executed through different pathways. For example, for a patient with poor motor control and decreased sensory feedback, cognitive attention to movement tasks may be required to enhance motor learning. Depending on the areas that remain intact, some patients may use added visual cues, whereas others may need detailed auditory commands to supplement sensory input. As the patient's status improves and internal feedback mechanisms can increasingly be relied on, this additional feedback can be gradually reduced.[2]

Environmental, Social, and Cultural Factors

The environmental factors that seem to influence the patient's ability to maximize functional capability include the accessibility of the home and community. Because many patients will not achieve complete independence in ambulatory and activities of daily living (ADL) skills, environmental constraints need to be eliminated or minimized. The status of the patient's personal environment is an integral part of a complete evaluation. A home and occupational assessment will provide the therapist with the information necessary to ensure optimal functioning when the patient is discharged from the hospital or rehabilitation setting.

Many hemiplegic patients are elderly; thus many of the factors that pertain to that age group must be taken into consideration during evaluation and treatment (see Chapter 9).[3] For example, healthy elderly persons commonly ambulate at a slower pace than younger individuals and may have increased difficulty on uneven ground or at night. Hemiplegic patients share these base-line limitations and are also further limited by additional physical impairments. Impaired communication skills and limitations in ambulation within the community may make interaction with others difficult.

Medical and Psychological Factors

The initial incident from an embolus, thrombosis, or hemorrhage may result in acute medical problems as well as in the neurological event. Depending on the cause, the patient may be taking medication to prevent additional infarcts. Stability of vital functions is of primary concern immediately poststroke. If the patient has difficulty swallowing, aspiration may occur.

Visceral functions including bowel and bladder control may be affected as a result of decreased sensory awareness, altered tone, or involvement of the autonomic nervous system.

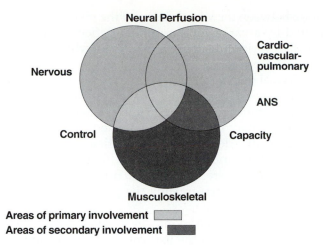

Figure 10–1. Areas of primary and secondary involvement.

The patient may be depressed, anxious, or emotionally labile. The extent of functional limitation and the potential for returning home may influence the patient's psychological state. The ease with which the person adapts to the altered role that may accompany the functional limitation will influence the outcome.

Physical Systems

The evaluation of the physical systems usually begins with the systems directly involved: the autonomic nervous, the central nervous, and cardiovascular–pulmonary systems, as well as movement control (Fig. 10–1). The evaluation also should assess the musculoskeletal system and the area of movement capacity (Fig. 10–2). The extent of the lesion, the patient's premorbid status, and chronicity of involvement will influence the extent to which these latter areas are involved.

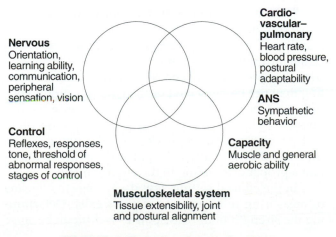

Figure 10–2. Evaluation of physical systems.

Autonomic Nervous System

In addition to somatic dysfunction, damage to higher centers may influence the autonomic nervous system and affect homeostasis.[4] Patients may demonstrate responses that could be considered sympathetic in nature: discrimination among many sensory inputs may be difficult, the patient either may not respond at all or may attempt to respond to all stimuli; movements may frequently lack purpose; distal circulation may be affected, as evidenced by a lower-than-normal temperature in the hands and feet. Procedures selected to increase parasympathetic control will help to promote a balance between these antagonistic systems and achieve the goal of homeostasis (see Chapter 3).

Cardiovascular–Pulmonary System

Breathing patterns may be impaired owing to altered tone of intercostal and abdominal muscles.[5] Reduced muscular control may result in both a decreased ability to expand the chest walls equally and an ineffective forced expiration. Respiratory evaluation and treatment are essential, particularly for the patient remaining on bed rest for an extended period of time because of medical complications.

The patient's heart rate and blood pressure may be unstable. The postures that are included in treatment may be limited by these values, and hypotension may occur as the patient moves between postures.[6]

Central Nervous System

Assessment of the patient's awareness of the disability and orientation with respect to time and place is important. Confusion, depression, and realistic concern for the future should also be noted.

The patient's ability to follow commands needs to be assessed. The difficulty can be progressed from one-step tasks such as "lift your arm" to more complicated three-step commands. Some patients may have less difficulty performing goal-directed movements, such as "reach for this glass" or "walk to the bathroom." Cues from different intact sensory modalities such as visual, verbal, or sensory may be needed to augment the response, depending on intact systems. Although a complete language evaluation should be performed by a speech therapist, the physical therapist must have an awareness of the patient's ability to understand and express simple or more complex verbal communication. If verbal input is to be used effectively, the patient's ability to receive information and then transfer stimuli into a motor response must be assessed. Written and verbal, receptive and expressive communication may be differentially affected.

Nonverbal communication relies on the patient's ability to accurately process different modes of sensory input, such as visual and perceptual. Although communication through these inputs can be assessed in a number of ways, a common method is to ask the patient to mimic the therapist's movement patterns. The use of alternative means of communication may be necessary with patients with aphasia as well as when a common language is not shared.

Exteroceptive sensation is evaluated by touch, pressure, and thermal stimuli. The more refined sensory abilities of two-point discrimination and stereognosis also should be noted. Depending on the area of the lesion, the patient may be unable to discriminate among various types of sensory inputs. Localization of sensation on the involved side may be possible but the sensation may be extinguished when the input is presented bilaterally.[7] Testing position sense, kinesthesia, and the patient's appreciation of tension in a muscle will provide the therapist with general information concerning proprioceptive feedback.

The results of the evaluation of both the exteroceptive and proprioceptive sensations help to determine the use of sensory inputs such as manual contacts, cold or warmth, vibration, joint traction, or compression to facilitate or inhibit motor responses. Even if the patient is not aware of the sensory input, however, elicitation of a reflex response may still be possible. If the stimulus response pathway is purely reflexive or is mediated by intact portions of the central nervous system (CNS), conscious awareness of the sensation may not be necessary to obtain the desired response. For example, joint compression may facilitate activity in postural muscles even though the patient may not sense the stimulation. Perception of sensation may be critical, however, if the response is to be sustained, learned, and made functional. In the standing position, an awareness of weight bearing and of proper joint position may be needed before ambulation can become a skilled function. Intact sensory modalities such as vision or pressure on the sole of the foot may be used initially to compensate for diminished segmental awareness (lack of joint sensation).

As discussed in Chapter 3, the effects of many sensory stimuli such as vibration may vary when applied to people with CNS deficits. Therefore, the initial and summated responses and any rebound effects must be carefully monitored.

Although body image and perceptual awareness can be assessed by the physical therapist, a more thorough evaluation of perception is usually performed by the occupational therapist. Many abilities such as rolling, dressing, moving in space, locating the brake on the wheelchair, or perceiving the distance between the wheelchair and the mat may be impaired by a variety of perceptual deficits. The functional severity may be compounded when sensory and visual problems also are present.

Visual field tests help the therapist determine the patient's visual awareness of the environment. The patient's ability to respond to and navigate in the environment may be adversely affected by visual impairments. If a deficit exists, the patient's bed should be strategically placed in relation to other objects in the room to ensure optimal visual input. The therapist's position when treating the patient should also be adjusted.

Vertical orientation may be evaluated by asking the patient to assess the verticality of objects and by observing the patient's posture. A discrepancy may exist between the patient's perception of his or her vertical orientation and the actual vertical posture. This is usually related to an imbalance of sensory input from the two sides of the body.[8]

Movement Control

Reflexes and Reactions. A reflex assessment can be used to determine the dominance of reflexes that should normally be integrated and the presence of postural reactions that will help orient the patient to the environment. The results of this assessment help determine the sequence of postures that would be most advantageous during the intervention. For example, if the patient demonstrates a dominance of the symmetrical tonic labyrinthine reflex (STLR) and increased extensor tone in supine, sidelying may be the position of choice to initiate flexor movements of the lower extremity. In the bridging position, the patient's ability to maintain the knee in flexion may be reduced as a result of an increase in extensor tone with weight bearing on the foot; an alternative weight-bearing posture such as kneeling may be indicated with such patients and included in treatment until extensor tone is diminished.

The righting and postural control reactions involve another level sensory–motor integration. The inability of a patient to respond to a change in the center of gravity (CoG) might indicate either a sensory or motor deficit. The sensation of altered position may not be perceived or the patient's motor control may be so impaired that a response is not possible. The disparity between the exteroceptive and proprioceptive feedback from the two sides of the body may also affect the patient's ability to maintain a proper orientation to the environment.

In the clinical setting, few if any objective means of measuring reflexes and reactions exist. Determining the strength of these responses is difficult because they may be affected by many variables, such as medication, positioning, and psychological status. It is important, however, to assess the presence of all these reflexes, as they can impact the effectiveness of an exercise procedure.

Tone. Abnormal muscle tone interferes with the ability to: alter the intensity and speed of the contraction, maintain or hold a posture or segment at various points in the range, reverse movements, or relax. Muscle tone can range from flaccidity to hypertonia. Abnormalities may be due to alterations in neural control and changes in the contractile and noncontractile portion of the muscle.[9] In some situations the tone may appear to be related to hyperactive stretch reflexes, whereas in other conditions stiffness may best describe the muscle response. The clinical assessment of muscle tone is largely subjective. Tone can be measured by testing deep-tendon reflexes, resistance to passive stretch, and the excursion of movement in and between postures. However, a lack of consistency in applying these tests, for example, variations in the speed of the passive movement, can reduce objectivity. Furthermore, muscle tone, like reflexes and reactions, may be affected by environmental and autonomic changes such as head and body position, medication, and anxiety, as well as by previous voluntary effort and rhythmic passive movement.[9] In spite of the many variables affecting tone and the lack of objectivity in its assessment, the distribution of altered tone both in specific muscle groups, such as the biceps or finger flexors, and in total movement patterns, such as mass extension of the lower extremity, should be evaluated. Reliability can be optimized when the patient is evaluated over time by the same therapist, who is consistent with measurement criteria.

Chewing and Swallowing. Chewing and swallowing functions are most commonly depressed in patients with cranial nerve involvement. Both decreased sensory awareness and diminished motor control in the facial, tongue, hyoid, laryngeal, and pharyngeal muscle groups may result in reduced function. (Evaluation and treatment of these vital functions are addressed later in this chapter.)

Stages of Control. Assessed in this chapter are the movement characteristics described by the stages of control. Specific attention is focused on the amount of head and neck control, types of movement patterns, range of control, and the threshold of abnormal reactions. Because a cerebral hemisphere influences contralateral as well as ipsilateral body parts, many hemiplegic patients present with bilateral symptoms even though one side may be more severely involved.[1] Thus, it is not unusual for a patient to demonstrate subtle tonal abnormalities and a lack of coordination on the "intact" side.

The therapist assesses the level of exercise that the patient can tolerate without causing an excessive increase in abnormal tone, lower-level reflexes, or associated reactions. Initially, any voluntary or cortical effort, or simply movement of the limb against the resistance of gravity may result in unwanted responses. Increased tone or associated movements in the involved upper limb may occur if too difficult a procedure is attempted for the lower extremities. As tone decreases, these abnormal responses may be evident only when higher level postures are assumed. The persistence of abnormal reactions may indicate that the procedure is too stressful for the patient. Stress can be produced by any or all components of the intervention procedure: performance of an **activity** with a raised CoG, such as standing or modified plantigrade, application of a **technique** that requires controlled movement in a posture before stability has been established, or changing the **parameters** of movement, such as increasing intensity of resistance while the patient's threshold for abnormal movement is low. The level of patient effort should not be allowed to reach a point at which abnormal reactions interfere with function.

Mobility. Mobility refers to the availability of range of motion (ROM) to assume postures and the ability to initiate movement. During the initial stages, when the patient is partially flaccid or hypotonic, ROM may be full; later joint or muscle stiffness or increased tone may limit movement. For example, limited extensibility in the wrist or hand flexors may reduce the ability to assume postures such as modified plantigrade; stiffness in the lower trunk and hips may decrease the ability to sit with an erect posture or move between sitting and standing. An increase in abnormal reactions during the assisted assumption of a posture is an indication that the patient does not have free mobility into the posture. In early stages of recovery, initiation of active movement may be difficult. Movements in certain muscles may occur only with reflex support, as in the initiation of wrist extension with the shoulder raised above 90° (Souques' phenomenon).[10] Voluntary initiation of movement usually improves, allowing an entire movement pattern to be performed. This movement may be limited, however, to synergistic patterns. Progress may continue so that the patient may combine movements of the major synergistic patterns before being able to isolate movement.[10] Proximal and distal movements should be differentially assessed as control of these segments may vary.

Stability. Muscle stability refers to the ability to sustain an isometric contraction in the shortened range against gravitational resistance. Of concern with hemiplegic patients is an inability of weakened muscle groups, such as the triceps and wrist extensors, to perform controlled isometric contractions. Holding of muscles, such as the quadriceps, which demonstrates an increase in tone, is equally problematic. Increased tone cannot be equated with strength, stability or control. Weakness of hypertonic muscles may be due in part to inappropriate and insufficient activation of motor units.[11,12] Controlled low-intensity isometric contractions are an important component of stability and are performed to promote a normal recruitment of slow-twitch to fast-twitch muscle fibers.

Postural stability implies a controlled, simultaneous contraction of muscles on both sides of a joint during maintenance of all postures. Altered sensory input from visual, vestibular, and proprioceptive receptors can affect the muscle, righting, and postural responses that contribute to postural stability.[13]

Head and neck stability may be affected by a brain-stem stroke. Although the specific details of head and neck control are discussed in the next section, we should note here that the ability to stabilize the head and rotate it across the midline needs to be evaluated.

Controlled Mobility. The ability to perform trunk rotational movements and to move or weight shift in weight-bearing postures requires an interaction of the two sides of the body and a reversal of antagonists, which seem to be difficult for hemiplegic patients. Rotational movements of the head, neck, and trunk require crossing of the midline and may be impeded by perceptual deficits. As movement through increments of range is performed in weight-bearing postures, righting and postural reactions are assessed as well as the patient's ability to assume various postures. The hemiplegic patient may have difficulty performing these tasks with bilateral equality. For example, the patient may have difficulty assuming the sitting posture from sidelying on both the right and left sides.

Static–Dynamic Activities. This intermediate step between controlled mobility and skill emphasizes unilateral weight bearing on the involved limb. This activity requires some level of proximal dynamic stability and postural control. The increase in body-weight resistance makes unilateral weight bearing

more difficult than the previous stages which examine control during non–weight-bearing and bilateral weight-bearing activities.

Skill. At the skill stage the patient's ability to function within the environment is assessed including locomotion, manipulation/ADL, and communication. Skill requires sufficient proximal dynamic stability for the patient to perform postural adjustments in response to extremity movement. In the extremities, the skill level of control implies appropriate timing and sequencing of reversing movements to perform goal-directed functional movements. Many patients may be able to perform skill level activities such as ambulation or dressing but not with normal sequencing, timing, or bilateral equality. Evaluation of the amount of assistance required and the speed of the task should be included.

Musculoskeletal

Mobility of both the noncontractile as well as contractile tissues is assessed. ROM can vary as a result of fluctuations in tone reducing the reliability of goniometric measurements. Some motions become limited more frequently, and those that are critical for function include: scapula protraction, shoulder flexion with external rotation, elbow extension, forearm supination, wrist and finger extension, and ankle dorsiflexion. These impairments of range are associated with the common patterns of increased tone and typical resting postures.

In the lower extremity, the inability to passively dorsiflex the ankle may be one of the impairments leading to hyperextension of the knee during the stance phase of gait.

An increase in osteoporosis or osteopenia may result from the increased sedentary behavior, necessitating caution during ROM procedures. Exercise, particularly in weight-bearing postures, is important to prevent bone loss.[14]

Movement Capacity

The patient's capacity to participate in an exercise program needs to be assessed. Such assessment will help with the projection of goals and outcomes. Both muscle and general body endurance are needed during the performance of therapeutic procedures and functions such as ADL skills and ambulation. Because the patient may be less efficient in performing these tasks, a tendency to conserve energy by moving more slowly may result.[6] As capacity improves, so may the speed of movement, which may promote a more normal timing and sequencing of functional tasks.

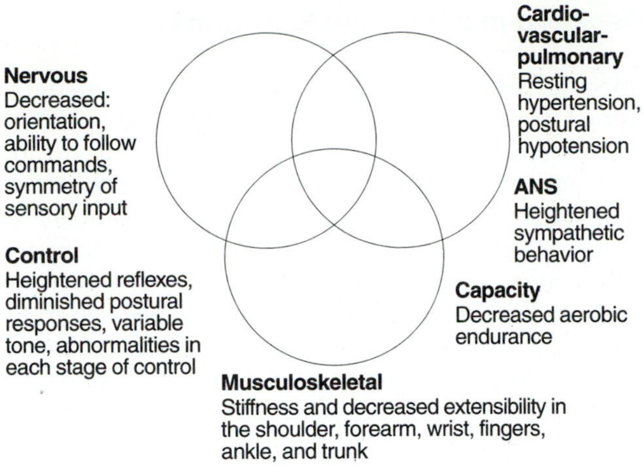

Nervous
Decreased: orientation, ability to follow commands, symmetry of sensory input

Cardio-vascular-pulmonary
Resting hypertension, postural hypotension

ANS
Heightened sympathetic behavior

Control
Heightened reflexes, diminished postural responses, variable tone, abnormalities in each stage of control

Capacity
Decreased aerobic endurance

Musculoskeletal
Stiffness and decreased extensibility in the shoulder, forearm, wrist, fingers, ankle, and trunk

Figure 10–3. Common evaluative findings.

EVALUATIVE FINDINGS

The findings of the evaluation that can contribute to limited function in the hemiplegic patient will change over time (Fig. 10–3). Following is a brief description of patient characteristics that may be found at three stages of recovery. Depending on the extent of the lesion, the patient may plateau at any stage.

Initial Stage

Movement Control. Initiation of movement may be restricted to associated reactions or minimal initiation of synergistic patterns. Ability to sustain isometric contractions or stabilize in postures is impaired. Muscle tone may progress from flaccidity to increasing hypertonia, with a dominance of phasic or tonic reflexes and diminished postural responses. The patient commonly has impaired cognition and may have difficulty following multiple-step commands.

Movement Capacity. Muscle and exercise endurance is poor. Contractions cannot be maintained for prolonged periods. The patient may tire easily.

Functional Ability. Assistance is needed to perform most ADLs; the patient may be limited to assisted locomotion in a wheelchair.

Middle Stage

Movement Control. All synergistic movements can be initiated, as well as some movements out of synergy. More challenging postures can be maintained and weight shifting can be controlled through wider ranges. Increased tone of antigravity muscles may be combined with decreased ability to contract opposing muscle groups. Lower-level reflexes are more integrated than in the initial stage and increased control over postural responses is emerging.

Movement Capacity. The tolerance for activity is improving, as evidenced by decreased fatigue during treatment and daily activities.

Functional Ability. Some ADL skills may be independent or require moderate to minimal assistance. Tasks may be performed primarily with the uninvolved limbs. Gait may require assistive devices for balance and lower-limb positioning. Gait abnormalities such as circumduction, knee hyperextension, and poor ankle control may be evident.

Advanced Stage

Movement Control. The patient may be able to combine most movements but may still have difficulty with the normal timing and speed of movement. Abnormal tone interferes less with function and the patient is able to respond to postural challenges under most conditions.

Movement Capacity. Ambulatory distance and speed are improving. Increased intensity of exercise can be performed with demonstration of fewer abnormal responses.

Functional Abilities. Most ADL skills should be performed independently and with increasing bilateral dexterity. Ambulation may require assistive devices only in challenging environmental conditions. Gait deviations are less predominant, although poor ankle control may persist.

Recovery of other functions, such as sensation, perception, and communication, may follow a pattern similar to the one described for the motor system. The extent and location of the lesion and the amount of neural recovery will influence the progression and the time required to attain the functional outcome.

INTERVENTION

The intervention plan is organized to ensure a comprehensive and coordinated sequencing of events. Interaction with other professions including medicine, occupational therapy, nursing, speech therapy, social service, and vocational therapy is usually indicated.

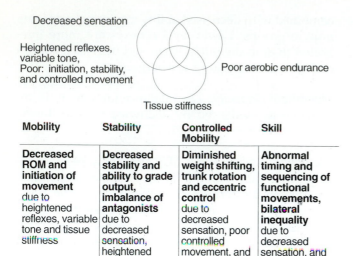

Mobility	Stability	Controlled Mobility	Skill
Decreased ROM and initiation of movement due to heightened reflexes, variable tone and tissue stiffness	**Decreased stability and ability to grade output, imbalance of antagonists** due to decreased sensation, heightened reflexes, and variable tone	**Diminished weight shifting, trunk rotation and eccentric control** due to decreased sensation, poor controlled movement, and poor aerobic endurance	**Abnormal timing and sequencing of functional movements, bilateral inequality** due to decreased sensation, and poor endurance

Figure 10–4. Relationship between findings and movement characteristics.

The physical therapy treatment plan is developed based on these general intervention principles: *Intervention encompasses a progressively more challenging sequence of therapeutic procedures designed to rectify physical impairments and to promote functional outcomes. The difficulty of the procedure is continuously advanced as the threshold of abnormal responses is raised.*

Decision-making Considerations

Specific findings and functional limitations are determined from the evaluation. The findings are then transposed into and delineated according to the movement characteristics of the intervention model (Fig. 10–4). Each finding may have an influence on more than one characteristic. A movement characteristic that is deemed to be restricted is termed an **impairment** (Table 10–1). Only those impairments that limit function need to be considered when developing the treatment plan. The interpretation of an impairment as associated with a functional deficit is based on the therapist's knowledge of the biomechanical and physiological properties of functional movement and the proportional contribution of each impairment to the deficit, as well as the therapist's clinical experience. Once the impairments are identified, goals can be set. **Treatment goals,** which are stated in positive terms, represent the anticipated improvements in the impairments and the prevention of further dysfunction (Table 10–2). The **functional outcomes** are projections of the patient's ability to ambulate, perform ADL and occupational and recreational tasks, and communicate. To achieve optimal functional outcomes, the treatment strategies can include: a change in the patient's abilities, use of compensatory aides and movement strategies, and modifications in the environment. In choosing among these

TABLE 10–1. CLASSIFICATION OF IMPAIRMENTS

Mobility	Stability	Controlled Mobility	Skill
Decreased ROM shoulder, forearm, wrist, fingers, ankle, trunk	Decreased muscle holding and ability to grade output	Diminished weight shifting, trunk rotation and eccentric control	Abnormal timing and sequencing of functional movements, bilateral inequality
Decreased initiation of reflexive and voluntary movement	Poor postural stability, imbalance of antagonists, decreased sensory input		

TABLE 10–2. CLASSIFICATION OF TREATMENT GOALS

Mobility	Stability	Controlled Mobility	Skill	Intensity	Duration/Frequency
Maintain or gain functional ROM	Promote graded isometric contractions	Promote movement within and between postures	Promote functional ambulation and ADL	Increase intensity of effort to raise threshold of abnormal responses and increase strength	Longer sessions distributed throughout the day and week to improve learning and enhance endurance
Promote voluntary initiation of movements in a variety of combinations	Improve ability to maintain all postures	Improve reversal of antagonists and eccentric contractions	Improve timing and sequencing of movement		

strategies, the therapist considers the time since onset, the influence of comorbid diseases and dysfunctions, the immediate needs, and the patient's desires. The functional outcomes, treatment goals and procedures, and projected date of discharge are set according to the likelihood of success of these strategies. By translating the evaluative findings into impairments, the relationship between deficits in movement characteristics, goals, and functional outcomes can be more clearly determined.

Using this process enables development of a logical treatment plan and sequence of procedures.

The following example illustrates this process. A common evaluative finding in a hemiplegic patient is stiffness in the posterior tissues of the ankle. This finding may be translated as a deficit in mobility–ROM. The therapist determines that this impairment in mobility will contribute to a limitation in the function of ambulation. The tissue limitation also is assessed for its potential to change within a reasonable length of time. If the therapist determines that the ankle range can be increased to a level required for functional activities, increasing ankle ROM becomes a treatment goal and therapeutic procedures are developed. If the stiffness is chronic and a change in the tissue does not seem possible, compensatory mechanisms or environmental modifications need to be considered. In this example, if increasing ankle range does not seem feasible, an ankle-foot orthosis (AFO) and a heel wedge may be considered.

Treatment procedures consisting of activities, techniques, and parameters are developed on the basis of treatment goals and intervention principles (Fig. 10–5). In the remainder of this chapter, the sequence of treatment procedures is divided into three stages that correspond to the initial, middle, and advanced levels of the patient's abilities. The findings, impairments, goals, and specific treatment principles as they relate to each level are described in depth at the beginning of each stage of treatment, followed by specific procedures designed to achieve the stated goals.

The stages of treatment and the intervention procedures discussed in the following sections are based on the most common pattern and rate of recovery. Individual variations occur for many reasons, including the site and extent of the lesion. Although in this chapter treatment procedures have been linked to different stages, the therapist must evaluate the individual patient's needs and apply the appropriate procedures. For example, within the same treatment session the therapist may choose advanced procedures for the trunk and initial procedures for the extremities.

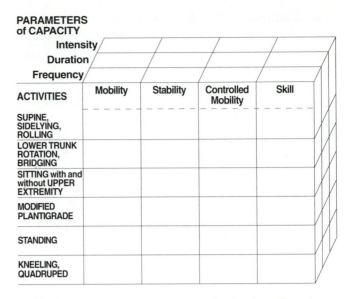

Figure 10–5. Treatment procedures can be developed based on the classifications of the intervention model.

Initial Stage

Patient Findings. The evaluation at this stage may reveal flaccidity or minimal hypertonia. The patient may be unable to isolate movement out of synergistic patterns. A predominance of spinal and tonic reflexes may interfere with normal movement patterns. Perceptual deficits combined with the increase in reflexes may diminish trunk rotation and crossing of the midline. Vital functions, including respiratory, swallowing, and feeding abilities, may be impaired.

Impairments

▶ **Mobility:** Wrist extension and ankle dorsiflexion ROM may be decreased. The patient may be unable to initiate voluntary movement of the limbs or trunk out of synergistic patterns. The initiation of respiratory and oral movements is difficult.

▶ **Stability:** There may be inability to perform isometric contractions without increasing abnormal tone. Low-level postures can be maintained for a limited duration. A list to one side may be evident during attempts at maintaining postures.

▶ **Controlled mobility:** There may be inability to rotate the trunk, to move within postures more than 25% of full range, or to control eccentric contractions.

▶ **Skill:** Functional activities are performed with uninvolved limbs and require assistance.

▶ **Endurance:** It is decreased and movements are slow, with poor capacity for functional tasks.

▶ **Intensity:** Increasing patient effort accentuates abnormal responses.

The abilities leading to functional outcomes that may be anticipated at this phase include:

▶ Improved breathing patterns and effective swallowing;

▶ rolling from supine to sidelying;

▶ maintenance of sitting and standing postures;

▶ transfer from bed to chair with assistance.

The treatment goals to achieve these outcomes include:

▶ Improve respiratory, swallowing, and feeding functions;

▶ maintain mobility of the trunk and upper and lower extremities;

▶ initiate trunk and limb movement out of synergy;

▶ improve muscle and postural stability in the trunk and proximal limbs;

▶ improve weight shifting ability in weight-bearing postures.

Intervention Principles and Implications

Activities: Postures and Movements

▶ The activities are progressed to promote proximal-to-distal control in the trunk and upper and lower extremities.

▶ Postures are chosen to afford the patient a large base of support (BoS) and low center of gravity (CoG) to minimize the level of difficulty and decrease the need for postural responses.

▶ Trunk and proximal control are initiated in postures in which the effects of gravity and tonic reflexes are diminished.

▶ Movements are performed with a short lever arm to decrease the amount of resistance.

▶ Rotational movements are incorporated to decrease lower-level reflexes, promote rotational righting responses, assist the patient in crossing the midline, reduce primitive movement patterns, improve body awareness, and enhance segmental trunk motions.

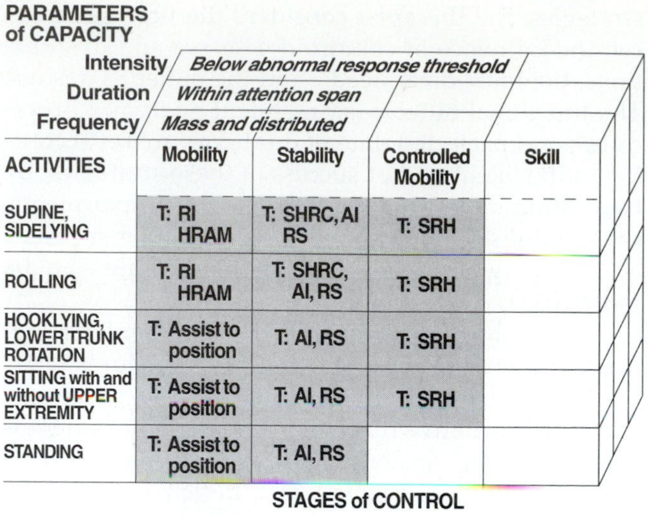

PARAMETERS of CAPACITY

Intensity / *Below abnormal response threshold*
Duration / *Within attention span*
Frequency / *Mass and distributed*

ACTIVITIES	Mobility	Stability	Controlled Mobility	Skill
SUPINE, SIDELYING	T: RI HRAM	T: SHRC, AI RS	T: SRH	
ROLLING	T: RI HRAM	T: SHRC, AI, RS	T: SRH	
HOOKLYING, LOWER TRUNK ROTATION	T: Assist to position	T: AI, RS	T: SRH	
SITTING with and without UPPER EXTREMITY	T: Assist to position	T: AI, RS	T: SRH	
STANDING	T: Assist to position	T: AI, RS		

STAGES of CONTROL

Figure 10–6. Intervention model, initial stage.

▶ Various combinations of movement patterns are promoted to allow for the variety of motions needed for function.

▶ Limb movements are enhanced by increasing sensory input within the involved limb and promoting sensory input from the uninvolved extremity.

Experimentation on brain-damaged animals suggests that exercise of the uninvolved extremity may result in decreased functioning of the contralateral involved limb.[15] Although contralateral inhibition may occur in some experimental conditions, empirical findings indicate that bilateral facilitation, especially in proximal areas, improves the sensory experience of movement and enhances motor learning.

Based on these principles and goals, the postures used in the initial stage include sidelying, supine, hooklying, sitting, and standing (Fig. 10–6). The extremity movements include trunk and bilateral combinations performed in the D1 direction to avoid synergistic patterns. However, if the patient remains flaccid for a prolonged period of time, the expectation of independent functional outcomes may need to be lowered. In addition, the therapist may need to initiate synergistic patterns to achieve function with compensatory movements.

Stages of Control: Techniques

▶ Techniques are applied to first promote homeostasis. Balancing the autonomic nervous system (ANS) will increase the effectiveness of subsequent techniques chosen to: reduce excessive tone, emphasize the initiation and relearning of movement, normalize the pattern of motor unit recruitment, and enhance the reversal of antagonists.

▶ During initial phases of rehabilitation, many sensory inputs may be required to facilitate responses. Later, as motor responses improve, these inputs may be withdrawn.

▶ The enhancement of low-intensity voluntary contractions may enhance a normal recruitment pattern.

Employing these principles, techniques are chosen to achieve the treatment goals: homeostasis is promoted with rhythmic initiation (RI); passive and guided movement are used to maintain mobility–ROM and active movement is initiated with RI, hold relax active movement (HRAM), and repeated contractions (RC); stability and the isometric reversal of antagonists are promoted with shortened held resisted contractions (SHRC), alternating isometrics (AI), and rhythmic stabilization (RS); movement within postures and the isotonic reversal of antagonists are promoted with slow reversal hold (SRH) and slow reversal (SR). Within a segment these techniques are applied to improve control of all muscles.

Verbal commands are simple and direct. If the patient is confused or aphasic, verbal communication must be carefully selected. The patient may be able to follow only one- or two-step commands and may require assistance in carrying out goal-directed cues. Manual contacts will be most effective if placed on areas that are sensitive to touch and pressure. Certain stimuli, when applied to a nervous system that is still in flux, may not produce the desired responses and a detrimental effect may result (see Chapter 3). Therefore, inputs such as ice and vibration should be used judiciously.

Parameters

▶ The intensity of patient effort is dependent on the status of the CVP and neurological systems and the extent to which voluntary effort produces associated reactions. Intensity is gradually increased to improve strength and proprioceptive feedback and to match the changing threshold of abnormal responses.

▶ Careful attention to the frequency, duration, and timing of sensory inputs is required for learning or relearning motor tasks.

In accordance with these principles, the duration and frequency of treatment procedures are controlled, be-

ginning with short treatment sessions resulting in mass practice, extending to sessions distributed throughout the day and eventually the week and month to enhance automatic motor behavior, the generalization of movement skills, and improve the internalization of functional tasks.[2,16] The treatment setting and other environmental conditions should be structured sufficiently to encourage the safe practice of functional tasks and also varied sufficiently to discourage situation-specific learning. Resistance is kept within the patient's level of tolerance. Transient increases in tone may be anticipated with increased patient effort.[17] However, persistent increases in tone may necessitate modifications to the appropriate level of difficulty.

Treatment Procedures

A: Supine, sidelying; limbs positioned and moved out of synergistic patterns
T: Positioning, passive movement, RI

The goal of maintaining mobility in the trunk and extremities is an important consideration during the initial aspect of treatment and may be encouraged by proper bed positioning to avoid synergistic muscle patterns and to optimize joint mobility.[10,18] In the most comfortable postures for the patient, supine and sidelying, appropriate pillow or towel supports are used to position the trunk and involved limbs out of the most common synergistic patterns. The shoulder should be abducted with the elbow extended and forearm supinated; the pelvis should be protracted with the hip in abduction, external rotation, and the knee in flexion. Because the finger and wrist flexors usually become hypertonic, a firm object is placed in the hand.[19] In addition, maintaining the wrist in slight extension and the fingers in extension and abduction will help to decrease tone.[18] The foot should be positioned in dorsiflexion with a splint.

Passive ROM should be normal during the initial stage and should not become limited unless moderate to marked increases in tone or prolonged immobilization occur. The main goal achieved by ROM exercises at the initial stage is to provide the patient with the sensation of movement.[20] Because shoulder pain is a common secondary impairment, range of that joint should be performed very carefully. Passive shoulder movement is most frequently performed in supine. The scapula elevation and upward rotation that normally accompany shoulder motion should always be incorporated into ROM shoulder exercises. Glenohumeral motion without scapulothoracic movement may overstretch capsular structures and impinge on the supraspinatus tendon resulting in subsequent shoulder pain and increased dysfunction. Nursing staff and family members who will be involved in the patient's care need to understand the ramifications of poor technique. It is the responsibility of the therapist to ensure proper implementation of this passive movement.

A. Supine, sidelying, semisitting; oral and
   respiratory functions
T. Active, guided movement, AI, SR, RC

Vital Functions. Although the procedures discussed in this section focus on the treatment of the patient with hemiplegia, the reader is reminded that this series of exercises may be adapted to the treatment of any patient who has hypotonia and dysphagia as a result of CNS deficit, peripheral nerve involvement, or surgical complications.

The goal of improved respiratory function can be promoted in the three postures of supine, sidelying, and sitting emphasized during the initial stage of treatment. Respiratory output is often decreased significantly in hemiplegic patients, making breathing exercises especially important.[21] Weakness in intercostals and other trunk muscles, combined with prolonged immobilization, can be contributing factors. In supine, apical and lateral expansion can be promoted with manual contacts on the sternum and lateral chest wall, respectively (Fig. 10–7). In sidelying, with the involved side uppermost, lateral and posterior expansion can be increased. The technique of RC can be used in all positions to stretch the intercostal muscles and to enhance inspiration. By varying the placement of manual contacts, all areas of segmental expansion can be emphasized.[22]

Mastication and Deglutition. Evaluation of a patient who has suffered a massive CVA or brain-stem stroke often reveals deficits in chewing (mastication) and swallowing (deglutition). Treatment should facilitate these important functions, which may be impaired from either sensory or motor dysfunction. Because the physical therapist does not receive extensive training in the facilitation of chewing and swallowing mechanisms, this important aspect of treatment is often ignored. The purpose of the following paragraphs is to acquaint the reader with the prerequisites of deglutition and to offer suggestions for the facilitation and activation of this complex activity. The procedures to be discussed may be initiated a few days post insult, when the patient is still confined to bed, and should be continued until the patient can swallow without danger of aspiration. Whenever possi-

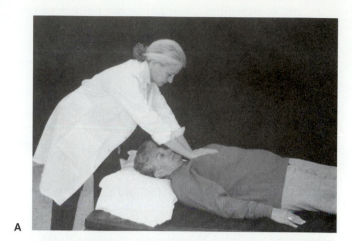

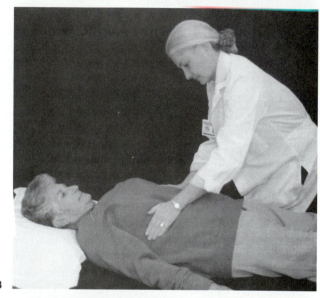

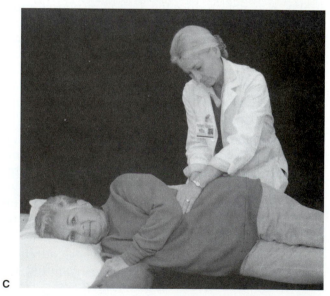

Figure 10–7. (A) A: Supine; apical breathing; T: RC. **(B)** A: Supine; lateral chest expansion; T: RC. **(C)** A: Sidelying; lateral chest expansion; T: RC.

ble, all the procedures should be performed with the head of the patient's bed elevated. This position makes swallowing easier and reduces the risk of aspiration.[23]

The first and most important treatment goal is head and trunk control. Without proximal control, normal swallowing patterns and intelligible speech are difficult, if not impossible, to attain. Therefore the focus during initial treatment sessions should be on the reestablishment of axial control with techniques to increase stability. When beginning stability is evident, attention can then be directed to the facilitation of the musculature of mouth and jaw, tongue, soft palate, pharynx, and larynx.

In order to chew properly, the patient must first be able to perform fundamental jaw opening and closing and must be able to close his or her lips around the feeding utensil. Unresisted jaw opening is the function of the pterygoideus externus and suprahyoid muscles, while jaw closing is accomplished by the other muscles of mastication: the pterygoideus internus, masseter, and temporalis.[24] Resistance to jaw opening strengthens the suprahyoid musculature, which plays an important role in the movement of the hyoid bone and the base of the tongue during deglutition as the bolus of food is driven from the mouth into the posterior pharynx.[25] Ice can be used effectively to stimulate the orbicularis oris, hyoid muscles, and the muscles of mastication (Fig. 10–8). Ice application can be followed by quick stretch and resistance to further facilitate movement and to strengthen the responses of lip closure and jaw opening and closing (Fig. 10–9). Facial muscles are composed primarily of fast-twitch or phasic muscle fibers and appear to respond well to phasic exteroceptive input. According to some authorities, facial muscles are devoid of muscle spindles.[26,27] Because of the lack of the Ia fiber, quick stretch would not appear to be a viable treatment option for facial muscles. Clinical observations indicate, however, that stretch does effectively elicit lip closure and other facial movements. Whether it is the actual stretch or the cutaneous stimulation that is responsible for the positive effects is open to speculation.

The tongue is an intricate and complex structure that is vital for speech, taste, mastication, and deglutition. It is composed of both extrinsic and intrinsic muscles, which contain muscle spindles that are dissimilar to those found in the extremity and trunk musculature.[28] Multifibrous and tendinous interconnections exist between the tongue and the mandible, soft palate, pharynx, epiglottis, and hyoid bone. To perform all of its varied functions, the tongue must be able to achieve all levels of control: **Mobility** is the initiation of movement in all directions; **Stability** is holding a groove, as occurs with sucking. The tongue must also be able to maintain a bolus of food in the front of the oral cavity prior to initiation of a swallow.[25] **Controlled mobility** is the fixation of the tip of the tongue on the teeth while the proximal portion elevates during swallowing. When tongue elevation is restricted because of paralysis of the tongue, palate pressures are changed and the bolus of food cannot be moved with normal speed through the oral cavity. Consequently, material may remain in the front of the mouth, on the tongue, or collect along the palatal vault.[25] **Skill** is the sequencing of movement within the tongue to promote proximal dynamic stability while the distal portion is used for speech (S.A. Stockmeyer, unpublished notes on procedures for improvement of motor control, 1979).

Physical therapy treatment of the tongue facilitates the first three levels of motor control. For **mobility,** a moist tongue depressor can be used to stimulate a combination of forward, lateral, and rotatory tongue movements by quickly stretching, then guiding or resisting these movements with the tongue blade (Fig. 10–10). As with the facial muscles, tongue mobility may be preceded by quick swabs with an ice cube to the different areas of the tongue. If the tongue depressor method does not produce results, the therapist can grasp the tongue with gloves and gently stretch and resist the movements.[29] Such stimulation may not be comfortable for the patient, but it is an effective means of eliciting tongue movement when other methods fail.

Stability of the tongue can be facilitated by having the patient suck through an empty straw that is placed against any object, such as his fingertip. In addition to facilitating tongue stability, resisted sucking can facilitate stability of the neck and jaw musculature in sitting. This can be accomplished in children in a prone-on-elbows posture.[19] Sucking on a nonsugary lollipop enhances both the mobility and stability levels of tongue control and will facilitate lip and jaw musculature.[23] This exercise should be supervised, however, and should be discontinued if the patient is not able to cope with the increased saliva production.

Controlled mobility, elevation of the posterior tongue to the soft palate, may also be stimulated with a dampened tongue depressor. If the direction of the resistance of the depressor is downward and backward, the base of the tongue will respond to the stimulation with an upward and forward movement. Stretch stimuli to the posterior tongue may result in the activation of the gag reflex which, although uncomfortable for the patient, may be a goal of treatment. Many hemiplegic patients lack the protection of the gag reflex and can easily aspirate liquids or

Figure 10–8. A: Semisitting; **(A)** orbicularis oris; **(B)** suprahyoid; **(C)** muscles of mastication; T: Quick ice.

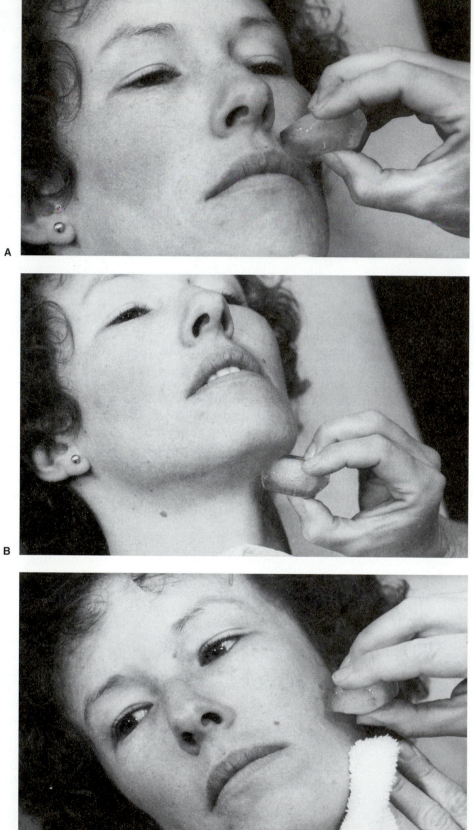

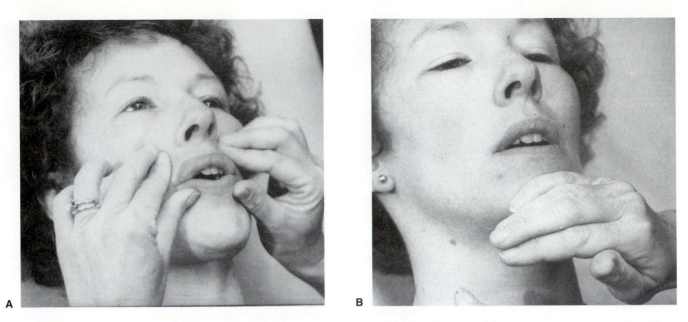

Figure 10–9. A: Semisitting; **(A)** lip closure; **(B)** jaw closure; T: RC.

solid foods. Controlled mobility tongue exercises are important, therefore, to facilitate a tongue movement that is an integral component of swallowing, to facilitate a hypoactive gag reflex, and lastly, because of fibrous interconnections, to indirectly stimulate contraction of the soft palate and pharyngeal muscles.

During swallowing the muscles of the soft palate interact with those of the pharynx and larynx. The larynx elevates anteriorly and the soft palate ascends to prevent passage of food into the nasopharynx.[30] The pharynx is simultaneously drawn upward and dilates to receive the bolus of food from the mouth. Subsequently, the vocal cords adduct and the entrance to the larynx closes, preventing aspiration into the trachea; the pharyngeal elevator muscles relax; and the pharyngeal constrictors contract to move the food into the esophagus.[25] Once the food is in the esophagus, the soft palate and the larynx return to their resting positions.

Elevation of the soft palate may be directly achieved by bilateral stretching of the folds of the soft palate with moistened cotton swab sticks (Fig. 10–11).

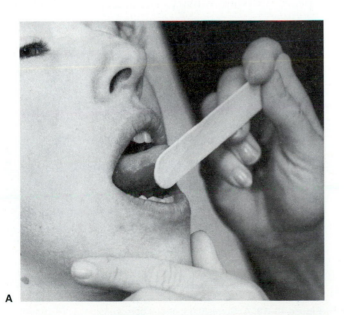
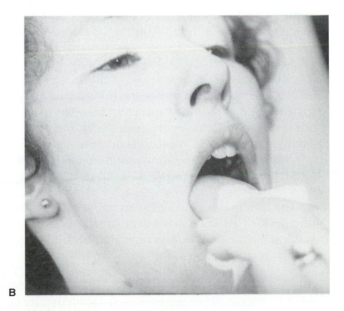

Figure 10–10. A: Semisitting; tongue mobility; T: RC; **(A)** tongue blade; **(B)** sterile gauze pad.

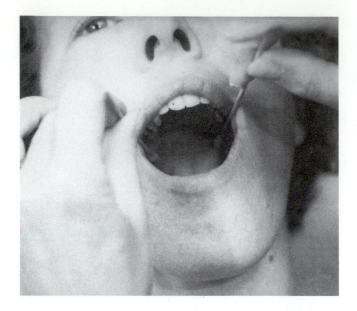

Figure 10–11. A: Semisitting; soft palate elevation; T: RC; cotton swab sticks.

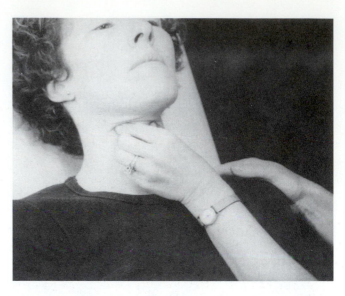

Figure 10–12. A: Semisitting; laryngeal elevation; T: RC.

While the stimulus is applied, the patient should be instructed to phonate with a series of staccato "ahs" performed at both low and high pitches.[29,30] This repeated stretching and phonating sequence should result in contraction of the soft palate and pharyngeal musculature, upward mobility of the larynx, and abduction and adduction of the vocal cords.

Vocal cord adduction can also be stimulated by having the patient hum.[31] Performance of Valsalva maneuver is yet another means of achieving laryngeal adduction, but obviously should be used with caution or even avoided in many cases. Manual elevation of the larynx can assist the patient with swallowing and provide the appropriate sensory feedback (Fig. 10–12).[30]

As stated, pharyngeal muscles may be stimulated indirectly by contractions of the tongue. They also may be stimulated by contractions of the orbicularis oris and buccinator muscles. Like the tongue, both of these muscles interconnect with the pharyngeal muscle group. Contractions of either the orbicularis oris or buccinator will therefore result in stretch and facilitation of the muscles of the posterior pharynx.[19]

The buccinator is an accessory muscle of mastication. Besides its reflexive effect on the pharyngeal muscles, buccinator stimulation is important because of the role it plays in holding food within the oral cavity. Facilitation of this muscle can easily be achieved by means of a quick ice application, followed by repeated contractions that are bilaterally resisted with tongue depressors (Fig. 10–13).

Areas of decreased sensory innervation can be determined by testing with a cotton swab. Facilitation techniques that emphasize those areas with optimal sensitivity have the greatest chance for success. Intraoral exercises are also indicated for patients who exhibit a hyperactive gag reflex and tongue thrust. The eventual goals for these patients are similar to those for patients with hypotonia, but the methods used to accomplish the goals differ.[32] Treatment should be coordinated with other allied health professionals who may be involved in this aspect of care such as speech, nursing, dietary, and occupational therapy.

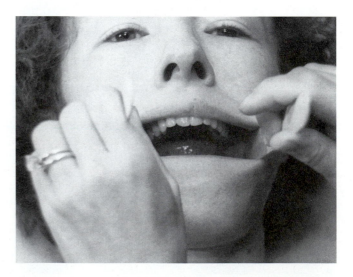

Figure 10–13. A: Semisitting; cheek compression; T: RC; tongue depressors.

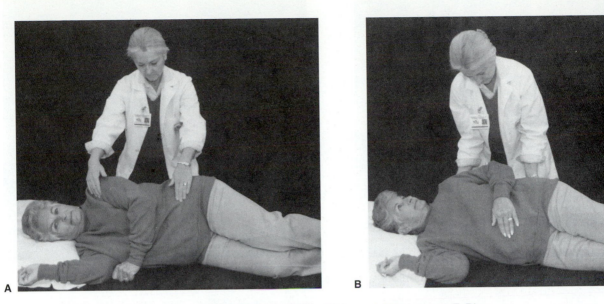

Figure 10–14. A: Rolling; **(A)** forward; **(B)** backward; T: RI.

Procedures to Improve Trunk and Proximal Control

A: Rolling: sidelying toward supine and toward
  prone; upper- and lower-trunk rotation.
T: RI, HRAM; manual contacts scapula and pelvis.
P: Low-intensity assisted movement.

The goal of this procedure is to initiate trunk and proximal limb movement. The activity of rolling may be performed in the patient's bed, beginning in sidelying where the effects of gravity and tonal influences are minimized; movement progresses through larger excursions of range (Fig. 10–14). Segmental rolling movements may precede total body rotation to decrease the difficulty of the active movement and to enhance learning. Upper and lower trunk protraction and retraction can be initiated with RI. The technique of RI begins with passive movement; the patient then assists in the movement before finally participating more actively (see Chapter 3). The forward protraction motion may need to be emphasized with the technique of HRAM to balance the increased activity commonly seen in the retractors. If abnormal responses occur HRAM can be modified by reducing the amount of range, the speed of the movement, and the intensity of the stimuli. In addition, forward rotation of the lower trunk in sidelying and in other more advanced activities may help to promote the lower trunk control needed for gait.

A: Rolling; upper-trunk patterns
T: RI progressing to SRH and SR

Proximal movement can also be enhanced by rolling in combination with upper-trunk patterns (Fig. 10–15). Trunk combinations with the limb moving in the D1 direction are particularly effective activities during early stages of treatment to promote body awareness, crossing the midline, an interaction of trunk and limb antagonists, and the initiation of movement out of synergistic patterns. The involved extremity aided by the uninvolved limb moves into D1F, which will promote scapular protraction and shoulder flexion with adduction. The elbow can remain straight throughout the movement or can move into extension as the shoulder flexes. The reverse

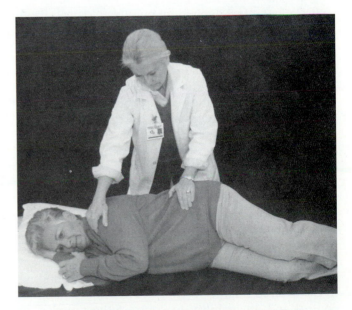

Figure 10–15. A: Rolling; upper-trunk rotation; T: RI.

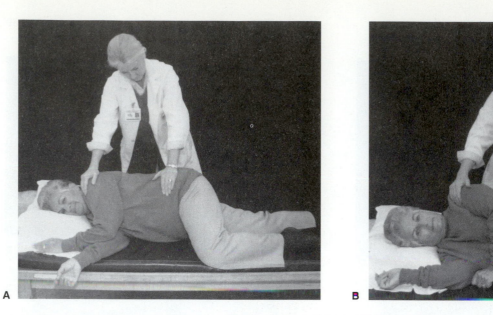

Figure 10–16. A: Sidelying; T: **(A)** AI; **(B)** RS.

trunk movement, in which the involved limb moves in D1E out of the synergistic pattern, combines shoulder extension with abduction. Upper-trunk patterns can also be performed in supine to focus on proximal limb function. As the patient is able to initiate movement, more resistance can be applied throughout range and at the ends of the range with the techniques of SR and SRH. Once active movement can be initiated, techniques to promote stability can be emphasized.

> A: Sidelying; limbs positioned out of synergistic positions.
> T: SHRC, AI, RS to the trunk segments or entire trunk.
> P: Patient effort dependent on physiological stress and threshold of associated reactions.

The goal of promoting muscle and postural stability in the trunk can be initiated in sidelying (Fig. 10–16). The patient can be positioned with the involved side uppermost to focus on direct activation or positioned lying on the involved side to improve sensory awareness. A SHRC with low-intensity resistance is applied to promote isometric activation and to encourage a normal motor unit recruitment pattern of the postural extensors without excessive associated reactions. AI is then applied to promote a smooth reversal of isometric contractions of trunk extensors and abdominals. The difficulty is progressed with RS to enhance counterrotational isometric control. Although RS may be attempted during early treatment stages, the patient may not be capable of responding in the desired manner because of a lack of rotational control and an inability to contract the muscles on both sides of the trunk simultaneously. Trunk stabil-

ity is necessary to maintain all higher-level postures and should be a goal of treatment during all stages of recovery.

> A: Supine; lower-trunk patterns with the involved limb in D1F and D1E.
> T: SHRC.

Supine affords a large BoS and low CoG from which to promote the goal of initiating trunk and proximal movements. Lower-trunk patterns incorporate limb–trunk rotation with mass flexion and extension movements (Fig. 10–17). As with the upper-trunk

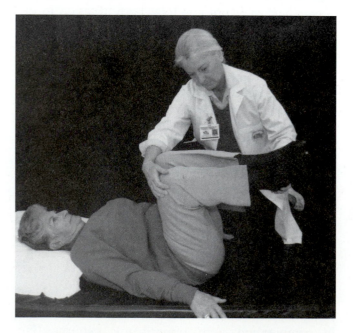

Figure 10–17. A: Supine; lower-trunk pattern; T: SHRC.

combinations, the involved extremity moves in the D1 direction, which combines flexion with adduction and extension with abduction. If lower-extremity extensor tone is dominant, flexion can be emphasized by isometrically contracting the flexors first in the shortened ranges, progressing to more lengthened ranges in which the effects of gravity, the length of the lever arm, and the tendency toward extension are increased. Conversely, for patients who present with a generalized decrease in tone or a predominant flexor withdrawal response, the extensor rather than the flexor phase should be emphasized. For all hemiplegic patients, the combination of hip extension with abduction is important for the stance phase of gait[10,18] and can be enhanced by facilitation of isometric contractions in the shortened range of the trunk extensor pattern to promote hip stability.

A: Hooklying and lower-trunk rotation (LTR); upper extremities positioned in shoulder extension, abduction, elbow extension, and forearm supination

T: RI progressing to AI progressing; to SR; manual contacts (MC) knees

P: Low intensity and slow speed, depending on patient's response.

The goal of these procedures is to further promote the initiation and control of movement. As in sidelying, the lower-trunk rotational motion may help to balance tone and promote the pelvic forward rotational movement necessary for ambulation (Fig. 10–18).[33] In comparison to sidelying, however, hooklying in-

creases the length of the lever arm, the number of joints involved, and the influence of tonic reflexes. If increased extensor tone, a dominance of the symmetrical tonic labyrinthine reflex (STLR), an extensor thrust, or proximal weakness reduce the patient's ability to maintain hip and knee flexion, the feet may need to be supported by the therapist. The upper extremity is positioned at the patient's side to discourage abnormal posturing.[18] The technique of RI is performed through increments of range to promote the initiation of lower-trunk rotation. AI can then be applied with MC on the knees in the midline position to promote initial aspects of stability of the trunk and hips. SR applied through small increments of range is used to initiate an isotonic reversal of trunk and hip antagonists.

A: Sitting; upper extremities weight bearing, feet in contact with supporting surface.

T: AI, RS progressing to SRH; MC head, scapula, or arm.

In sitting, postural stability in the trunk and proximal limbs is further enhanced in a posture with a smaller BoS, higher CoG (Fig. 10–19 A,B). The resistance to trunk and limbs is varied due to the different orientation of the body to gravity requiring the need for postural responses. Patients are frequently positioned sitting in a chair but may have difficulty maintaining sitting independently because of decreased muscle stability, reduced postural responses, or imbalances in sensory feedback from the two sides of the body. Promoting postural stability in various directions

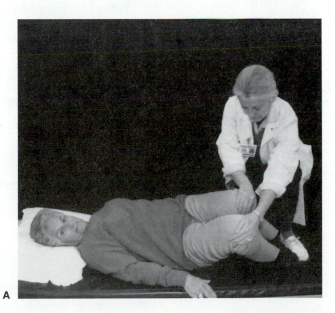

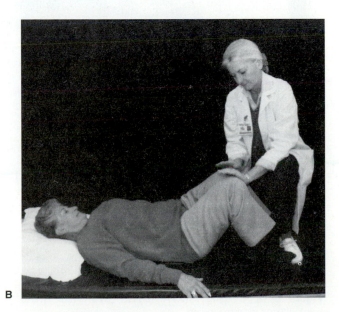

Figure 10–18. A: Hooklying; T: **(A)** RI; **(B)** AI.

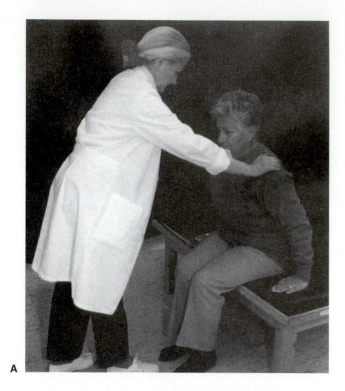

A

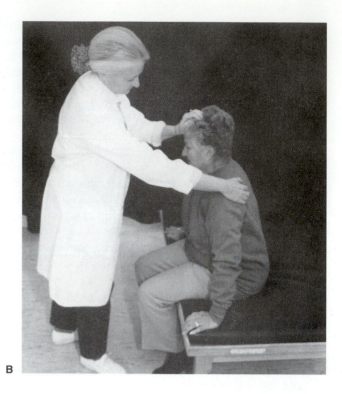

B

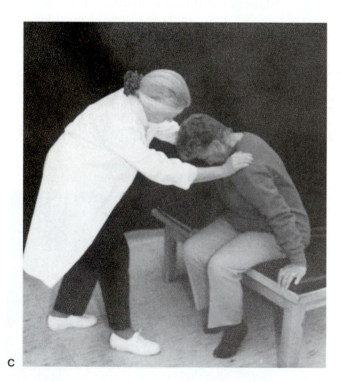

C

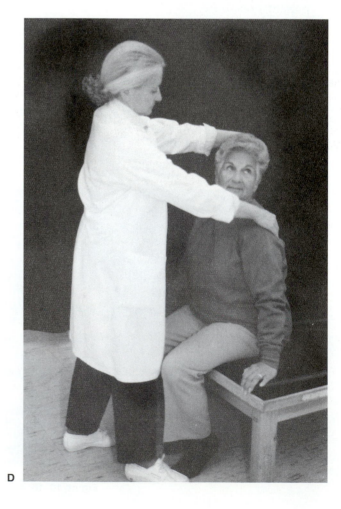

D

Figure 10–19. A: Sitting; T: **(A)** AI; **(B)** RS; **(C)** and **(D)** SRH, to trunk, flexion, and extension.

may help to prevent falling backward, forward, or to either side. AI performed in one or two planes is usually followed by RS. The placement of MC and the position of the involved arm can be altered to emphasize the head, neck, trunk, and upper extremity. When sitting balance is extremely poor, muscle stability should first be emphasized in the lower-level postures of sidelying and supine, as previously indicated.

Weight shifting in sitting helps promote the goal of improved dynamic postural control (Fig. 10–19 C,D). Movements in the directions of flexion and extension are combined with rotation and enhanced with the techniques of SRH or SR through increments of range. The techniques are initiated by guiding the patient through small ranges to teach the movement, RI, before applying resistance. Movement between postures is assisted as the patient is transferred from the bed to a chair.

A: Standing.
T: Assist to position, progress to AI; MC scapula and pelvis.
P: Short duration.

For many patients, standing early in the treatment progression is necessary for psychological support and enhancement of physiological systems even though adequate trunk and lower-extremity stability has not fully been established. As often occurs throughout the sequence of procedures, the patient may be capable of maintaining the position and weight shifting within small ranges before being able to independently assume the posture (Fig. 10–20). Beginning stability may be promoted with AI applied to the trunk. Equal weight bearing through both lower extremities is encouraged, even though sufficient stability has not been developed in the lower extremity. Unsuccessful attempts at ambulation may indicate the need to develop control in less stressful, lower-level postures. Emphasis on ambulation with maximal assistance and external supports can tend to frustrate the patient and may result in poor gait patterns. More importantly, prolonged ambulation with gait deviations often leads to the development of orthopedic problems, such as hip, knee, and low-back pain. Sequencing of procedures to build in appropriate control may help to prevent the development of such problems, which will eventually require additional care.

Summary. The procedures in the initial stage of recovery focus on the goals of improving vital functions, maintaining passive ROM, initiating active movement in the trunk and proximal segments, and promoting stability and controlled movement through

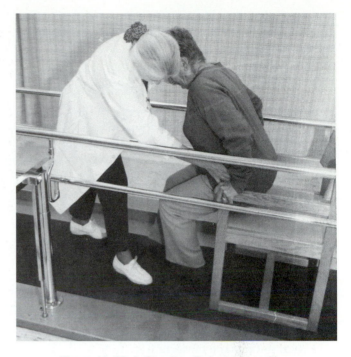

Figure 10–20. A: Standing; T: Assist to position.

increments of range in low-level postures. The goals are developed to achieve the functions of improved rolling, the maintenance of sitting and standing, and safe transfers. The procedures have combined the postures of supine, sidelying, and sitting with trunk and proximal limb movements and the techniques of RI, SHRC, AI, RS, and SRH. The intensity, duration, and frequency have been modified according to physiological tolerance and learning needs.

Middle Stage

Patient Findings. The patient commonly demonstrates more return in the trunk and extremities. Synergistic movements predominate, with the strongest components noted as shoulder adduction, elbow, wrist, and finger flexion, hip adduction, hip and knee extension, plantarflexion and inversion.[10] Some movement out of synergy may be performed. Increased tone and tissue stiffness may be moderate to marked, with extensor tone typically predominating in the trunk and lower extremity and flexor tone in the upper extremity. Compared to the initial stage, the dominance of tonic reflexes usually is reduced, and righting and postural reactions are more prominent. At the beginning of this stage the patient may have difficulty assuming most postures and moving independently between postures, such as from sitting to standing and back to sitting. Although ambulation occurs at this stage the patient cannot walk with the normal timing and sequencing that characterizes skilled movement.

Impairments

▶ **Mobility:** ROM may be limited in the shoulder, wrist, hand, and ankle; there may be difficulty with initiation of movement in varying combinations.

▶ **Stability:** There may be inadequate stability of the proximal and intermediate segments; difficulty maintaining postures without a list to one side; inability to bear weight equally on both lower extremities.

▶ **Controlled mobility:** There may be difficulty with trunk rotation, eccentric muscle contractions, and postural transitions.

▶ **Skill:** There may be difficulty performing functional activities with both extremities. Perceptual deficits may interfere with ADL.

The **functional abilities** that may be anticipated at this phase of recovery include:

▶ Independent transfers to and from bed, wheelchair, mat, toilet and car;

▶ independent dressing although assistive devices may be required;

▶ ambulation approximately 40 feet on level surfaces, with supervision or assistance required on stairs.

The **treatment goals** to achieve these functions include:

▶ Maintain or gain functional ROM;

▶ improve initiation of all movements;

▶ improve stability of postural muscles within various postures;

▶ improve trunk and proximal rotational and eccentric control;

▶ improve dynamic stability within various postures.

Intervention Principles and Implications

Activities

▶ Postures are chosen that progressively increase the biomechanical challenge and enhance postural control responses by decreasing the size of

the BoS and increasing the height of the CoG, the number of joints involved, the length of the lever arm, and the effect of gravity.

▶ Voluntary control of proximal and intermediate limb segments is promoted by increasing the variety of movement combinations and recombining synergistic patterns in non–weight-bearing and weight-bearing postures.

▶ Properly directed overflow from the intact segments may enhance motor unit recruitment.

▶ Weight bearing through a joint may enhance the balance of antagonistic muscle groups and postural stability around that segment.

Based on these principles, sidelying, hooklying, bridging, sitting, modified plantigrade, and standing are the postures included at this stage of treatment (Fig. 10–21). Bilateral D1 extremity patterns are performed in both supine and sitting. In the lower extremity, mass flexion and advanced combinations are emphasized. Care must be taken when attempts are made to decrease lower-extremity extensor tone and increase flexion. Depending on the location and extent of the lesion, the patient may not regain volitional control. In such instances, extensor tone—which can be useful in supporting the limb during transfer and gait activities—may be more beneficial to the patient than a predominance of flexor tone.

Techniques

▶ Techniques are applied to maintain functional ROM, further enhance a balance of muscle tone,

Intensity / Moderate to increase strength				
Duration / Longer and more often to improve				
Frequency / Endurance and learning				
ACTIVITIES	Mobility	Stability	Controlled Mobility	Skill
SUPINE, SIDELYING; LIMB MOVEMENTS	T: HRAM		T: SRH, SR	
HOOKLYING, LOWER TRUNK ROTATION		T: AI, RS	T: SRH, SR	
BRIDGING		T: AI, RS	T: SRH, AR ➡ RC, TE	T: SRH, SR
MODIFIED PLANTIGRADE		T: AI, RS	T: SRH, SR AR	
SITTING; LIMB MOVEMENTS	T: RI, HRAM		T: SRH, SR, RC	T: AR Active Mov't
STANDING		T: AI, RS	T: SRH, SR	T: SRH, RP

Figure 10–21. Intervention model, middle stage.

initiate all combinations of movement, and promote dynamic stability.

▶ Techniques are modified according to the amount of voluntary movement and abnormal tone.

▶ Eccentric contractions and the reversal of trunk and limb antagonists with minimal time delay are required for movement within and between postures and for the performance of functional tasks.

A balance of tone and the initiation of movement are continued at this stage with RI and HRAM. SHRC, AI, and RS will further increase stability. Controlled mobility is best achieved with SRH applied through increments of range to enhance a balance of antagonists and postural responses. The combination of stability and controlled mobility techniques will promote the development of dynamic stability. The patient's CNS may better tolerate various types of sensory input at this stage in treatment. Neutral thermal stimuli, rather than heat or ice, may be used to decrease tone to avoid a rebound effect.[34] Vibration may be effective in improving the patient's ability to initiate a movement or hold a muscle contraction and may also be effective in producing reciprocal relaxation of an antagonist. However the anticipated inhibitory response may not occur in hypertonic muscles if reciprocal inhibitory mechanisms are not intact.[35]

Parameters

▶ The threshold of abnormal responses increases as neural recovery and a more normal motor unit recruitment pattern occurs.

▶ Increasing the intensity, duration, and frequency of procedures improves total body and muscular endurance as well as the learning of motor abilities.

These principles are applied by augmenting the intensity of patient effort by increasing manual, body-weight, reflexive, and mechanical resistance. Procedures are performed more frequently throughout the day, including independent practice sessions.

Selected Procedures

A: Sidelying, supine, rolling; trunk and proximal rotation, limbs in D1F, involved lower extremity in mass, progressing to advanced pattern.
T: HRAM progressing to SRH, SR.
P: Intensity within threshold of abnormal responses, increasing duration, frequency, and speed.

Upper-trunk forward rotation can be combined with scapula protraction and shoulder flexion; backward rotation can be combined with scapula retraction and shoulder extension (Fig. 10–22). Initiation of these movements in sidelying, rather than supine, reduces gravitational and tonal resistance.

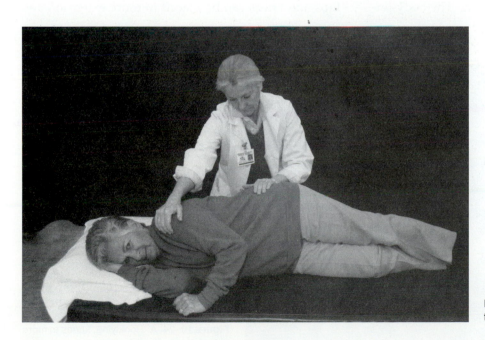

Figure 10–22. A: Sidelying; upper-trunk forward rotation; T: HRAM.

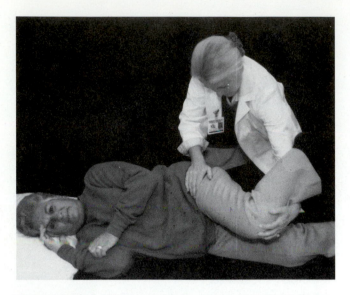

Figure 10–23. A: Sidelying; pelvic forward rotation with hip flexion; T: HRAM.

In the initial stage, pelvic rotation and hip flexion were initiated in sidelying as separate motions. Once proximal control is evident in this posture, pelvic, hip, and knee motions can be combined in preparation for the swing phase of gait.[36] In sidelying, isometric contractions can be performed in shortened and mid ranges, progressing to isotonic movement through range (Fig. 10–23). When the combined mass flexion can be initiated with HRAM, emphasis can shift to a controlled reversal of movements with SRH. Mass extension is avoided by combining hip extension with abduction and knee flexion.

Initiation of unilateral hip and knee flexion in supine is a progression from sidelying. The body-on-body contact incorporated into the trunk combinations performed during the initial stage is eliminated, and the gravitational and tonal resistance is increased. The therapist has greater control of unilateral movements and can more accurately adjust the amount of stretch and resistance than with trunk or bilateral patterns.

To achieve the goal of improved trunk rotational control, rolling can be facilitated both to the involved and uninvolved sides with or without extremity combinations. Segmental trunk motions can be performed with the technique of SRH. The smooth reversal of upper or lower trunk rotation is a prerequisite to the more advanced counterrotational movement needed during ambulation.[37]

A: Hooklying; lower-trunk rotation; knees positioned at 90° progressing to more extension.
T: AI, RS progressing to SRH, SR; MC knees progressing to ankles.

The goal of improved stability in the lower trunk and lower extremities can be enhanced in the hooklying position. The sequence may be initiated with the lower extremities in contact with each other, a trunk combination, progressing to a bilateral combination with limbs separated, then finally progressing to a unilateral pattern. To reduce the tendency toward a mass extensor motion, the hips and knees are positioned near full flexion to place the quadriceps on prolonged stretch; the foot position can be modified so that only the heel is in contact with the mat. The techniques of AI and RS can be performed with MC on the knees, then ankles. When the patient can control isometric contractions in this flexed position the hips and knees can be placed in more extension and

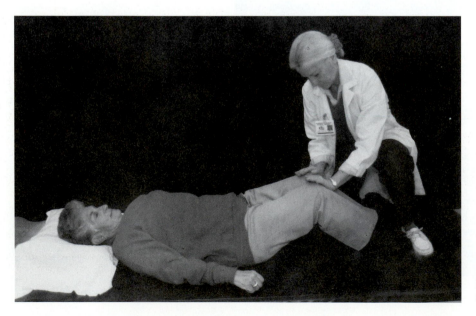

Figure 10–24. A: Hooklying, knees in more extension; T: AI.

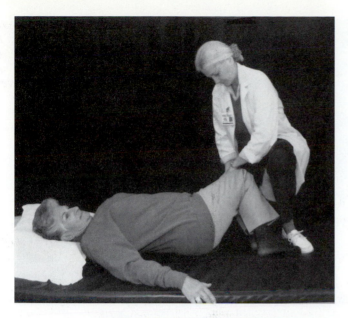

Figure 10–25. A: LTR; T: SRH.

A: Bridging; knees in increasing ranges of extension, bilateral to unilateral support.

T: AI, RS → SRH, agonistic reversals (AR) → RC, timing for emphasis (TE); MC pelvis → knees → ankles.

Many procedures can be applied in bridging to further develop dynamic stability in the lower trunk and extremities. The patient may need assistance in assuming the posture against gravity but, once attained, the posture should be able to be maintained independently. In bridging, the low-back and hip extensors contract in shortened ranges, which enhances the muscle stability needed to maintain upright postures. As with hooklying, the knees initially are positioned in flexion, then gradually extended (Fig. 10–26). The stability techniques of AI and RS with proximal or distal MC can be followed by SRH or SR to promote lateral weight shifting and rotation of the pelvis. RC or TE may be added to strengthen any weak components of the movement. The application of AR is important to promote the eccentric control of the hip extensors needed for the transition between standing and sitting, and for eccentric control of the hamstrings in preparation for terminal swing and stance. Manual contacts can be altered to promote control of various segments: on the pelvis for the trunk, on the knees for the hip, and on the ankles for the emphasis of knee musculature (Fig. 10–27). Static–dynamic activities are performed to increase body-weight resistance and simulate the weight bearing produced during the stance phase of gait. During

the techniques repeated (Fig. 10–24). As full knee extension is approached, the tendency toward an abnormal quadriceps response increases; hamstring control is required to counteract this tendency. The intensity of resistance must be increased gradually and adjusted as the difficulty of the activity and technique is increased. The resistance is first applied slowly and rhythmically and then accelerated to facilitate faster responses.

SR and SRH are used to promote the goal of improved trunk rotational control and the reversal of movement through range (Fig. 10–25). SRH also enhances stability of the hip extensors and abductors in the shortened range of the extensor phase in preparation for the stance phase of gait. Forward rotation of the pelvis on the involved side is an important aspect of the swing phase of gait and can be facilitated during movement and resistance of the knees toward the uninvolved side.

Summary. In hooklying (1) the activity progresses from a trunk pattern with the limbs together, to a bilateral pattern with the legs separated, then to a unilateral hip and knee combination; the hips and knees progress from flexion toward extension; (2) the techniques progress from AI to RS to increase stability, to SR and SRH to increase controlled mobility; MC progress from the knees to the ankles; (3) the intensity and speed are gradually increased. The purpose of these procedures is to achieve the treatment goal of improved muscle stability around the trunk, hips, and knees in increasing ranges of knee extension and to promote pelvic rotation in preparation for the functional activity of gait.

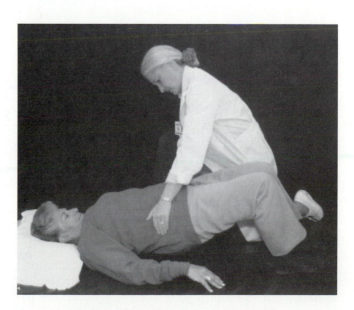

Figure 10–26. A: Bridging; T: AI; MC pelvis.

Figure 10–27. A: Bridging; T: AI; MC **(A)** knees, **(B)** ankles.

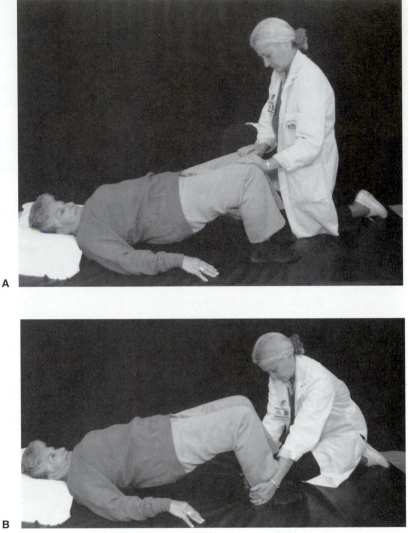

all these procedures the amount of patient effort is monitored for excessive abnormal reactions in either the upper or lower extremity. If these occur, the difficulty of the procedure may need to be decreased by altering the position of the lower extremities, the placement of MC, or the intensity of the technique. The patient may independently be able to practice maintaining the posture and abducting the hips against elastic resistance.

Summary. The procedures in bridging can be used to achieve the treatment goal of improved lower-trunk and lower-extremity dynamic stability in preparation for the functional outcome of ambulation. The difficulty of the activity can be altered by increasing knee extension and decreasing the BoS with unilateral weight bearing; the techniques can be progressed to enhance both isometric and isotonic control; the parameter of intensity can be altered by the proximal-to-distal placement of MC in conjunction with alterations in the speed and duration of resistance.

A: Modified plantigrade; weight bearing on upper extremity.
T: AI, RS progressing to SRH; MC scapula and arm.

In modified plantigrade, the goal of improved proximal dynamic stability in the upper trunk and extremity can be progressed from that initiated in sidelying and sitting. More weight bearing occurs through the upper extremity than in sitting and the proximal muscles are further challenged by the increase in the angle of shoulder flexion (Fig. 10–28). As in sitting, the hand is opened and in prolonged contact with the supporting surface, which may lead to inhibition of excessive tone in the finger flexors (S.A. Stockmeyer, unpublished notes, 1979). If the patient does not have complete distal mobility, the heel of the hand can be

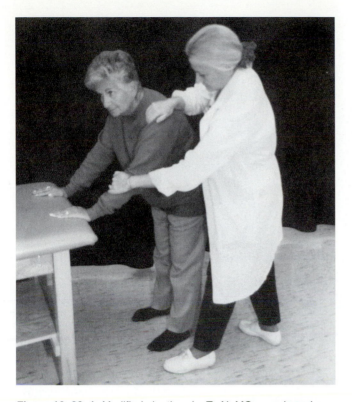

Figure 10–28. A: Modified plantigrade; T: AI; MC scapula and arm.

placed on the edge of the table. Stability techniques in the posture are followed by weight shifting, which further increases ROM, enhances proximal dynamic stability, and promotes upper-trunk and extremity postural reactions. MC can be positioned proximally to promote scapula control and can be progressed more distally as control improves. The intensity of weight-bearing resistance can be increased as the limb responses warrant.

> A: Modified plantigrade; lower extremities symmetrical or in stride.
> T: AI, RS progressing to SRH, SR, AR; MC on pelvis progressing to knee.

With less weight-bearing resistance than occurs in standing, but more than occurs in bridging, weight can be shifted onto the involved lower extremity to promote the knee and ankle dynamic stability needed during the stance phase of gait. The lower extremity is maintained in an advanced position with the hip minimally flexed, the knee extended, and the ankle dorsiflexed. The lower-extremity position can be varied, with the feet placed symmetrically or in stride with the involved limb positioned either anteriorly or posteriorly.

Knee hyperextension during procedures in the weight-bearing postures of modified plantigrade and standing may be due to: (1) increased tone in the triceps surae or stiffness in the ankle joint, leading to inability of the tibia to roll over the talus; (2) increased tone or weakness of the quadriceps, leading to a reliance on ligamentous or capsular stability; (3) decreased isometric and eccentric control of the hamstrings in lengthened ranges; or (4) diminished position sense.[10] Procedures are designed to increase ankle mobility, eccentric control of the triceps surae, improve quadriceps and hamstrings stability, and enhance lower-extremity controlled mobility. In both modified plantigrade and standing, the range at the knee should be carefully monitored and the procedures adjusted so that extension, not hyperextension, occurs. For example, rocking may be modified by slowly moving through increments of range while maintaining the proper knee alignment. Proximal stability and improved position sense can be enhanced with contacts on the pelvis or directly placed on the involved knee (Fig. 10–29).

Following the application of stability techniques, weight shifting in anterior–posterior, lateral, and rotational directions can be performed with SRH to promote several goals: during anterior weight shifting the tibia dorsiflexes over the talus while the triceps surae lengthens, promoting the ankle mobility and the eccentric control needed for the mid to late stance phase of gait; lateral shifting over the involved limb will increase the resistance of body weight and dynamic stability of that limb which can be increased even further by lifting the uninvolved limb; control of forward rotational pelvic movement practiced in lower-level postures can be emphasized with RC. Short-arc squats are performed with AR to enhance eccentric quadriceps and hamstring control. Elastic or pulley resistance with the force applied at the knee will allow independent practice of this procedure (Fig. 10–30).

The three pelvic motions performed as separate movements with the feet symmetrical can be combined into one smooth diagonal rocking motion with the involved limb positioned forward in stride to simulate the weight acceptance that occurs during stance. The combined motion incorporates forward and lateral shifting over the stance limb with forward rotation of the contralateral pelvis. The involved limb also can be positioned posteriorly to simulate the transition between late stance and swing. Stabilization of the upper trunk on the supporting surface, coupled with verbal instruction, will help to isolate movement to the lower trunk during all of these preparatory gait activities.

A: Sitting, prone, supine; lower extremity bilateral or unilateral movements.
T: AR.

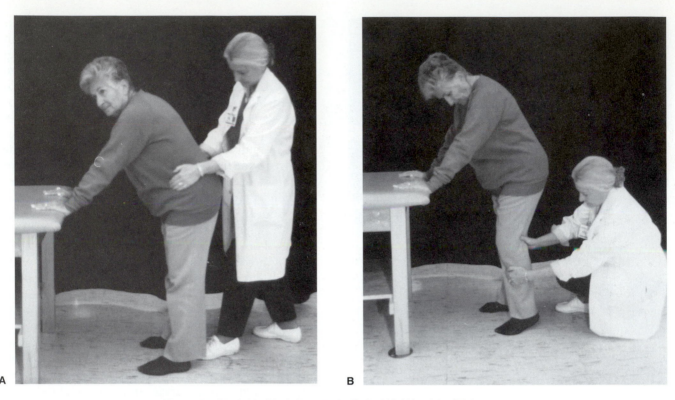

Figure 10–29. A: Modified plantigrade; T: AI; MC **(A)** pelvis, **(B)** knees.

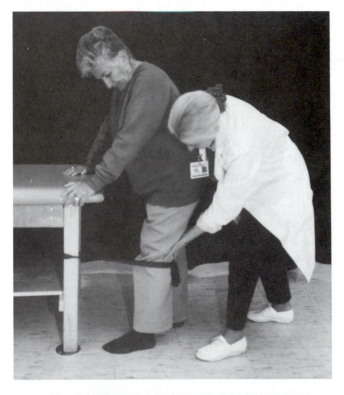

Figure 10–30. A: Modified plantigrade; short-arc squats; T: AR; elastic resistance.

Eccentric hamstring control, which is essential during the terminal swing and stance phase of gait, also can be emphasized in sitting, prone, or supine. The advantages and disadvantages of each posture need to be considered when selecting activities. In sitting, visual input can enhance the response, but because the hamstrings are more lengthened than occurs during ambulation, passive insufficiency may limit range (Fig. 10–31). In prone, the length of the muscle more closely simulates that which occurs in standing, but visual input is eliminated. In both postures, overflow from the uninvolved limb can be used to enhance the response and augment sensory input. In supine, hamstring control can be promoted unilaterally with an advanced combination of hip extension with knee flexion (Fig. 10–32). Resisted knee flexion should not be encouraged beyond 40° to 45° in this advanced pattern to emphasize functional range and to avoid muscle cramping as a result of active insufficiency. In conjunction with focusing on the specific muscle control in these postures, hamstring activity needs to be promoted in the weight-bearing postures of bridging, modified plantigrade, and standing. The proper sequencing of quadriceps and dorsiflexor activity can be initiated in an advanced combination.

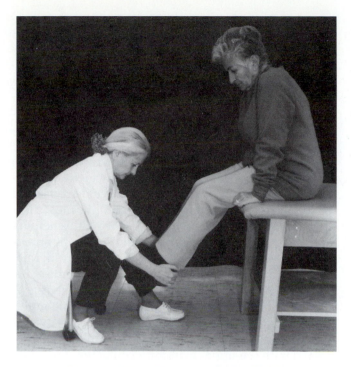

Figure 10–31. A: Sitting; knee flexion; T: AR.

A: Sitting; upper-trunk and bilateral patterns.
T: RI, HRAM progressing to SR and RC.

Upper-extremity movements can be promoted with trunk and bilateral combinations in sitting. Compared to procedures performed in supine during the initial stage, the overall challenge is greater: the CoG is raised, the BoS is decreased, and the effects of grav-ity are increased. The trunk and bilateral combinations continue to be performed to increase the sensation of movement with the involved limb moving in the D1 direction (Fig. 10–33). The bilateral movements performed in sitting promote the trunk and extremity control needed for ADL. As in other postures, RI and HRAM are applied to balance tone and initiate movement, SR is performed to promote a smooth reversal of antagonists, and RC is included to strengthen specific portions of the range.

A: Standing in parallel bars, with cane, or with upper extremities on the stall bars.
T: AI, RS progressing to SRH, SR progressing to RP; MC on various segments.
P: Tracking resistance to guide the movement.

Promoting the goal of proximal dynamic stability in the standing posture may be the most difficult because of the progression of the biomechanical factors and consequently the need for increased postural control. The sequence of procedures in standing is similar to the order described in the modified plantigrade posture. Stability techniques of AI and RS can be performed with MC on the pelvis, shoulder, on both shoulders and pelvis, or the knees to alter areas of emphasis. As in modified plantigrade, controlled mobility can be practiced with the lower extremities

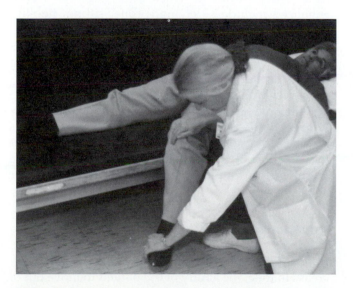

Figure 10–32. A: Supine; unilateral advanced pattern; T: RI → SR.

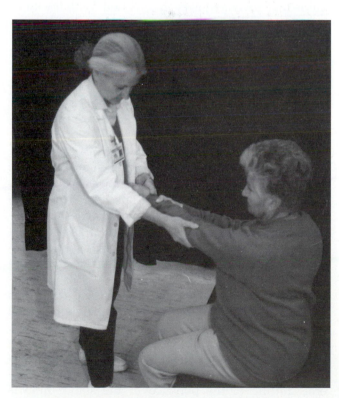

Figure 10–33. A: Sitting; D1 thrust assisted; T: RI.

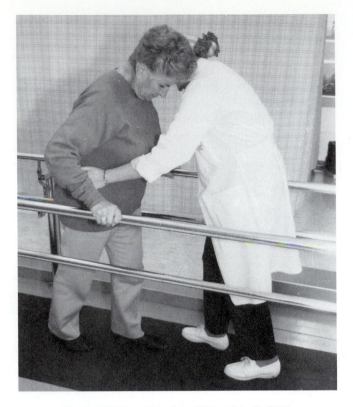

Figure 10–34. A: Standing; LE in stride; T: SRH.

movement combination of hip extension and knee flexion.[18] Sidewalking should be performed in both directions: sidewalking toward the uninvolved side requires stabilization of the pelvis and trunk by the abductors on the involved side; walking toward the involved side requires dynamic proximal control of the involved limb. The patient may attempt to substitute hiphiking or lateral trunk flexion for hip abduction during this procedure. Patients may also attempt to turn their trunk and flex and abduct their leg with the tensor fascia lata, rather than abduct with the gluteus medius. Such compensatory movements should be discouraged. Braiding is considered the most difficult activity in the gait sequence. During this activity the lower extremities cross the mid line both anteriorly and posteriorly, encompassing lower-trunk rotation and a reversal of antagonistic movements.[38] Because of the narrowed BoS, speed of movement, and combination of movement patterns, multijoint, multidirectional responses are required.

In standing, upper-extremity control can be promoted with the upper extremity contacting the parallel bars or holding onto stall bars if possible. At the stall bars the angle of the shoulder can be gradually increased (Fig. 10–36). Stability and controlled mobility of the scapula, shoulder, and elbow can be promoted by varying the techniques and the placement of MC.

in a symmetrical position with MC on the pelvis to guide the movement in each direction. With the limbs in stride the pelvic motions are combined to encourage forward and lateral weight shifting over the anterior foot and forward rotation of the contralateral pelvis (Fig. 10–34). If trunk rotational movements appear to be particularly difficult, a return to less stressful procedures in sidelying, hooklying, bridging, or modified plantigrade may be indicated to further reinforce the rotational response.

Exaggerated movements that are not part of normal gait, such as knee flexion on the stance limb, are avoided. Although slight knee flexion at heel strike is normal, excessive knee flexion may result in a more forceful hyperextension movement. By constant evaluation during all phases of gait training, the therapist will be able to assess areas of deficiency and thus determine the procedures to be emphasized during the program.

Slow, deliberate walking in different directions can be performed with MC on the pelvis to guide the proper sequencing of proximal movement (Fig. 10–35). Circumduction and mass extensor movements that reinforce synergistic patterns are discouraged. During forward walking, the forward and lateral shifting of the pelvis over the stance limb is reinforced. Walking backward requires an advanced

Summary. The procedures of the middle stage have been chosen to achieve the treatment goals of maintaining mobility–ROM, facilitating the initiation of all movements, and improving dynamic stability in the trunk and proximal extremities to attain the functional outcomes of safe, independent ambulation and ADL. The postures in which these goals have been enhanced include sidelying, prone, sitting, hooklying, bridging, modified plantigrade, and standing. Ambulation may be performed with assistive devices but may lack the components of a skilled activity (see the next section). As specific aspects of control, capacity, and learning are being developed, transfers, ambulation on flat surfaces, dressing and other functional activities are practiced. During these activities feedback is gradually withdrawn to increase the internalization of abilities. Environmental conditions are altered to improve the generalization of motor skills.

Advanced Stage

Patient Findings. This stage is characterized by a decrease in tone, the ability of the patient to move out of synergistic patterns, increased control of proximal

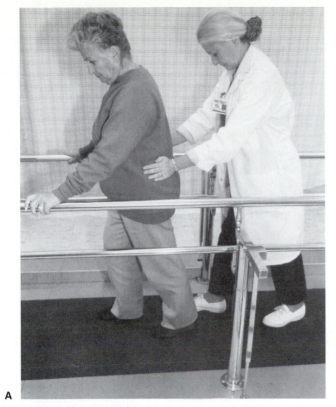

A

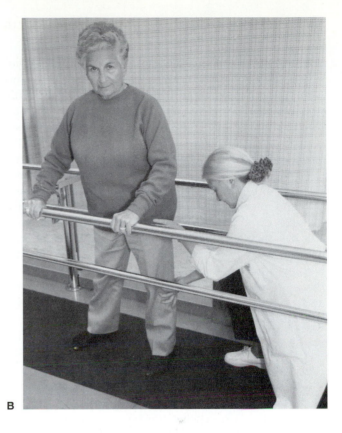

B

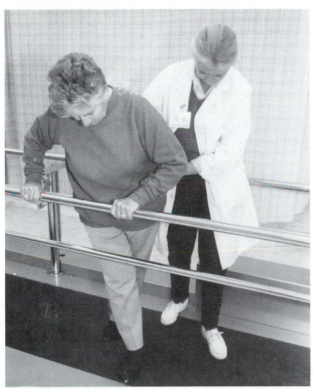

C

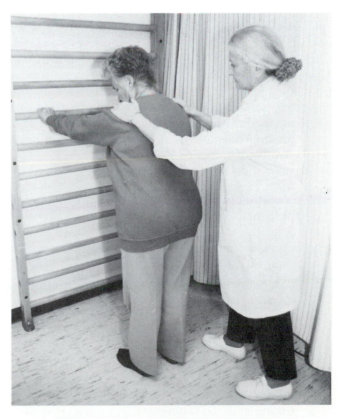

Figure 10–35. A: Walking; T: RP; **(A)** backward, **(B)** sideward, **(C)** braiding.

Figure 10–36. A: Standing at stall bars; T: AI.

dynamic stability, and reversal of antagonistic movements. Muscle imbalances in the distal segments and difficulty with movements that recombine synergistic patterns may persist. The normal timing of distal movements, eccentric control of extensors, and quick reciprocating movement may be difficult.[39] By this stage, ambulation is usually a functional activity, but abnormalities in the gait pattern are often evident. Because of the location and extent of the lesion, many patients may not be able to perform the procedures suggested for this stage of recovery. Volitional distal control, particularly fractionalization of movement, is primarily a cortical function and may be permanently lost owing to damage in the motor or sensory strip or the internal capsule.[40] The extent of motor, sensory, and perceptual return will influence the extent of independence achieved.

Impairments

▶ **Mobility:** ROM into ankle dorsiflexion may be limited if excessive tone persists in the triceps surae; initiation of wrist and finger extension and ankle eversion may be difficult.

▶ **Stability:** muscle and postural stability are deficient in the distal segments.

▶ **Controlled mobility:** inability to shift weight in all directions through full range; poor eccentric control of the lower-extremity muscles particularly in mid to lengthened ranges.

▶ **Skill:** abnormal sequencing and timing during the performance of functional activities, including gait. Decreased trunk counterrotation and delayed muscular contraction can contribute to unequal step length, decreased upper extremity swing, and slow cadence.

The functional outcomes that may be anticipated at this phase include:

▶ independent ambulation on all surfaces with a cane and AFO as needed;

▶ independent dressing and ADL with minimal compensatory strategies.

The treatment goals to achieve these outcomes include improvement of:

▶ postural and eccentric control

▶ timing of distal segments

▶ reciprocation and speed of movement

▶ strength and endurance

▶ trunk counterrotation

Treatment Principles and Implications

Activities

▶ Advanced combinations will promote a recombination of synergistic movements and promote the motions needed during many functional tasks.

▶ Skilled movement incorporates proximal dynamic stability to maintain the posture, appropriate sequencing of responses to guide the limb in space and normal timing of distal movement to manipulate the environment.

▶ Functional movement requires sufficient control and capacity to perform and sustain the response.

▶ Postural responses and skilled upper extremity movements require a distal-to-proximal sequencing of movement.

On the basis of these principles and to achieve the treatment goals, sidelying, bridging, sitting, modified plantigrade, standing, quadruped, and kneeling are the postures included in treatment (Fig. 10–37). The extremity patterns emphasize unilateral movements in both diagonal directions. Bilateral patterns may still be used to enhance overflow.

Intensity: *Increasing to funtional needs*			
Duration: *Long bouts to increase endurance*			
Frequency: *Distributed throughout the day*			
ACTIVITIES	Mobility	Stability	Controlled Mobility	Skill
SIDELYING, SUPINE				T: SRH, SR
BRIDGING; KNEES NEAR EXTENSION		T: AI, RS	T: SRH, SR, AR	T: Active Mov't
SITTING; LIMB MOVEMENTS			T: SRH, SR, AR	T: NT, AR
MODIFIED PLANTIGRADE			T: SRH, SR AR	
STANDING			T: SRH, SR AR	T: RP, NT
KNEELING, QUADRUPED		T: AI, RS	T: SRH, SR AR	

Figure 10–37. Intervention model, advanced stage.

Techniques

▶ Techniques are introduced to promote the normal timing and sequencing of movement.

▶ Proximal dynamic stability continues to be promoted by techniques to enhance stability, controlled mobility, and static–dynamic stages of control.

▶ The strength and sequence of muscle responses can be improved by facilitating motor unit recruitment with overflow from intact segments and by guiding the limb through the proper movement.

▶ As voluntary control increases, the external stimuli that may have been necessary in earlier procedures can be eliminated.

Consistent with these principles, the following techniques are used: normal timing (NT) to promote the sequencing and timing of skilled movement, resisted progression (RP) to guide the proper sequencing of ambulation, and RC and TE to strengthen specific responses.

Parameters

▶ As neural recovery continues to occur, the threshold of abnormal responses increases.

▶ The stress and difficulty of movement can be decreased by improving the body's capacity to respond.

▶ Repetitive practicing of movements and functional activities will enhance motor learning, aerobic endurance, and aid in the prevention of another CVA.[41]

These principles can be applied by: increasing the intensity of the resistive force and positioning MC more distally; increasing the duration, frequency, and intensity of many of the procedures included during the initial and middle stages of treatment and during the practice of functional activities. Total body movement capacity is improved by ambulation on a treadmill or the performance of upper or lower body ergometry. Strengthening and eccentric control can be achieved with a pulley or isokinetic program and isokinetic devices may help to improve timing of reciprocal movements.[39]

Specific Procedures

A: Sidelying, supine; trunk counterrotation: upper-trunk combination and lower-trunk rotation.
T: RI, SR.

The goal of improving trunk counterrotation may be promoted in sidelying with the technique of RI progressing to SR. Because trunk counterrotation requires coordinated sequencing of trunk movements it may need to be initially performed in the low-level postures of sidelying and supine. Slow, deliberate movements are gradually increased in speed to facilitate a smooth reversal of antagonists similar to that needed during the gait cycle. Counterrotation also can be promoted in supine by combining upper-trunk patterns with lower-trunk rotation. The addition of the limb movements may improve the coordination of arm swing during gait. The procedure in supine is more difficult than sidelying because the trunk patterns incorporate a longer lever arm and involve more joints. The emphasis on lower-trunk rotation is continued as procedures in higher-level postures are performed.

A: Bridging; increasing knee extension, unilateral weight bearing.
T: AI, RS progressing to SRH, SR, AR progressing to active movement.

The bridging activity is repeated in the advanced stage to further enhance weight acceptance and to increase the speed and reciprocation of movement needed during gait. With the knees positioned near full extension and MC at the ankles, stability and eccentric control of the hamstring can be promoted with the techniques of AI, RS and AR (Fig. 10–38). To improve the timing of muscle contraction and relaxation, the speed of altered resistive forces is gradually increased. Lateral weight shifting with the knees in more extension can be followed by static–dynamic activities in preparation for unilateral weight bearing. Alternating control is progressed by actively marching in place with increasing speed to match the cadence of gait.

A: Standing, modified plantigrade, kneeling, half-kneeling; short-arc squats, hip and knee extension.
T: AR through increments of range.

Sitting from standing and descending stairs requires eccentric control of the quadriceps and hip extensors into mid and lengthened ranges. Eccentric control in shortened to mid ranges can be performed in standing or modified plantigrade with elastic or pulley resistance as part of the patient's independent or home program. These procedures may be made more difficult by progressing to unilateral weight bearing. Eccentric control in more lengthened ranges can be enhanced with AR in the kneeling-to-heelsitting activity.

Figure 10–38. A: Bridging; knees near full extension; T: AI.

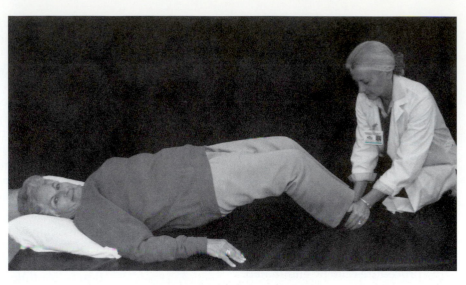

Kneeling is incorporated late in the treatment sequence because the BoS, which is positioned under and posterior to the CoG, requires postural responses in the trunk and hip extensors and knee flexors to keep the patient from falling forward. The hamstrings, which are holding in the shortened range, may have difficulty responding to postural disturbances. Although improving eccentric control of the hip and knee extensors is the primary goal, stability and weight shifting may need to precede the eccentric procedure (Fig. 10–39). Small-range flexion–extension and lateral pelvic movements can be enhanced with SRH. Because the upper trunk is not stabilized in kneeling, the patient may substitute total trunk motion for the desired isolated lower-body movement. The patient's arms can be positioned on the therapist's shoulders or one hand placed on the therapist's knee to discourage total body substitution. If isolated movement is difficult to achieve even though upper-trunk stability is provided, a return to less stressful postures is appropriate.

Moving between kneeling and half-kneeling may be the most difficult mat activity for hemiplegic patients and is practiced to assume standing from lower-level postures in case of a fall. In half-kneeling the involved limb can be positioned either anteriorly or posteriorly to enhance different aspects of control of different muscle groups. Rocking with the involved limb positioned anteriorly is performed to increase dorsiflexion: stretch of the gastrocnemius is reduced while eccentric control of the soleus is emphasized. Because the position of the involved limb is one of mass flexion, this forward position should be avoided with patients who are still demonstrating an increase in flexor tone. When the involved limb is posterior, the hip is extended and the knee flexed in an advanced combination, a position at the hip similar to the stance phase of gait. Rocking through increments of range will challenge eccentric hip and knee control (Fig. 10–40).

Ankle Control

Imbalances in ankle musculature are common in a variety of patients with musculoskeletal as well as neurological dysfunction: patients with ankle sprains may have overstretched everters and lateral ligaments; patients with ankle fractures that have been casted present with decreased mobility and disuse atrophy; patients with hemiplegia and multiple scle-

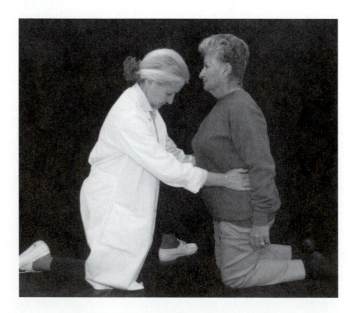

Figure 10–39. A: Kneeling; T: AI; MC pelvis.

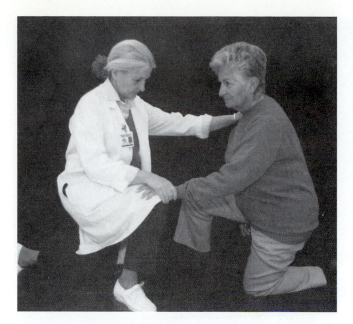

Figure 10–40. A: Half-kneeling; T: AR.

rosis demonstrate imbalances of stability, strength, and control. All these patients may exhibit some degree of proprioceptive loss. Normal timing of movement combined with balanced dorsiflexion is necessary for a skilled gait pattern. Balanced dorsiflexion can be defined as a normal synergistic action of the inverters and everters that allows flexion of the ankle to occur without a dominance of either movement.[42] Because inversion is incorporated into both the flexor and extensor pathological synergistic patterns, eversion is a very difficult movement to facilitate and therefore is emphasized during treatment of the hemiplegic patient.

The following procedures can be applied in both non–weight-bearing and weight-bearing postures to improve movement control with the functional outcome of restoring or improving ambulatory activities.

A: Sitting, supine, modified plantigrade, bridging, standing; D1, D2 movements.
T: HR, passive positioning progressing to SHRC, AI, RS progressing to SRH, AR.

Range into dorsiflexion has been promoted during all phases of treatment. Passive positioning, inhibitory casting, and splinting may be needed if abnormal tone or tissue stiffness limits range. Active and passive techniques to restore muscle and joint mobility may be applied in non–weight-bearing postures of supine or sitting. Tissue extensibility can be maintained by stretching in modified plantigrade or half-kneeling postures. Both ankle stability and controlled mobility can be promoted in supine or sitting with

manual contacts positioned on the foot and ankle (Fig. 10–41). The timing and sequencing of the distal segment can be emphasized during the performance of skilled non–weight-bearing activities. In bridging, modified plantigrade, standing, and half-kneeling techniques can be applied to promote postural stability, controlled weight shifting, and eccentric contractions if the patient has a sufficient amount of distal return. For some patients isometric contractions in the shortened range of plantar flexion can be made more difficult by increasing the weight borne through the limb and then controlling eccentric movement.

A: Supine, sitting; mass progressing to advanced limb movements.
T: SHRC, AI, RS progressing to TE, RC progressing to NT.

Eversion is most easily facilitated by application of resistance to a mass flexor pattern, which combines hip and knee flexion with dorsiflexion and eversion. Once eversion is initiated, flexion of the proximal components can be gradually reduced until the distal movements can be performed with the hip and knee in extension.[10] In conjunction with increasing the difficulty of the movement by extending the limb, the stage of control can be progressed by promoting stability in various ranges of dorsiflexion and eversion with the techniques of SHRC, AI, and RS. Of major

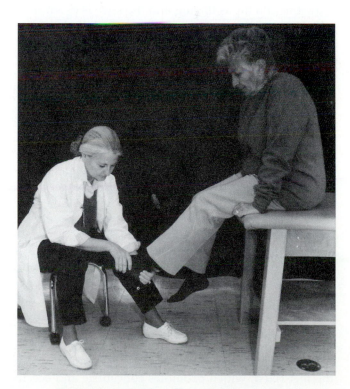

Figure 10–41. A: Sitting; T: AI; MC ankle and foot.

Figure 10–42. (A), **(B)** A: Supine; mass flexion in the lower extremity; T: TE ankle flexion.

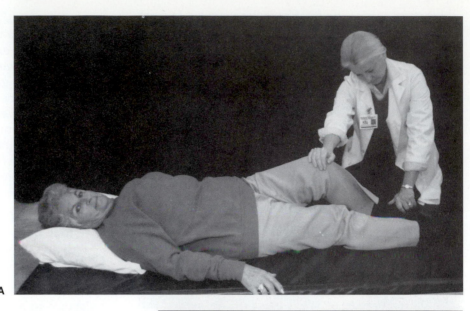

A

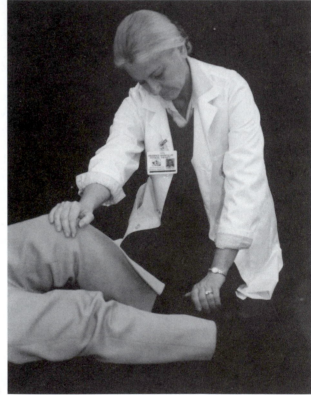

B

concern during these procedures is improvement of position sense of the ankle musculature. Verbal cues to enhance the awareness of limb position are gradually withdrawn as internal feedback improves. TE, RC, and AR can be applied to increase both concentric and eccentric control of dorsiflexion with inversion and eversion with the limb both flexed and extended (Fig. 10–42). Promoting balanced dorsiflexion while the hip is flexing and the knee is extending, an advanced combination, is the most skilled activity for the ankle and can be promoted in supine, sitting, standing, and during ambulation. The technique of NT in combination with an advanced pattern enhances the sequencing of segments needed at toe-off and during the swing phase of gait.

A: Modified plantigrade, standing, half-kneeling.
T: AR, NT.

Balanced medial–lateral ankle control between posterior tibialis and peroneal muscles is also required during the stance phase of gait and may be enhanced most effectively in weight-bearing postures, such as modified plantigrade, with techniques to promote stability and controlled mobility. To enhance proprioception, these procedures are performed first with, then without, visual feedback. Other important functions of the ankle, including eccentric control of the soleus, can be promoted in half-kneeling, modified plantigrade, and standing as previously described. To promote postural control with an ankle strategy, weight shifting can be performed in standing with the feet fixed, which promotes concentric and eccentric dorsiflexor control (Fig. 10–43). Activities on a moveable surface such as a balance board or a mini trampoline will further challenge dynamic control

by promoting faster sensori-motor responses (Fig. 10–44).

Selected Procedures: Upper Extremity

The most advanced level of control for the upper extremity is required for the performance of ADL skills. During skilled movements, the hand is free while the shoulder and scapula muscles provide the dynamic stability needed to guide the limb in space.[19] The therapist observes the patient's performance of functional activities to determine the aspects of control that need to be improved (see Chapter 5).

> A: Quadruped, standing at stall bars.
> T: AI, RS progressing to SRH.

The procedures performed at earlier phases of rehabilitation focused on the initiation of movement and an isometric and isotonic balance of antagonists in weight-bearing postures. At this more advanced phase of intervention, the goal of improving proximal dynamic stability may be further promoted in quadruped.

The quadruped position is the most difficult weight-bearing posture in which upper extremity control can be gained because of the amount of weight borne through the limb and the range in which the muscles are functioning (Fig. 10–45). In quadruped, as in modified plantigrade and sitting, triceps isometric and eccentric control can be enhanced by weight shifting onto an extended elbow, then gradually allowing the elbow to flex. Performance of static–dynamic activities will further increase the weight bearing on the involved limb. Many patients, however, may have difficulty with the amount of wrist and finger extension required to maintain this posture. For this and other reasons, such as inadequate postural responses, procedures in quadruped may produce an increase in unwanted tone. Patients for whom the position is too stressful

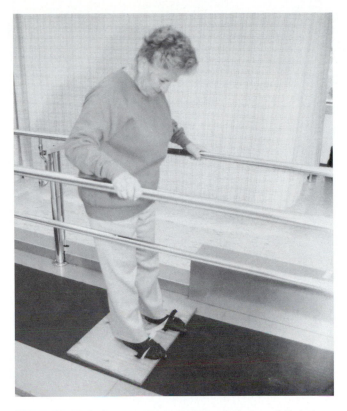

Figure 10–43. A: Standing on controlled mobility board; T: Active AR.

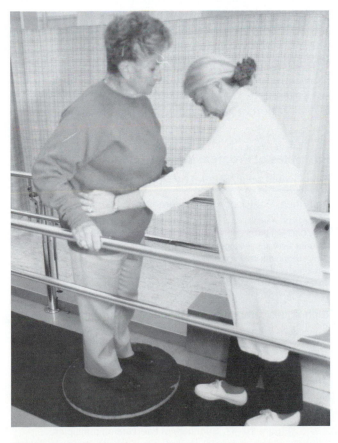

Figure 10–44. A: Standing on a balance board; T: Active movement.

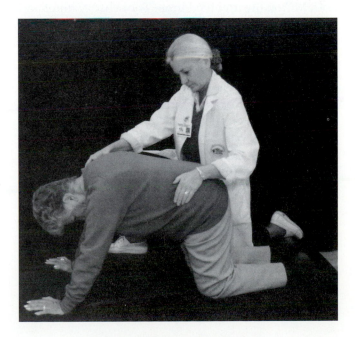

Figure 10–45. A: Quadruped; T: AI.

may find that weight bearing in previously mentioned postures, such as modified plantigrade or sitting is more appropriate. Controlled movement of the entire limb during the performance of non–weight-bearing functional activities can be overlapped with these procedures in weight-bearing postures.

> A: Supine, sitting; trunk, bilateral and unilateral upper extremity movements, in D1F progressing to D2F.
> T: SRH, SR, AR, NT.

The goal of these procedures is the normal timing and sequencing of movement needed for functional tasks. As discussed in the previous stages, movement should be initially enhanced in the D1 pattern. Because abnormal tone and synergistic movements are reduced at this advanced stage, movement into the D2 pattern can also be encouraged. In both supine and sitting, the sequencing of movements may progress from trunk combinations, during which the involved limb performs D1 and D2 flexion, to bilateral combinations that enhance both diagonal directions. During unilateral movement, D1 and D2 flexion and extension can be performed with the elbow remaining straight, flexing, or extending. The D1 thrusting pattern, which is one of the easiest movements for the patient to perform, combines shoulder flexion and adduction and encourages finger, wrist, and elbow extension. These movements recombine the dominant synergistic patterns, and, if successful, provide the patient with a greater variety of movement options (Fig. 10–46).

The finer aspects of proximal and distal control can best be promoted with unilateral patterns with both MC on the involved limb. The sensory input and overflow from the uninvolved limb is eliminated during the performance of unilateral patterns and the demand on the proximal shoulder muscles is increased.

Various techniques can be used to facilitate many aspects of control that may still be lacking: a smooth reversal of antagonists can be enhanced by SRH or SR and can be performed with increasing speed; strengthening may be best accomplished with the techniques of RC or TE; eccentric control is promoted with AR; and the normal sequencing of wrist and fingers movement can be enhanced with NT.

In this advanced stage, the goals of the procedures of treatment are: (1) initiation and control of movement in all muscles, (2) improved proximal dynamic stability and postural responses, (3) movement of distal segments with a normal timing of activity, and (4) increased speed of movement.

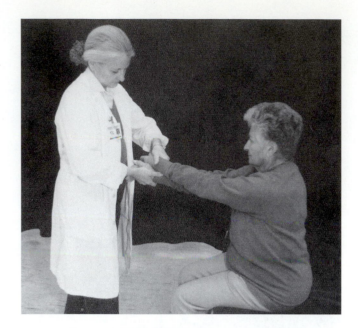

Figure 10–46. A: Sitting; BS D1 thrust; T: SRH.

► SUMMARY

All procedures are aimed at promoting the functional outcomes of ambulation, ADL, and communication. Components of the procedure can be progressed to enhance movement control and capacity (Fig. 10–47). Procedures are sequenced in order of difficulty corresponding with the patient's level of recovery. This sequencing allows the patient to achieve and practice progressively more difficult tasks and promotes internalization of goal-directed movements.

Principles of Progression ⟷ Intervention Choices

Impairment best rectified by a progression of procedures

Activities, Postures and Movements

Large BoS ➡ small Low CoG ➡ high Shorter lever arm ➡ longer Many segments involved ➡ few Proximal ➡ distal Integrating synergistic movement ➡ functional movements	Supine ➡ sitting ➡ modified plantigrade ➡ standing Trunk ➡ bilateral ➡ unilateral movements D1 ➡ D2 Hooklying ➡ bridging ➡ kneeling ➡ half-kneeling

Techniques, Stages of Movement Control

Promote the initiation of all movements Balance tone and strength Promote proximal dynamic stability Promote learning of functional tasks	RI + HRAM to initiate movement and balance tone SHRC ➡ AI + RS = isometric strength and stability SRH, SR, AR = dynamic stability NT + RP = functional movement Varying sensory inputs to alter feedback

Figure 10–47. Summary of intervention principles.

▶ **REVIEW QUESTIONS**

1. Why would you want to promote mass movements before advanced movements in the lower extremity? In which postures can each be promoted?

2. Normal timing of ankle control is needed for ambulation. Describe a sequence of procedures that can be used to promote the stages of control preliminary to the normal timing of movement.

3. How might you determine that a patient is lacking eccentric control of the lower body? Which muscle groups are involved with each functional limitation? Which procedures would you choose to improve control?

4. What sequence of procedures would best promote functional movement without reinforcing abnormal movement of the upper extremity?

5. In standing, the patient demonstrates marked increase in lower-extremity tone and an associated reaction of the upper extremity during attempts to increase unilateral weight bearing. How might you alter the components of this procedure to avoid these unwanted responses?

REFERENCES

1. Caronna JJ. Coma in ischemic cerebral vascular disease. In Russell RWR, ed: *Vascular Disease of the Central Nervous System*. 2nd ed. New York, NY: Churchill Livingstone, 1983.

2. Salmoni AW, Schmidt RA, Walter CB. Knowledge of results and motor learning: a review and critical appraisal. *Psycho Bull*. 1984;95:355–386.

3. Guccione AA. *Geriatric Physical Therapy*. St. Louis, Mo, CV Mosby Co, 1993.

4. Brooks CM, Koizumi K, Sato AY, eds. *Integrative Functions of the Autonomic Nervous System*. Amsterdam, Elsevier, North-Holland Biomedical Press, 1979.

5. Irwin S, Tecklin J. *Cardiopulmonary Physical Therapy*. 2nd ed. St. Louis, Mo, CV Mosby Co; 1990:515–516.

6. Cohen M, Hoskins MT. *Cardiopulmonary Symptoms in Physical Therapy Practice*. New York, NY: Churchill Livingstone, 1988.

7. Scott AD. Evaluation and treatment of sensation. In: Trombley CA, ed. *Occupational Therapy for Physical Dysfunction*. 2nd ed. Baltimore, Md: Williams and Wilkins, 1983.

8. Cloning K, Hoff H. Cerebral localization of disorders of higher nervous activity. In: Vinken PJ, Bruyn GW, eds. *Handbook of Clinical Neurology*. New York, NY: American Elsevier Publishing Co, Inc., Vol 3, 1969.

9. Carey JR, Burghardt TP. Movement dysfunction following central nervous system lesions: a problem of neuromuscular or muscle impairment. *Phys Ther*. 1993; 73:538–547.

10. Brunnstrom S. *Movement Therapy in Hemiplegia*. New York, NY: Harper & Row Publishers Inc; 1970.

11. Katz RT, Rymer WZ. Spastic hypertonia: mechanisms and measurements. *Arch Phys Med Rehabil*. 1989;70:144.

12. McComas AJ, Sica RE, Upton AR, et al: Functional changes in motoneurons of hemiplegic patients. *J Neurol Neurosurg Psychiatry*. 1973;36:183–193.

13. Badke MB, Difabio RP. Balance deficits in patients with hemiplegia; considerations for assessment and treatment. In: Duncan PW, ed. *Balance Proceedings of APTA Forum*. Alexandria, Va: American Physical Therapy Association; 1990.

14. Marcus R, Drinkwater B, Dalsky A, et al. Osteoporosis and exercise in women. *Med Sci Sports Exerc*. 1992;24(6 suppl):S301–S307.

15. Taub E, Berman AJ. Movement and learning in the absence of sensory feedback. In: Freedman SJ, ed: *The Neuropsychology of Spatially Oriented Behavior*. Homewood, Ill: Dorsey Press, 1968.

16. Winstein CJ: Motor learning considerations in stroke rehabilitation. In: Duncan PW, Badke MB, eds: *Stroke Rehabilitation*. Chicago, Ill: Year Book Medical Publishers, 1987.

17. Rose DK, Guiliani CA, Light KE: The immediate effects of isokinetic exercise on temporal-distance characteristics of self-selected and fast hemiplegic gait. *Proceedings of the Forum on Physical Therapy Issues Related to Cerebral Vascular Accident*. Alexandria, Va, American Physical Therapy Association, 1992.

18. Bobath B. *Adult Hemiplegia: Evaluation and Treatment*. London, England: William Heinemann Medical Books Ltd, 1978.

19. Stockmeyer SA: An interpretation of the approach of Rood to the treatment of neuromuscular dysfunction. *Am J Phys Med*. 1966;46:900–956.

20. Brodal A. Self-observations and neuroanatomical considerations after a stroke. *Brain*. 1973;96:675–694.

21. Haas A, Rusk HA, Pelosof H, et al: Respiratory function in hemiplegic patients. *Arch Phys Med Rehabil*. 1967; 48:174–179.

22. Frownfelter D: Breathing exercise and retraining—chest mobilization exercises. In: Frownfelter D, ed: *Chest Physical Therapy and Pulmonary Rehabilitation*. 2nd ed. Chicago, Ill: Yearbook Medical Publishers, Inc, 1987.

23. Zimmerman JE, Oder LA. *Swallowing Dysfunction in the Acutely Ill Patient*. Read at the Midwinter Section Meeting of the American Physical Therapy Association; 1980; New Orleans, La.

24. Kendall FP, McCreary EK, Provance PG: *Muscles-Testing and Function*, 4th ed. Baltimore, Md: Williams and Wilkins, 1993.

25. Logeman J. *Evaluation and Treatment of Swallowing Disorders.* San Diego, Calif: College-Hill Press, 1983.

26. Shahani B. The human blink reflex. *J Neurol Neurosurg Psychiatry.* 1970;33:792–800.

27. Young RP. The clinical significance of exteroceptive reflexes. In: Desmedt JE, ed. *New Developments in Electromyography and Clinical Neurophysiology.* Basel, Switzerland: Karger, 1973:3.

28. Bowman JP. *The Muscle Spindle and Neural Control of the Tongue.* Springfield, Ill: Charles C Thomas Publisher, 1971.

29. Knott M, Voss DE. *Proprioceptive Neuromuscular Facilitation.* 2nd ed. New York, NY: Harper & Row Publishers Inc, 1968.

30. Adkins HV, Winstein C. *Swallowing Dysfunction: Assessment and Management.* Read at the Annual Conference of the American Physical Therapy Association; June, 1980, Phoenix, Ariz.

31. Schultz AR, Niemtzow P, Jacobs SR, et al. Dysphagia associated with cricopharyngeal dysfunction. *Arch Phys Med Rehabil.* 1979;60:381–382.

32. Mueller HA. Facilitating feeding and speech. In: Pearson PH, Williams DE, eds. *Physical Therapy Services in the Developmental Disabilities.* Springfield, Ill: Charles C Thomas, 1972.

33. Konecky C. *An EM Study of Abdominals and Back Extensors During Lower-Trunk Rotation.* Boston, Mass: Boston University, Sargent College of Allied Health Professions; 1980. Thesis.

34. Rood M. The rise of sensory receptors to activate, facilitate and inhibit motor response, autonomic and somatic, in developmental sequence. In: Sattely C, ed. *Approaches to the Treatment of Patients with Neuromuscular Dysfunction.* Dubuque, Iowa: Wm C Brown, 1962.

35. Bishop B. Spasticity: its physiology and management. *Phys Ther.* 1977;57:385–395.

36. Lehman JF: Gait analysis: diagnosis and management. In: Kottke FJ, Stillwell GK, Lehmann, JF, eds. *Krusen's Handbook of Physical Medicine and Rehabilitation.* 3rd ed. Philadelphia, Pa: WB Saunders, 1982.

37. Trueblood PR, Walker JM, Perry J, et al: Pelvic exercise and gait in hemiplegia. *Phys Ther.* 1989;69:18–26.

38. Voss DE, Ionta MK, Myers BJ. *Proprioceptive Neuromuscular Facilitation Patterns and Techniques.* 3rd ed. Philadelphia, Pa: Harper & Row, Publishers, 1985.

39. Watkins MP, Harris BA, Koslowski BA: Isokinetic testing in patients with hemiparesis. *Phys Ther.* 1984;64:184–189.

40. Lawrence D. *Anatomical Localization of Descending Pathways and Their Contributions to Motor Control.* Harvard University Conference on Motor Control; Oct 7 1980; Sponsored by Harvard Medical School, Boston, Mass.

41. Hillegass EA, Sadowski HS. The well individual. In: *Essentials of Cardiopulmonary Physical Therapy.* Philadelphia, Pa: WB Saunders, 1994.

42. Rood M. *Treatment of Neuromuscular Dysfunction: Rood Approach.* Read at Conference on Neurological Dysfunction Sponsored by Massachusetts Chapter American Physical Therapy Association; June, 1976; Boston, Mass.

Glossary of Terms

REFLEXES AND REACTIONS

Tonic Neck Reflexes. Mediated by proprioceptors in the proximal cervical area.

Asymmetrical Tonic Neck Reflex (ATNR). A change in muscle tone of the extremities as a result of head rotation. When the head is turned to one side, extensor tone increases in the extremities on the chin side and flexor tone increases on the skull side.

Symmetrical Tonic Neck Reflex (STNR). Head flexion produces an increase in flexor tone in the upper extremities and extensor tone in the lower extremities; extension produces an increase in extensor tone in the upper extremities and flexor tone in the lower extremities.

Labyrinthine Reflexes. Mediated by the vestibular system.

Symmetrical Tonic Labyrinthine Reflex (STLR). Extension in supine produces an increase in extensor tone in all four extremities. Flexion in prone produces a decrease in extensor tone or an increase in flexor tone.

Asymmetrical Tonic Labyrinthine Reflex (ATLR). Side-lying produces an increase in flexor tone of the uppermost extremities and an increase in extensor tone of the lowermost extremities that are in contact with the supporting surface.

Righting Reactions. Orienting movements of the head, neck, and body to maintain the eyes horizontal, head vertical, and the body in proper relationship to the head. Stimulus may be optical, labyrinthine, proprioceptive, or tactile. Optical, labyrinthine, and body-on-head reactions orient the head and body in the coronal and sagittal planes. Neck and body-on-body righting reactions orient the head and body in the transverse plane.

Postural Control. Movements that attempt to maintain the center of gravity (CoG) within the base of support (BoS). Reactions are in response to input from vestibular, ocular, proprioceptive, and tactile receptors.

AUTONOMIC NERVOUS SYSTEM (ANS)

Autonomic Nervous System. Primarily a motor system that innervates smooth muscle and glands throughout the body. Autonomic control of blood sugar and blood supply can affect skeletal muscle responses.

Sympathetic Division. That portion of the ANS that gives rise to generalized responses, which include acceleration of heart rate and force of heartbeat, increased production by sweat glands, vasoconstriction of cutaneous and visceral blood vessels, and stimulation of adrenal glands. Sympathetic responses are greatest during stress situations. Increased sympathetic stimulation results in a high level of anxiety and a low threshold of pain and may produce an increase in muscle activity.

Parasympathetic Division. That portion of the ANS that gives rise to localized responses assigned to conserve and restore energy sources of the body. Parasympathetic stimulation is associated with a decreased level of anxiety and an increased threshold of pain. The interaction of the sympathetic and parasympathetic divisions results in the regulation of the body in such a way that homeostasis results.

Homeostasis. Coordination of the sympathetic and parasympathetic divisions of the ANS, resulting in a balance of excitatory and inhibitory responses and a consistency in the internal environment.

MUSCLE TERMINOLOGY

Muscles can be classified according to anatomical, physiological, and metabolic characteristics. Few muscles can be categorized as pure flexors or extensors because of the varying degrees in physiological and metabolic compositions. However, in this text flexor and extensor muscles are defined as follows:

Extensor–Tonic–Postural

▶ Located proximally—usually cross one joint—broad attachments.

▶ Composed primarily of small, slow-twitch, type I motor units that are resistant to fatigue. Type I motor units have a low threshold to stimuli.

▶ Low glycogen content with an abundance of oxidative enzymes.

▶ Best suited for performance of sustained contractions.

Flexor–Phasic

▶ Located superficially—usually cross two joints—long tendinous attachments.

▶ Composed primarily of large, fast-twitch, type II motor units that fatigue easily. Type II and IIA motor units have a higher threshold to stimuli than type I.

▶ High glycogen content with few oxidative enzymes.

▶ Best suited for performance of brief, forceful contractions.

Normal Recruitment Order. Activation of type I motor units before type II.

Proprioceptor. A receptor that is located deep within the tissues of the body (for example muscles, tendons, joints, inner ear) and that responds to changes in position, movement, or deep pressure.

Muscle Spindle. A proprioceptor located in skeletal muscle parallel to the extrafusal fibers (Fig. I). The main purpose of the muscle spindle is to provide information regarding muscle length to the CNS.

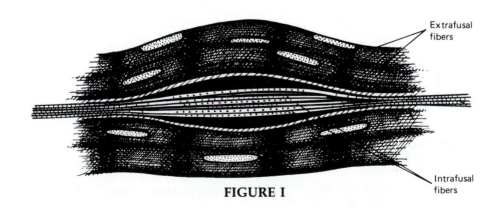

Extrafusal fibers

Intrafusal fibers

FIGURE I

Intrafusal Fibers. Muscle fibers located within the muscle spindle. Two main types exist: bag and chain (Fig. II). Both dynamic and static bag fibers have been identified.

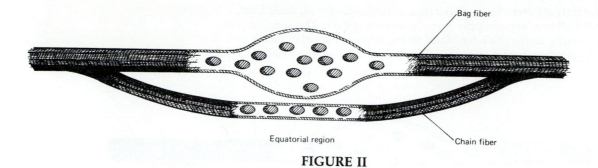

FIGURE II

Ia or Primary Afferent Fiber. A large nerve fiber that forms part of the afferent nerve
supply from the muscle spindle. The fiber receptor is located in the equatorial or
middle regions of both bag and chain fibers (Fig. III). Excitation of the Ia receptors

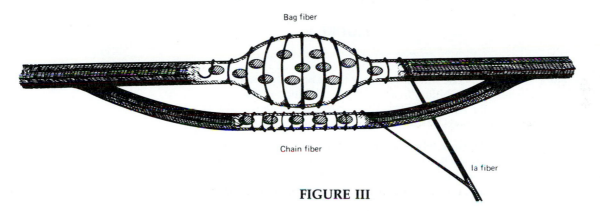

FIGURE III

by quick or maintained stretch results in autogenic facilitation (facilitation to
homonym and synergists) and reciprocal inhibition to antagonistic muscle groups
(Fig. IV). Small changes in movement, as well as rates of change or movement, are

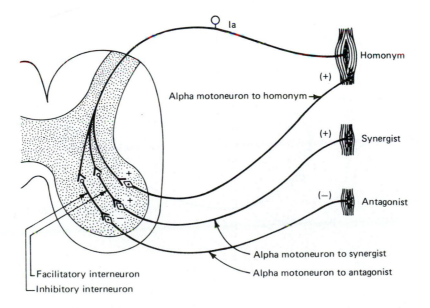

FIGURE IV

monitored by the Ia receptors on the dynamic bag fiber. More static states such as
maintained muscle stretch appear to be monitored by the Ia receptors on the static
bag and chain fibers.

II or Secondary Afferent Fiber. A nerve fiber that, in conjunction with the Ia fiber, makes up the afferent nerve supply from the muscle spindle. The fiber receptor, which is primarily on the chain intrafusal fibers, is located at either end of the equatorial region but is more laterally situated than the Ia receptor (Fig. V). Excita-

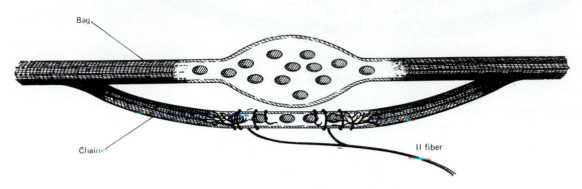

FIGURE V

tion of this receptor yields a response similar to that of the Ia fiber, that is, autogenic facilitation and reciprocal inhibition. In an extensor, inhibition to the homonym and facilitation to the antagonist may also occur. The II fiber receptor is highly sensitive to slow, maintained stretches in lengthened muscle ranges.

Fusimotor Fibers or Gamma Motoneurons. Nerve fibers that form the efferent or motor supply to the muscle spindle. The cell bodies of the gamma motoneurons are located in the ventral horn of the spinal cord, in close proximity to the cell bodies of the alpha motoneurons, and are under the influence of higher centers (Fig. VI).

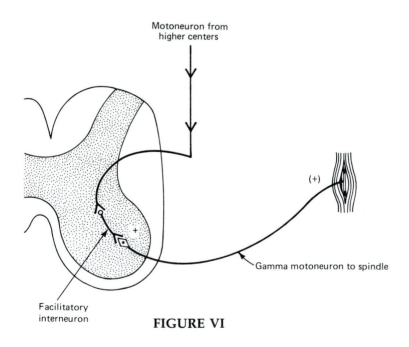

FIGURE VI

Dynamic Gamma Motoneurons. Motoneurons that innervate the polar or contractile regions, primarily of the dynamic nuclear bag fiber (Fig. VII). They are associated with increases of the dynamic response of the Ia fiber during changes in muscle length.

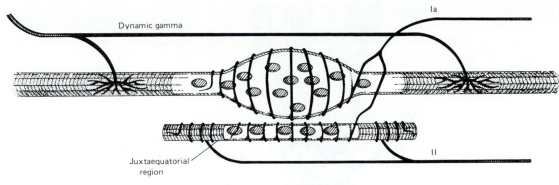

FIGURE VII

Static Gamma Motoneurons. Motoneurons that innervate the juxta- or quasiequatorial regions of both the static nuclear bag and the chain intrafusal fibers in close proximity to the receptors of the II fibers (Fig. VIII). They are associated with biasing or internally stretching the bag and the chain fibers, which keep the sensory endings responsive to change in muscle length.

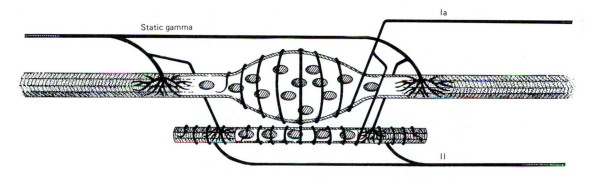

FIGURE VIII

Internal Stretch or Gamma Bias. The active contraction (stretch) of the intrafusal muscle fibers by the static gamma system. Excitation of the static gamma system keeps the spindle fibers taut or "loaded" and thereby responsive to externally applied muscle stretch. Internal stretch supports coactivation of alpha–gamma motor neurons. (See **Coactivation**.)

Slack or "Unloaded" Muscle Spindle. The passive shortening of the muscle spindle as a result of either extrafusal contraction or of positioning a muscle in shortened ranges. Because of the shortening, the tension on the spindle receptors decreases and consequently the spindle afferent excitation diminishes.

External Stretch. Stretch of both the extrafusal and intrafusal fibers by an outside force, for example, quick stretch applied in the lengthened range of a muscle or a pattern of movement. The application of external stretch may help to initiate a muscle contraction, but this contraction cannot be sustained unless internal stretch or maintained gamma efferent activity is present.

Golgi Tendon Organs (GTO). Proprioceptors that are located primarily at musculotendinous junctions in series with the muscle fibers (Fig. IX). These receptors are extremely sensitive to muscle tension, particularly when the tension is produced by an active muscle contraction. The response produced by GTO excitation is autogenic inhibition to the homonym and synergists and reciprocal facilitation to antagonistic muscle groups (Fig. X). The effects of GTOs are greater in tonic than in phasic muscles.

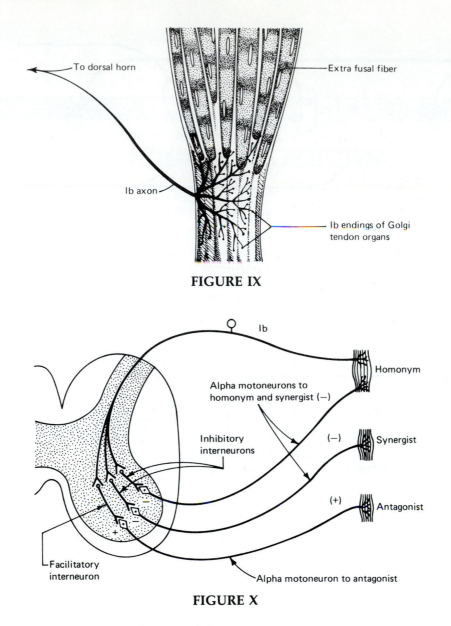

FIGURE IX

FIGURE X

Ib Fiber. The nerve fiber that forms the afferent nerve supply from the GTO. Unlike the muscle spindles, GTOs do not have efferent innervation.

Renshaw Interneuron. An interneuron that forms part of an inhibitory feedback circuit between the motoneurons to the homonym and their cell bodies in the anterior horn of the spinal cord. Renshaw cells also exert an inhibitory influence on the inhibitory interneuron that forms part of the final common pathway to the antagonistic musculature; the result of this disinhibition may be equivalent to facilitation of the antagonistic muscle groups (Fig. XI). Renshaw cells can be affected by impulses from higher centers. The effects of Renshaw cells are greater in tonic than in phasic muscles.

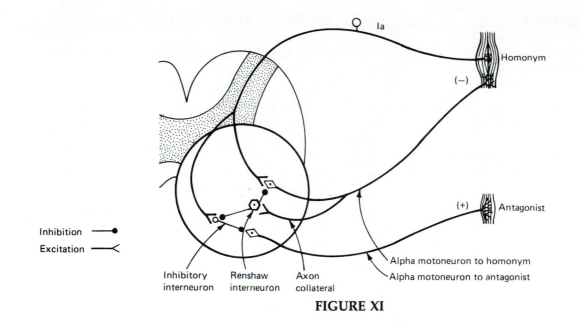

Inhibition —————●
Excitation —————≺

Inhibitory interneuron   Renshaw interneuron   Axon collateral

Homonym
(−)
(+) Antagonist

Ia

Alpha motoneuron to homonym
Alpha motoneuron to antagonist

FIGURE XI

Coactivation. The simultaneous activation of alpha and gamma motoneurons from higher centers for purposes of initiating or perpetuating muscle contractions.

Facilitation. Lowering the thresholds at synapses of motoneuron pools. Facilitation is not synonymous with activation or the actual firing of motor units.

Adaptation. A decline in the discharge frequency of a sensory receptor after the onset of stimulation. The mechanism of adaptation is not known and may differ for various sensory organs. Receptors such as pacinian corpuscles are said to adapt rapidly, whereas others, such as muscle spindle receptors, adapt slowly.

STAGES OF CONTROL _____

Mobility. The presence of a functional range of motion through which to move and the ability to initiate and sustain active movement through range.

Stability. The ability of both proximal and distal muscle groups to stabilize joints in both non–weight-bearing and weight-bearing postures.

Controlled Mobility. Weight shifting or movement in weight-bearing postures and rotation around the longitudinal axis.

Skill. Consistency in performing functional tasks with economy of effort. The upper limbs move freely in space (open chain) to perform ADL including occupational and recreational activities; the lower limbs combine and coordinate non–weight-bearing (open-chain) and weight-bearing (closed-chain) movements for functional ambulation.

Proximal Dynamic Stability. The ability of trunk and proximal segments to provide sufficient support during the performance of functional activities. The term indicates the presence of appropriate sequencing and timing of muscle contractions within and between segments to allow for coordinated movements. Attainment of dynamic stability begins with techniques to improve stability and improves as the patient moves through the controlled mobility, static–dynamic, and skill levels of control.

INTERVENTION TERMINOLOGY _____

Impairment. An alteration in anatomical or physiological structures or functions that may contribute to functional limitations.

Functional Limitation. A deficit in the ability to ambulate and perform activities of daily living (ADL), communication, and occupational and recreational activities.

Treatment Goals. Anticipated improvements in impairments and ways to prevent further dysfunction or maintain or improve existing function.

Functional Outcomes. Projections of the patient's ability to ambulate, communicate, and perform ADL and occupational and recreational tasks.

Procedure. A comprehensive term that includes all components of a specific exercise, that is, the activity, the technique, and the parameters of movement.

Activity. Any posture and the movements occurring within that posture.

Technique. Various types of muscle contractions and sensory inputs used to promote the stages of control.

Parameters of Movement. Intensity, duration, and frequency of exercise.

EXERCISE TERMINOLOGY _____

Direct Approach. The application of exercise techniques to an affected area.

Indirect Approach. The application of exercise techniques to an uninvolved area to gain overflow excitation or relaxation effects in an affected part. An indirect approach is appropriately used when the patient's involved limbs are either immobilized, weak, or painful.

Tracking. The tendency of a part to move in the direction of the sensory stimulus provided by a manual contact.

Mass Pattern. The proximal, intermediate, and distal joints of the lower extremity are simultaneously flexed or extended.

Advanced Pattern. The proximal and distal joints of the lower extremity are flexed or extended while the intermediate joint simultaneously performs the opposite movement.

Diagonal 1 Flexion Upper Extremity (D1F UE). Scapula elevation, abduction, upward rotation; combining movements of flexion, adduction, and external rotation occurring at the shoulder; elbow may move in flexion or extension or may remain extended throughout the movement pattern; wrist and fingers flex and deviate to the radial side and the thumb adducts.

Diagonal 1 Extension Upper Extremity (D1E UE). Scapula depression, adduction, and downward rotation; combining movements of extension, abduction, and internal rotation occurring at the shoulder; elbow may move in flexion or extension or may remain extended throughout the movement pattern; wrist and fingers extend and deviate to the ulnar side and the thumb abducts.

Diagonal 2 Flexion Upper Extremity (D2F UE). Scapula elevation, adduction, and upward rotation; combining movements of flexion, abduction, and external rotation occurring at the shoulder; elbow may move into flexion or extension or may remain extended throughout the movement pattern; wrist and fingers extend and deviate to the radial side and the thumb extends.

Diagonal 2 Extension Upper Extremity (D2E UE). Scapula depression, abduction, and downward rotation; combining movements of extension, adduction, and internal rotation occurring at the shoulder; elbow may move in flexion or extension or may remain extended throughout the movement pattern; wrist and fingers flex and deviate to the ulnar side and the thumb opposes the fingers.

Diagonal 1 Flexion Lower Extremity (D1F LE). Pelvic protraction; combining movements of flexion, adduction, and external rotation occurring at the hip; knee may move in flexion or extension or may remain extended throughout the movement pattern; ankles and toes dorsiflex and invert.

Diagonal 1 Extension Lower Extremity (D1E LE). Pelvic retraction; combining movements of extension, abduction, and internal rotation occurring at the hip; knee may move into flexion or extension or may remain extended throughout the movement pattern; ankles and toes plantar flex and evert.

Diagonal 2 Flexion Lower Extremity (D2F LE). Pelvic elevation; combining movements of flexion, abduction, and internal rotation occurring at the hip; knee may move into flexion or extension or may remain extended throughout the movement pattern; ankle and toes dorsiflex and evert.

Diagonal 2 Extension Lower Extremity (D2E LE). Pelvic depression; combining movements of extension, adduction, and external rotation occurring at the hip; knee may move into flexion or extension or may remain extended throughout the movement pattern; ankle and toes plantarflex and invert.

Bilateral Symmetrical Patterns (BS). The bilateral performance of one diagonal pattern (D1 or D2) by either both upper or both lower extremities. Movement of both extremities occurs simultaneously in the same direction—that is, both limbs flex or extend together.

Reciprocal Symmetrical Patterns or Bilateral Reciprocal (BR). The reciprocal performance of one diagonal pattern (D1 or D2) by either both upper or both lower extremities. Movement of both extremities occurs in different directions—that is, one limb flexes while the other extends in the same diagonal pattern.

Bilateral Asymmetrical Patterns (BA). The bilateral performance of the two diagonal patterns (D1 and D2) by either both upper or both lower extremities. Movement of both extremities occurs simultaneously in the same direction—that is, both limbs flex or extend together.

Reciprocal Asymmetrical or Crossed Diagonal Patterns (RA, CD). The reciprocal performance of the two diagonal patterns (D1 and D2) by either both upper or both lower extremities. Movement of both extremities occurs simultaneously in different directions—that is, one limb flexes in D1 while the other extends in D2.

Upper Trunk Flexor Pattern (UTF) (chop). An upper-trunk flexion pattern combines bilateral asymmetrical extensor patterns of the upper extremities—for example, D1 extension of the right upper extremity and D2 extension of the left upper extremity.

Upper Trunk Extensor Pattern (UTE) (lift). An upper-trunk extension pattern that combines bilateral asymmetrical flexor patterns of the upper extremities—for example, D2 flexion of the right upper extremity and D1 flexion of the left upper extremity.

Lower Trunk Flexion (LTF). A lower-trunk flexor pattern combines bilateral asymmetrical flexor patterns of the lower extremities—for example, lower trunk flexion to the right combines D2 flexion of the right lower extremity and D1 flexion of the left lower extremity.

Lower Trunk Extension (LTE). A lower-trunk extensor pattern combines bilateral asymmetrical extensor patterns of the lower extremities—for example, lower trunk extension to the right combines D1 extension of the right lower extremity and D2 extension of the left lower extremity.

Lower Trunk Rotation (LTR). A rotary pattern of movement of the lower trunk, performed in hooklying, that combines bilateral asymmetrical flexor patterns of the lower extremities from zero° to 90° of the movement pattern and bilateral asymmetrical extensor patterns from 90° to 180° of the movement pattern.

Trunk patterns may be easier for a patient to perform than bilateral patterns because of the contact between both sides of the body.

Braiding. The combination of all four lower-extremity and diagonal patterns performed in a side-to-side walking sequence.

JOINT TERMINOLOGY

Osteokinematic Movement. The bone motion occurring in a plane of movement, for example, shoulder flexion.

Athrokinematic Movement. The specific joint movements that occur during an osteokinematic movement. Depending on the joint and the degrees of freedom, a roll, glide, or spin may occur.

End Feel. The amount of resistance encountered when overpressure is applied at the end of the physiological range of motion. Each joint has a characteristic end feel that is physiologically normal for that movement and that depends on the soft tissue and bony anatomy of the joint. With abnormalities, the end feel may vary.

Joint Receptors. Sensory receptors located within the joint capsule and surrounding tissues. Although all of the functions of joint receptors have not been clarified, they appear to contribute to kinesthesia pain and the reflex support of movement. (Refer to Wyke in Bibliography for classification of joint receptors.)

Approximation. Compression of joint surfaces used to produce or enhance a sustained muscle response.

Traction. Separation of joint surfaces used to produce or enhance a phasic or dynamic muscle response.

► ABBREVIATIONS OF TERMS

The following terms are listed in alphabetical order.

ADL	activities of daily living
AI	alternating isometrics
ANS	autonomic nervous system
AR	agonistic reversals
ATLR	asymmetrical tonic labyrinthine reflex
ATNR	asymmetrical tonic neck reflex
BA	bilateral asymmetrical
BR	bilateral reciprocal
BS	bilateral symmetrical
BoS	base of support
CD	cross diagonal
CoG	center of gravity
CNS	central nervous system
CR	contract relax
CVA	cerebral vascular accident
CVP	cardiovascular–pulmonary
D1E	diagonal 1 extension
D1F	diagonal 1 flexion
D2E	diagonal 2 extension
D2F	diagonal 2 flexion
GTOs	Golgi tendon organs
HR	hold relax
HRAM	hold relax active motion
LE	lower extremity
LTE	lower trunk extension
LTF	lower trunk flexion
LTR	lower trunk rotation
MC	manual contacts
MMT	manual muscle test
MS	musculoskeletal
NS	nervous system
NT	normal timing
RC	repeated contractions
RI	rhythmic initiation
ROM	range of motion
RP	resisted progression
RR	rhythmical rotation
RS	rhythmic stabilization
SCI	spinal cord injury
SHRC	shortened held resisted contraction
SLR	straight leg raise
SR	slow reversal
SRH	slow reversal hold
SRH ↑↓ RANGE	slow reversal hold through increments or decrements of range
STLR	symmetrical tonic labyrinthine reflex
STNR	symmetrical tonic neck reflex
TE	timing for emphasis
UE	upper extremity
UBE	upper body ergometry
UTE	upper trunk extension
UTF	upper trunk flexion

Bibliography

Astrand PO, Rodahl K. *Textbook of Work Physiology.* New York, NY: McGraw-Hill Book Co; 1986.

Balance Proceedings of the APTA Forum. Alexandria, Va: American Physical Therapy Association, 1990.

Barnes MR, Crutchfield CA, Heriza CB, et al. *Reflex and Vestibular Aspects of Motor Control, Motor Development and Motor Learning.* Atlanta, Ga: Stokesville Publishing; 1990.

Bobath B. *Adult Hemiplegia: Evaluation and Treatment.* 3rd ed. London, England: Butterworth and Heinemann; 1990.

Bogduk N, Twomey LT. *Clinical Anatomy of the Lumbar Spine.* Melbourne, Australia: Churchill Livingstone; 1987.

Boissonault WG. *Examination in Physical Therapy Practice: Screening for Medical Disease.* New York, NY: Churchill Livingstone; 1991.

Brooks VB. *The Neural Basis of Motor Control.* New York, NY: Oxford University Press; 1986.

Brunnstrom S. *Movement Therapy in Hemiplegia.* New York, NY: Harper & Row Publishers Inc; 1970.

Claman PH. Motor unit recruitment and the gradation of muscle force. *Phys Ther.* 1993; 73:830–843.

Cohen M, Hoskins MT. *Cardiopulmonary Symptoms in Physical Therapy Practice.* New York, NY: Churchill Livingstone, 1988.

Crutchfield CA, Barnes MR. *The Neurophysiological Basis of Patient Treatment.* 2nd ed. Atlanta, Ga: Stokesville Publishing; 1975,1.

Cyriax JH. *Illustrated Manual of Orthopedic Medicine.* London, England: Butterworths; 1983.

Diener HC, Dichgans JT, Guschlbauer B, et al. The significance of proprioception on postural stabilizations assessed by ischemia. *Brain Res.* 1984;296:103–109.

Diener HC, Horak FB, Nashner LM. Stimulus parameters on human postural responses. *J Neurophysiol.* 1988; 59:1888–1905.

Duncan P, Badke MB. *Stroke Rehabilitation: The Recovery of Motor Control.* Chicago, Ill: Year Book Medical Publishers; 1987.

Feldman RG, Young RR, Koella WP, eds. *Spasticity: Disordered Motor Control.* Chicago, Ill: Year Book Medical Publishers; 1980.

Frankel VF, Nordin MA. *Basic Biomechanics of the Skeletal System.* Philadelphia, Pa: Lea & Febiger, 1989.

Guccione AA. Physical therapy diagnosis and the relationship between impairments and function. *Phys Ther.* 1991; 71:499–504.

Guccione AA, ed. *Geriatric Physical Therapy.* St. Louis, Mo: CV Mosby Co; 1993.

Gordon T, Mao J. Muscle atrophy and procedures for training after spinal cord injury. *Phys Ther.* 1994;74:50–60.

Gould MJ, ed. *Orthopedic and Sports Physical Therapy.* 2nd ed. St. Louis, Mo: CV Mosby Co; 1990.

Heiniger MC, Randolph SL. *Neurophysiological Concepts in Human Behavior—The Tree of Learning.* St. Louis, Mo: CV Mosby Co; 1981.

Henneman E. Peripheral mechanisms involved in the control of muscle. In: Mountcastle VB, ed. *Medical Physiology.* 13th ed. St. Louis, CV Mosby Co; 1974;1.

Higgins S. Motor control acquisition. *Phys Ther.* 1991; 71:123–139.

Hoppenfeld S. *Physical Examination of the Spine and Extremities.* 2nd ed. Norwalk, Conn: Appleton-Century Crofts; 1976.

Horak FB. Clinical measurement of postural control in adults. *Phys Ther.* 1987;67:1881–1885.

Inman VT, Ralston HJ, Todd F. *Human Walking.* Baltimore, Md: Williams & Wilkins; 1981.

Irwin S, Tecklin JS, eds. *Cardiopulmonary Physical Therapy.* 2nd ed. St Louis, Mo: CV Mosby Co; 1990.

Jette AM. Measuring subjective clinical outcomes. *Phys Ther.* 1989;69:580–584.

Joseph JA, ed. *Central Determinants of Age-Related Declines in Motor Function.* New York, NY: Academy of Sciences; 1988.

Kaltenborn FM, Evjenth O. *Manual Mobilization of the Extremity Joints: Examination and Basic Treatment Techniques.* Oslo, Norway: Olaf Norlis Borhandel; 1989.

Kandel ER, Schwartz JH, Jessell TM. *Principles of Neural Science.* 3rd ed. Norwalk, Conn: Appleton & Lange; 1991.

Kendall FP, McCreary EK. *Muscles: Testing and Function.* 4th ed. Baltimore, Md: Williams & Wilkins; 1993.

Kelso JAS. *Human Motor Behavior: An Introduction.* London, England: Lawrence Erlbaum Associates; 1982.

Kispert CP. Clinical measurements to assess cardiopulmonary function. *Phys Ther.* 1987;67:1886–1890.

Knott M, Voss DE. *Proprioceptive Neuromuscular Facilitation.* 2nd ed. New York, NY: Harper & Row Publishers Inc; 1968.

Langer S, Wernick J. *A Practical Manual for a Basic Approach to Biomechanics.* Wheeling, Ill: Langer Biomechanics Group; 1989.

Manual Therapy: Special Series. *Phys Ther.* 1992;72:839–967.

McComas AS, Sica REP, Upton ARM, et al. Functional changes in motoneurons of hemiparetic patients. *J Neurol Neurosurg Psychiatry.* 1973;36:183–193.

McGee DJ. *Orthopedic Physical Assessment.* Philadelphia, Pa: WB Saunders Co; 1987.

Michlevitz SL. *Thermal Agents in Rehabilitation.* 2nd ed. Philadelphia, Pa: F A Davis Co; 1990.

Mohr JP. *Manual of Clinical Problems in Neurology.* 2nd ed. Boston, Mass: Little, Brown; 1989.

Mooney V. On the dose of therapeutic exercise. *Top Rehabil.* 1992;15:653–656.

Nashner LM. Strategies for organization of human posture. In: Igarashi M, Black FO, eds. *Vestibular and Visual Control on Posture and Locomotor Equilibrium.* Basel, Switzerland: S Karger Publications; 1985.

Nashner LM. Organization of human postural movements during standing and walking. In: Grillner S, Stein P, Stuart D, et al, eds. *Neurobiology of Posture and Locomotor Equilibrium.* New York: Macmillan Press; 1986.

Norkin CC, Levangie PK. *Joint Structure and Function: A Comprehensive Analysis.* 2nd ed. Philadelphia, Pa: F A Davis Co; 1992.

Portney LG, Watkins MP: *Foundations of Clinical Research: Applications to Practice.* Norwalk, Conn: Appleton & Lange; 1993.

Proceedings of the 11-Step Conference. Alexandria, Va: Foundation for Physical Therapy; 1991.

Rothstein JM, ed. *Measurement in Physical Therapy.* New York, NY: Churchill Livingstone; 1985.

Rothstein JM, Lamb RL, Mayhew TP. Clinical uses of isokinetic measurements: critical issues. *Phys Ther.* 1987;67:1840–1844.

Schmidt RA. *Motor Control and Learning: A Behavioral Emphasis.* Champaign, Ill: Human Kinetics; 1988.

Skeletal Muscle: Special Series. *Phys Ther.* 1993;73:826–967.

Smidt GL. *Gait in Rehabilitation.* New York, NY: Churchill Livingstone; 1990.

Soderberg GL. *Kinesiology: Application to Pathological Motion.* Baltimore, Md: Williams & Wilkins; 1986.

Stewart DL, Abeln SH. *Documenting Functional Outcomes in Physical Therapy.* St. Louis, Mo: CV Mosby Co; 1993.

Sullivan PE, Markos PD, Minor MAD. *An Integrated Approach to Therapeutic Exercise: Theory and Clinical Application.* Reston, Va: Reston Publishing Co; 1982.

Sullivan PE, Markos PD. *Clinical Procedures in Therapeutic Exercise.* Norwalk, Conn: Appleton & Lange; 1987.

Tappan FM. *Healing Massage Techniques.* 2nd ed. Norwalk, Conn: Appleton & Lange; 1988.

Thompson LV. Effects of age and training on skeletal muscle physiology and performance. *Phys Ther.* 1994;74:71–81.

Umphred DA, ed. *Neurological Rehabilitation.* St Louis, Mo: CV Mosby Co; 1985.

Vaughan CL, Murphy GN, du Toit LL. *Biomechanics of Human Gait: An Annotated Bibliography.* Champaign, Ill: Human Kinetics; 1987.

Voss DE, Ionta MK, Myers BJ. *Proprioceptive Neuromuscular Facilitation Patterns and Techniques.* 3rd ed. New York, NY: Harper & Row Publishers Inc; 1985.

Watts NT. Clinical decision analysis. *Phys Ther.* 1989;69:569–576.

Winstein CL. Knowledge of results in motor learning: implications for physical therapy. *Phys Ther.* 1991;71:140–149.

Wolf SL. *Clinical Decision Making in Physical Therapy.* Philadelphia, Pa: F A Davis; 1985.

Wyke B. Articular neurology—a review. *Physiotherapy.* 1972;58:94–99.

Index

Also from Appleton & Lange

Patient Care Skills, 3/e
Mary A. Duesterhaus Minor, MS, PT; Scott Duesterhaus Minor, PhD, PT
1995, 512 pp., 732 illus., spiral, ISBN 0-8385-7709-1, A7709-7

Physical Agents
A Comprehensive Text for Physical Therapists
Bernadette Hecox, PT, MA; Tsega Andemicael Mehreteab, PT, MS; Joseph Weisberg, PT, PhD
1994, 473 pp., 180 illus., case, ISBN 0-8385-8040-8, A8040-6

Geriatric Physical Therapy
A Clinical Approach
Carole B. Lewis, PT, GCS, MSG, MPA, PhD; Jennifer M. Bottomley, PT, MS
1994, 635 pp., 120 illus., case, ISBN 0-8385-8875-1, A8875-5

Foundations of Clinical Research
Applications to Practice
Leslie Gross Portney, MS, PT; Mary P. Watkins, MS, PT
1993, 722 pp., illus., case, ISBN 0-8385-1065-5, A1065-0

Manual for Physical Agents, 4/e
Karen W. Hayes, PhD, PT
1993, 169 pp., illus., spiral, ISBN 0-8385-6143-8, A6143-0

Medical Terminology With Human Anatomy, 3/e
Jane Rice, RN, CMA-C
1995, 620 pp., illus., spiral, ISBN 0-8385-6268-X, A6268-5

Human Diseases
A Systemic Approach, 4/e
Mary Lou Mulvihill, PhD
1995, 496 pp., illus., paperback, ISBN 0-8385-3928-9, A2928-7

Introduction to Human Disease, 3/e
Thomas H. Kent, MD; Michael Noel Hart, MD
1993, 632 pp., illus., case, ISBN 0-8385-4347-2, A4347-9

Correlative Neuroanatomy, 22/e
a LANGE medical book
Stephen G. Waxman, MD, PhD; Jack deGroot, MD, PhD
1995, 384 pp., illus., paperback, ISBN 0-8385-1091-4, A1091-6

Available at your local health science bookstore
or call 1-800-423-1359 (in CT 838-4400).

Appleton & Lange • Four Stamford Plaza • PO Box 120041 • Stamford, CT • 06912-0041